Neurotoxicity - New Advances

Edited by Suna Sabuncuoglu

Published in London, United Kingdom

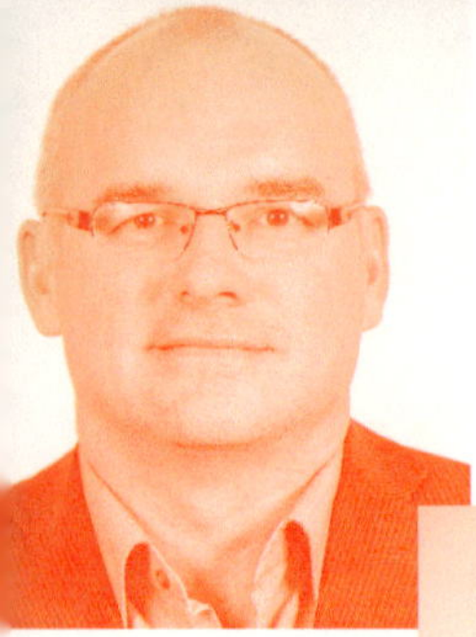
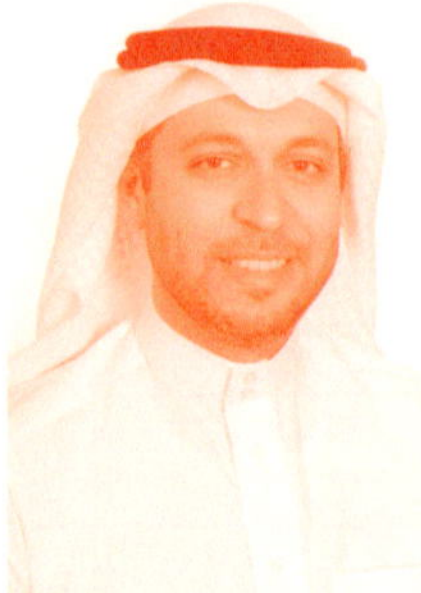
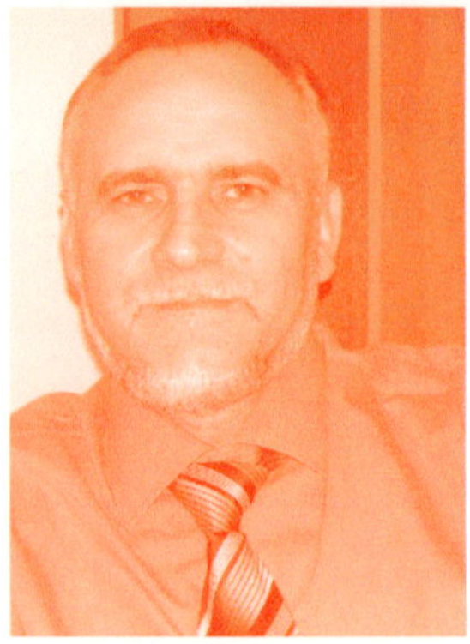
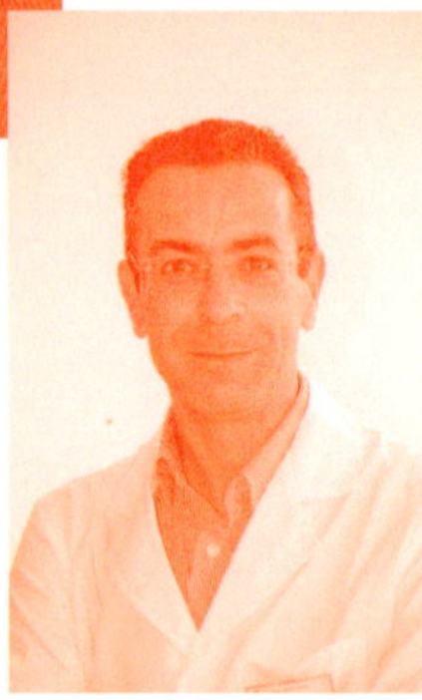
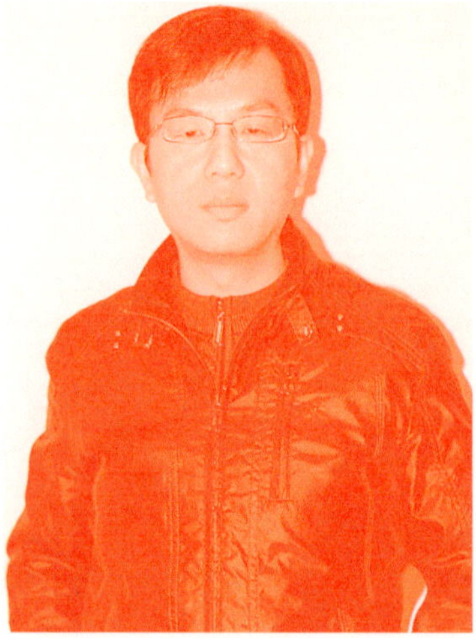
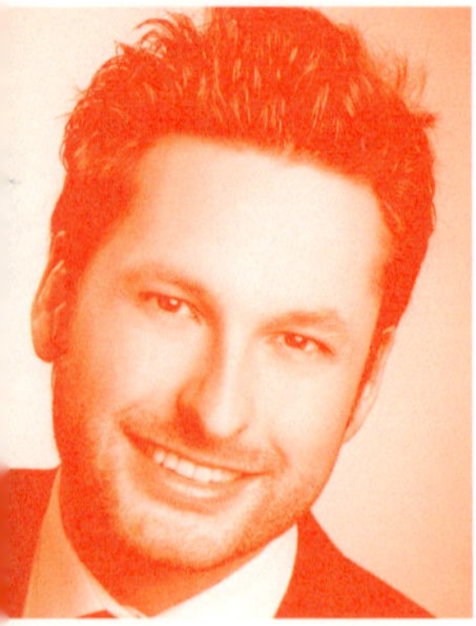
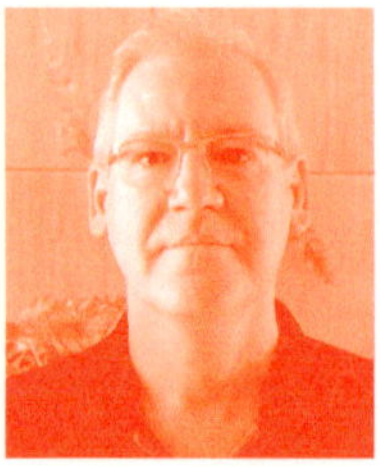

IntechOpen

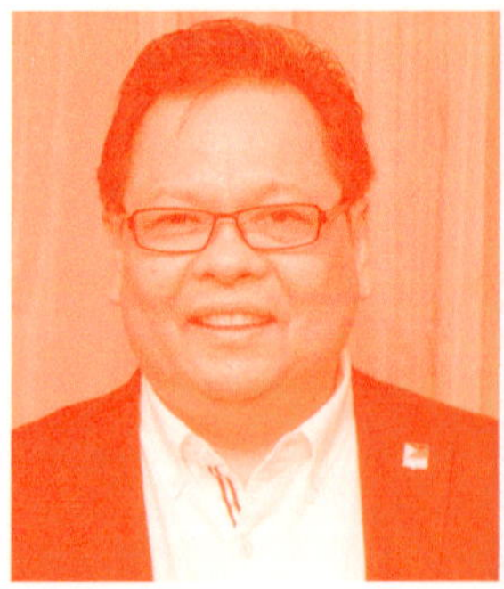
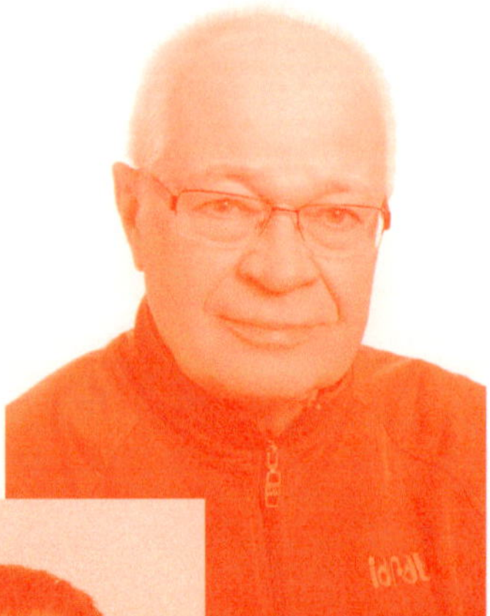
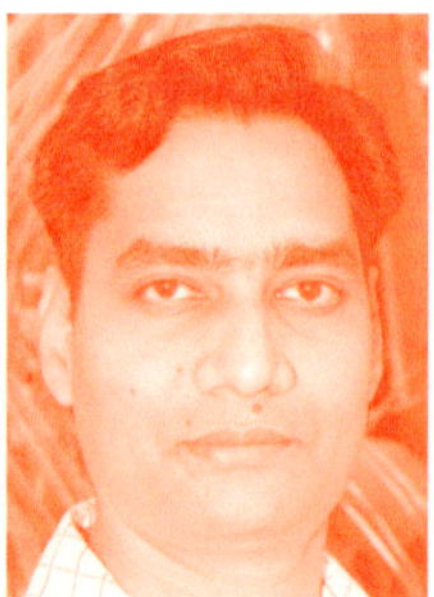
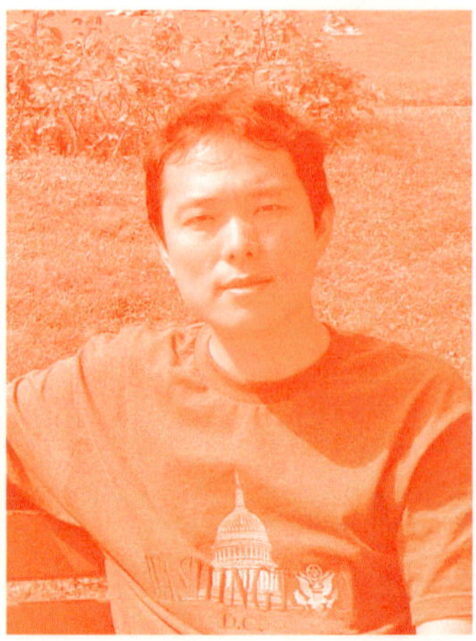
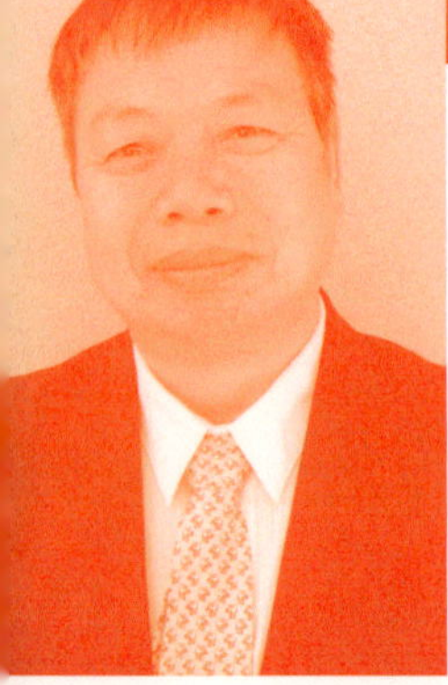
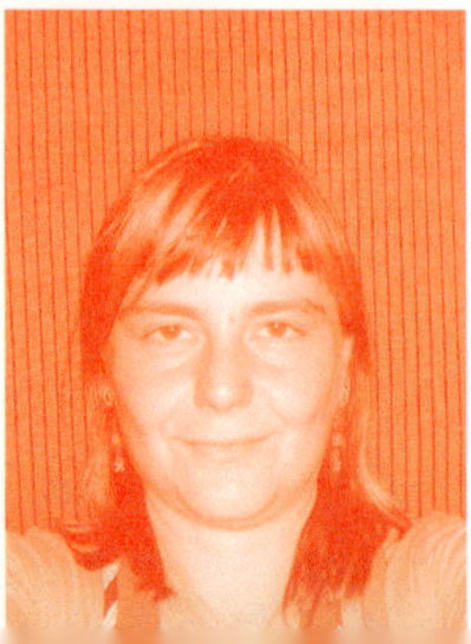

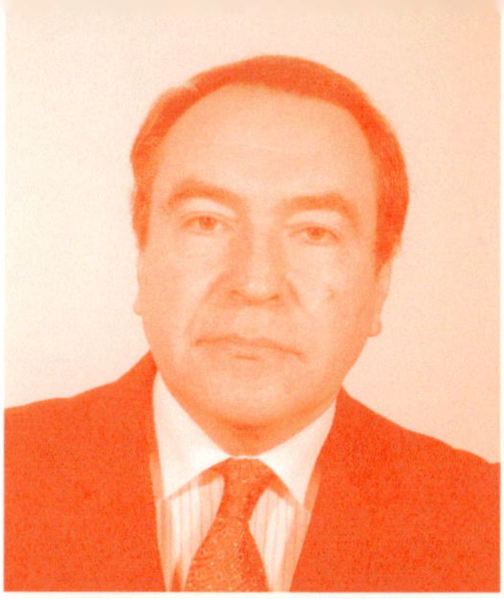

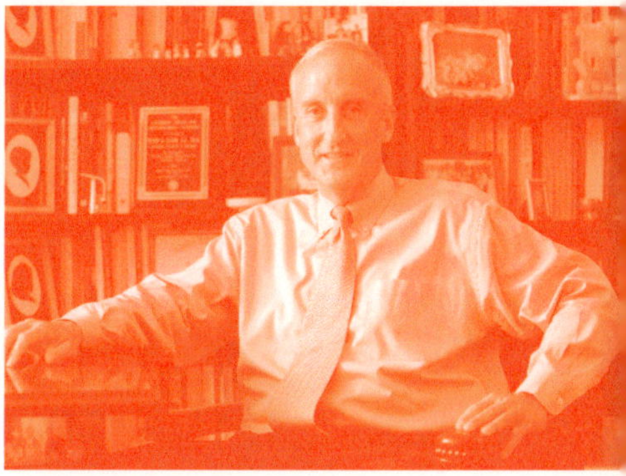

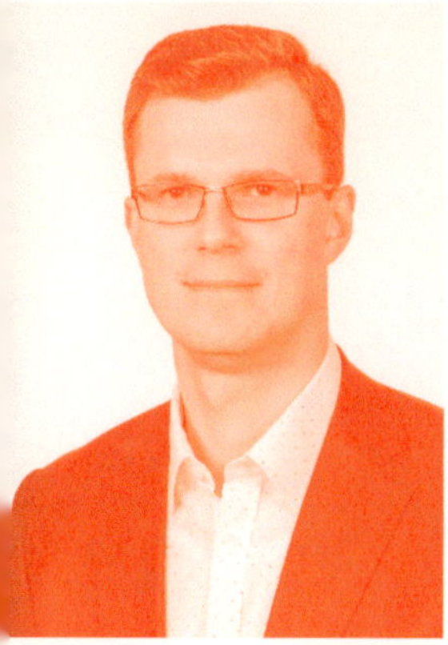

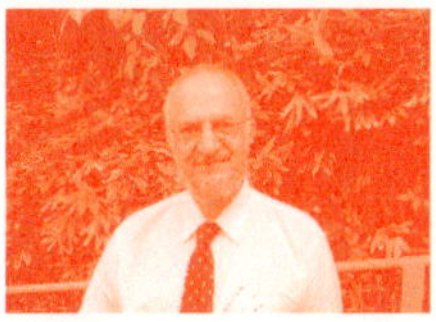

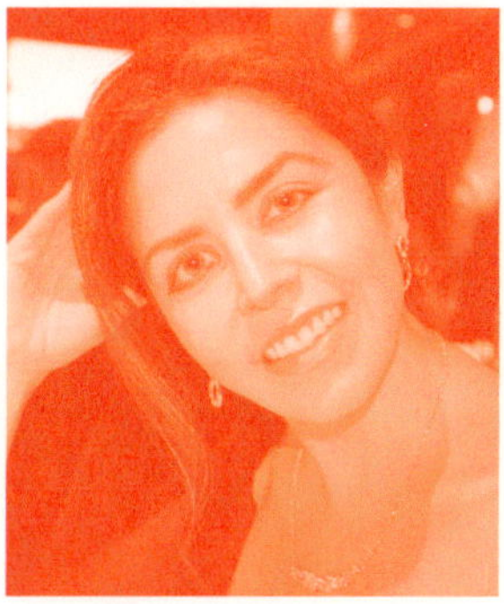

Supporting open minds since 2005

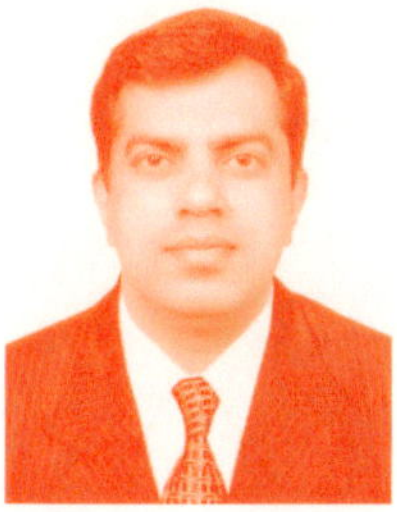

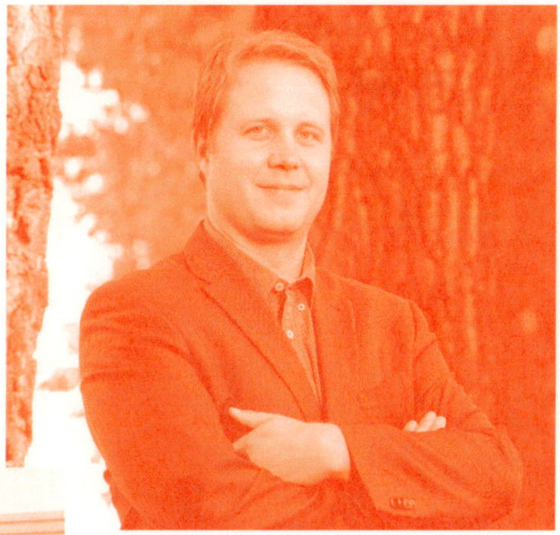

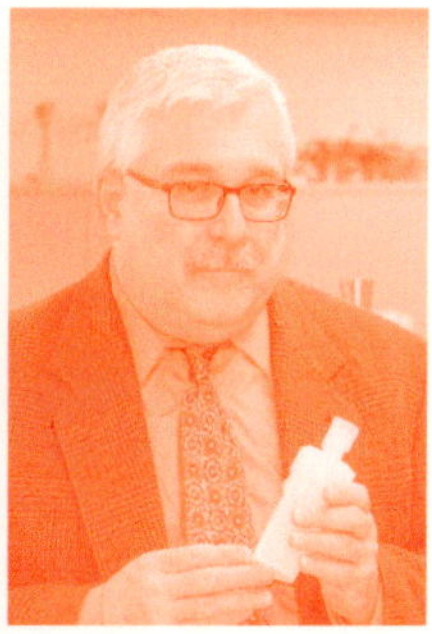

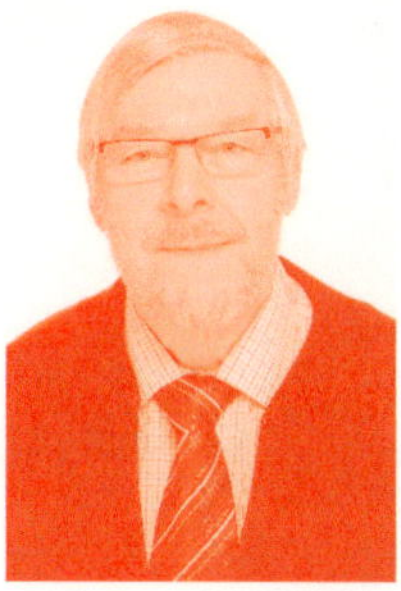

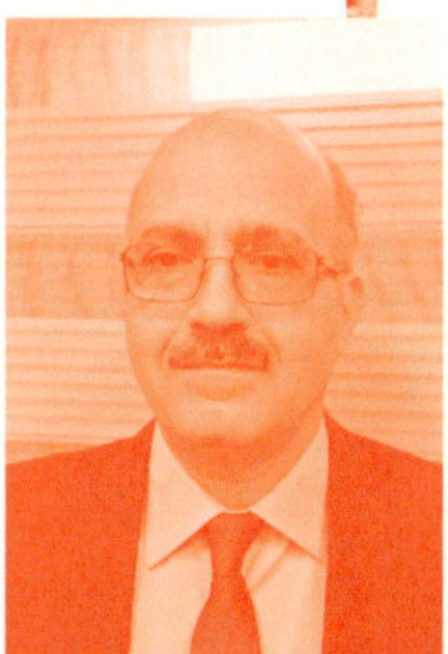

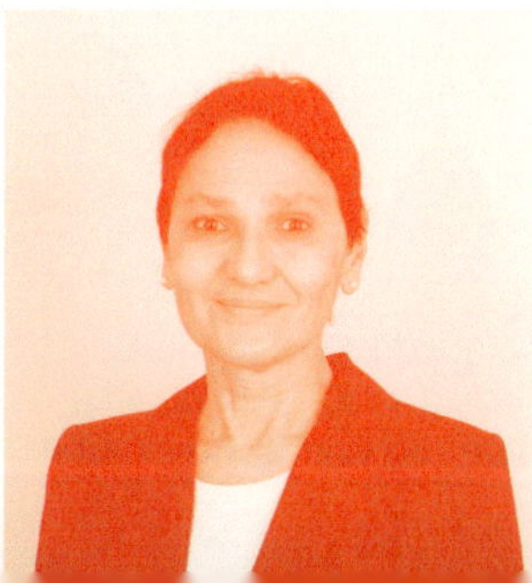

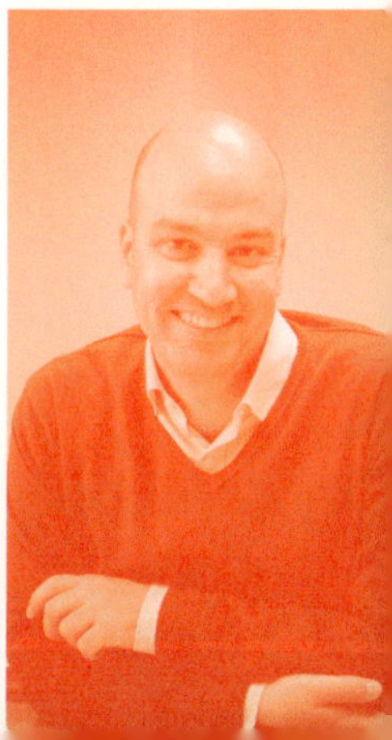

Neurotoxicity - New Advances
http://dx.doi.org/10.5772/intechopen.94708
Edited by Suna Sabuncuoglu

Contributors
Moisés Rubio-Osornio, Alejandra Mora-Gutiérrez, Carmen Rubio, Angel Alonso Romero-López, Jordi Casanova-Mollà, Yiling Hong, Neslihan Eskut, Asli Koskderelioglu, Nikhat J. Siddiqi, Sabiha Fatima, Bechan Sharma, Mohamed Samir Elrobh, Janneth Gonzalez, Felipe Rojas-Rodríguez, Andrés Pinzón, Daniel Fuenmayor, Tábata Barbosa, Diego Vesga Jimenez, Cynthia Martin, George E. Barreto, Andrés Aristizabal-Pachón, Maria Rosa Avila-Costa, Enrique Montiel-Flores, Oscar A. Mejía-García, Jose Luis Ordoñez-Librado, Ana Luisa Gutiérrez-Valdez, Jesús Espinosa-Villanueva, Claudia Dorado-Martínez, Leonardo Reynoso-Erazo, Rocío Tron-Alvarez, Vianey Rodríguez-Lara, Serap Bilge

First published in London, United Kingdom, 2022 by IntechOpen
IntechOpen is the global imprint of INTECHOPEN LIMITED, registered in England and Wales, registration number: 11086078, 5 Princes Gate Court, London, SW7 2QJ, United Kingdom
Printed in Croatia

British Library Cataloguing-in-Publication Data
A catalogue record for this book is available from the British Library

Additional hard and PDF copies can be obtained from orders@intechopen.com

Neurotoxicity - New Advances
Edited by Suna Sabuncuoglu
p. cm.
Print ISBN 978-1-83968-969-7
Online ISBN 978-1-83968-970-3
eBook (PDF) ISBN 978-1-83968-971-0

For EU product safety concerns:
IN TECH d.o.o., Prolaz Marije Krucifikse Kozulić 3, 51000 Rijeka, Croatia, info@intechopen.com or visit our website at intechopen.com.

Meet the editor

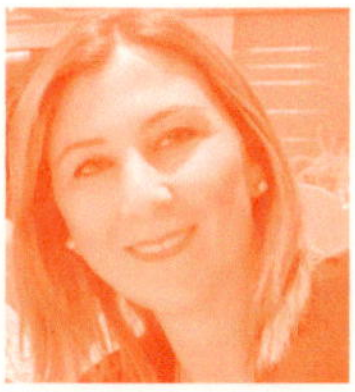

Suna Sabuncuoglu graduated from the Faculty of Pharmacy, Ankara, Turkey, where she obtained a Ph.D. in Pharmaceutical Toxicology. She worked as a Ph.D. student at the International Agency for Research on Cancer, Molecular Carcinogenesis Laboratory. She also had a postdoc position at the Department of Chemotherapy and Virology, Rega Institute, Catholic University of Leuven, Belgium. Dr. Sabuncuoglu became a lecturer in 2013 and an associate professor at Hacettepe University in 2014. She has been a European Registered Toxicologist (ERT) since 2018 and has served on many different boards, commissions, and centers.

Contents

Preface

Neurotoxicity refers to negative changes in the normal activity of the nervous system by endogenous and exogenous toxic substances. Many different chemical compounds or biological neurotoxins can cause neurotoxicity, including chemotherapy drugs, heavy metals, pesticides, and more. Studies on the neurotoxicity of substances are limited and the toxicity of many different substances is not fully known. For this reason, there is a need for neurotoxicologists specialized in this developing field as well as new prevention and treatment approaches against emerging toxicity.

Perturbations can come and go quickly, evolve slowly over days or weeks and regress over months or years, or result in chronic deficiencies. Although there may be a long delay between exposure and the emergence of neurotoxic consequences, neurotoxicity is usually self-limiting after exposure ends and rarely progressive in the absence of ongoing exposure.

Neurotoxicity - New Advances is an important and valuable resource for clinicians, toxicologists, and specialists in the field. It provides up-to-date information on neurotoxicity, behavior of neurotoxic agents, and prevention and treatment approaches.

Dr. Suna Sabuncuoglu
Associate Professor,
Faculty of Pharmacy,
Department of Toxicology,
Hacettepe University,
Sıhhiye, Ankara

Section 1

Nanoparticles and Neurotoxicity

Chapter 1

In-Utero Neurotoxicity of Nanoparticles

Nikhat J. Siddiqi, Sabiha Fatima, Bechan Sharma and Mohamed Samir Elrobh

Abstract

The unique physicochemical properties of nanoparticles (NPs) make them widely used in cosmetics, medicines, food additives, and antibacterial and antiviral compounds. NPs are also used in therapy and diagnostic applications. Depending on their origin, the NPs are commonly classified as naturally occurring and synthetic or anthropogenic NPs. Naturally occurring nanoparticles can be formed by many physical, chemical, and biological processes occurring in all spheres of the earth. However, synthetic NPs are specifically designed or unintentionally produced by different human activities. Owing to their nano size and special properties, the engineered NPs can enter the human body through different routes such as dermal penetration, intravenous injection and inhalation. NPs may accumulate in various tissues and organs including the brain. Indiscriminate use of NP is a matter concern due to the dangers of NP exposure to living organisms. It is possible for NPs to cross the placental barrier, and adversely affect the developing fetus, posing a health hazard in them by causing neurodevelopmental toxicity. Thus, NP-induced neurotoxicity is a topic that demands attention at the maternal-fetal interface. This chapter summarizes the routes by which NPs circumvent the blood-brain barrier, including recent investigations about NPs' neurotoxicity as well as possible mechanisms involved in neural fetotoxicity.

Keywords: nanoparticle, neurotoxicity, placental barrier, blood-brain barrier

1. Introduction

The term nanoparticle (NP) refers to particles with at least one dimension less than 100 nanometers [1]. NPs are an essential part of earth's biogeochemical system, produced by many physical and chemical processes including different natural and human activities. They are commonly classified as naturally occurring and synthetic or anthropogenic NPs, depending on their origin. Synthetic or anthropogenic NPs can be further categorized into two types: incidental and engineered nanoparticles [2]. Naturally occurring nanoparticles can be formed by chemical, photochemical, mechanical, thermal, and biological processes occurring in all spheres of the Earth. NPs such as alumina, iron oxide, gold, sulfur manganese oxide, and so on derived from natural sources can be found in volcanic ash, fine sand, ocean spray, and even some biological matter [1]. Incidental nanoparticles are unintentionally produced as a byproduct of human day-to-day activities involving combustion process such as running diesel engines, large-scale mining, and even starting a fire.

IntechOpen

On the other hand, the engineered or manufactured NPs such as silver, gold, zinc, metal oxides like manganese dioxide (MnO_2), aluminum oxide Al_2O_3, titanium oxide (TiO_2) of controlled shape, sizes, and compositions are specifically designed and deliberately synthesized by human beings [3]. Engineered NP include nonmetals like carbon nanotubes and quantum dots, polymers like chitosan, alginate, lipids like stearic acid, and metal sulfide like CuS, AgS, ZnS and so on [4]. Another classification of NP is their grouping into organic nanoparticles and inorganic nanoparticles. Organic nanoparticles include liposomes, dendrimers, micelles and so on. Examples of some of inorganic NP include metallic NP like gold, iron, silver, aluminum, titanium oxide (TiO_2), and zinc oxide (ZnO). Nanomaterials can also be classified based on their size for example zero-dimension, one dimension, two dimension, and three dimensions [5]. Silver, gold, copper, and platinum are some of the most commonly used metals NP. Metal-based NPs can be easily conjugated with various functional groups, like polylysine, polyethylene glycol (PEG) or bovine serum albumin [6, 7].

The technological advancements of human society as well as progress in the field of nanotechnology have shown a sharp rise in consumer products that deliberately include synthetic nanoparticles [8]. This has resulted in high levels of exposure to many types of synthetic NPs, and it is likely that this trend will continue in future. The easiest place to find these nano-enabled products in our own homes is in health care products, cosmetics, and food additives. In the past decade, many companies have used ZnO and TiO_2 NPs as sun block materials because these materials are very effective at absorbing UV radiation [9]. Some commonly used nanomaterials as food additives include silver, silicon dioxide (SiO_2), titanium TiO_2, and iron oxide (Fe_2O_3) [10]. Silver NPs are also commonly used as antibacterial and antiviral agents, while gold NPs are used for drug delivery, photothermal therapy and diagnostic applications, and polymeric NPs are used for controlled and targeted drug delivery [11].

Extensive use of engineered NP poses risk to human health. The health hazards are cause of concern in pregnant women and their unborn children. Therefore, it is important to study the toxic effect of NP on developing fetuses. In this chapter, we summarize the developmental toxicity of NP on the nervous system.

2. Factors affecting the toxicity of nanoparticles

The embryonic toxicity of nanoparticles depends on their bioaccumulation, which in turn depends on the following [12]:

- Chemical composition, particle size, shape, surface modification, and degree of agglomeration. Smaller NPs have been shown to induce more pronounced blood brain barrier (BBB) breakdown, brain edema and neuronal injuries, glial fibrillary acidic protein upregulation, and myelin vesiculation in young animals [13]. Similarly, different shapes of the same NP have been shown to induce different cellular responses by nonspecific uptake into cells [14]. In vivo animal studies have demonstrated that administration of higher doses of smaller particles NP caused their increased accumulation in placental and embryonic/fetal tissues [15].

- Type of coating, concentration of particles, surface charge of the particles, zeta potential, and crystal form. Unmodified fullerene NPs can generate reactive oxygen species (ROS) to damage cells, whereas surface-modified fullerene NPs have been demonstrated to enter cerebral microvessel endothelial cells and protect these cells by attenuating ROS-induced cellular damage, such as F-actin depolymerization [16].

- Other factors include the pH of the solution, salt concentration and the temperature [17], "protein corona," chemical characteristics, metal impurities, and degradation properties [18].
- Particle dissolution also alters the particle presence [15].
- Routes of exposure in in vivo studies. Inhalation is the main route of exposure in occupational and environmental settings. Experimental studies commonly use intravenous and intra peritoneal routes [15].
- The anatomical and functional state of the placenta [19, 20] and the critical period of exposure during gestation [15].
- Zeta potential of the NP. The charges on the NP determine their interactions with the biological system. Also, the zeta potential determines the stability of the NP in colloidal systems [21].

3. Entry of nanoparticles

The exogenous entry of engineered NP is mainly from hand-to-mouth contact in the workplaces. Nanoparticles enter the body through food, drinking water, drugs, or exposure during medical procedures. Inhalation of airborne nanoparticles is also an important point of entry into the body [22]. Larger particles are trapped in the nasopharyngeal region (5–30 μm), while the smaller particles (1–5 μm) get deposited in the tracheobronchial region. These particles can be removed by mucociliary clearance. Finally, the remaining submicron particles (< 1 μm) and nanoparticles (< 100 nm) with the smallest size distribution penetrate deeply into the alveolar region, where removal mechanisms may be insufficient. Nanosized particles can reach the alveolar region of the lungs where they get in contact with the alveolar epithelium. From the alveolar epithelium these particles can cross the blood-air-tissue barrier and enter the bloodstream to reach various organs [22]. Inhaled ultrafine particles may get deposited in the olfactory mucosa from where they can translocate in the central nervous system (CNS), which in turn might cause neurotoxicity. Studies have shown that the CNS may be a crucial target for nanoparticle inhalation or intranasal installation exposure [23, 24]. The third route of entry of NP into the body is through dermal penetration [22, 25].

The NPs enter the CNS through three main routes: (1) Transport through the lymphatic and circulatory system; (2) Activity of the mucocilliary escalator followed by oral exposure; and (3) Transport through the olfactory and trigeminal nerves [18, 26]. This pathway involves the passage of nanoparticles through the olfactory epithelium and the neurons associated with it to the brain [18]. Carbonaceous nanomaterials have been reported to show increased access to the brain via the facilitation of olfactory mucosa and olfactory nerve [23]. After uptake, NPs can permeate into other parts of the brain by simple diffusion and then travel along the direction of the convection of the interstitial fluid and the cerebrospinal fluid flow [27].

4. Barriers that restrict the entry of substances into the brain

4.1 Blood: Brain barrier (BBB)

The blood-brain barrier (BBB) is a term used to describe the unique properties of the microvasculature of the central nervous system (CNS). CNS is made of continuous and non-fenestrated vessels. These blood vessels function to regulate the movement of molecules, ions, and cells between the blood and the CNS [28, 29]. The central nervous system of vertebrates is isolated from the rest of the body by BBB. Normal functioning of BBB is essential for homeostasis. The BBB is made of two main types of cells, that is, endothelial cells (EC) and mural cells. ECs function to regulate the movement of ions, molecules, and cells between the blood and the brain. ECs are held together by tight junctions (TJs), which greatly restrict the paracellular movement of solutes [30]. The tight junctions hold CNS ECs in place forming a paracellular barrier to molecules and ions [30].

Mural cells are the cells surrounding the large vessels and pericytes, which are present on the abluminal surface of the endothelium [31]. Pericytes and astrocytes are considered the key cell types involved in BBB regulation through their interactions with brain endothelial cells. Astrocytes interact with brain endothelium and are thought to be involved in the maintenance of BBB endothelial cell properties [32] and regulate BBB permeability [33]. The BBB restricts the movement of molecules by forming a physical barrier, which is represented by tight junctions between the endothelial cells. The endothelial cells express two main types of transporters: the efflux transporters, which transport lipophilic substances toward the blood [34] and nutrient transporters, which transport nutrients into the CNS and remove waste products from the CNS to the blood [35]. The EC cells of the CNS are characterized by a higher number of mitochondria [36]. These mitochondria supply the BBB with Adenosine triphosphate to carry out their transport processes.

Other cell types of the BBB are astrocytes and immune cells, mainly macrophages and microglial cells [30]. Pericytes, astrocyte end-feet, and a discontinuous basal membrane support the functions of the BBB. The highly selective functionality of the BBB is due to endothelial tight junctions that are assisted by astrocytes and pericytes. The tight influx control is complemented by the efflux transport system, which rapidly eliminates classic xenobiotics and NMs buildup in the brain [37]. However, nanomaterials have been reported to cross the BBB via a transcytosis-mediated route [38].

4.2 Metabolic barrier

A second barrier observed in the nervous system is the metabolic barrier. The metabolic barrier is composed of enzymes and transport systems [39]. The metabolism of endothelial cells plays an important role in the function of BBB. L-Dihydroxyphenylalanine is the precursor of dopamine which enters the brain through the neutral amino acid-transport system. However, its entry is restricted due to L-Dihydroxyphenylalanine decarboxylase and monoamine oxidase inside the endothelial cells of the brain capillaries. This "enzymatic blood-brain barrier" limits the passage of L-Dihydroxyphenylalanine into the brain (https://nba.uth.tmc.edu/neuroscience/m/s4/chapter11.html). The brain capillaries contain enzymes that metabolize neurotransmitters. These enzymes include endopeptidases, cholinesterases, aminopeptidases, and Gamma-Aminobutyric acidtransaminases. The brain capillaries also contain drug and toxin-metabolizing enzymes found in the liver [40].

The endothelium of the BBB lacks pinocytic vesicles. This limits pinocytosis by the cells of BBB. The cells of BBB express many enzymes on the intra and extracellular surfaces, which restrict the movement of substances through the BBB. P-glycoproteins, and similar substances present on the endothelial cells also help to eliminate various endogenous and exogenous toxins [18]. P-glycoproteins cause multi-drug-resistant cancer cells to pump out the drugs. The endothelial cells have P-proteins, which help to pump some hydrophobic substances like cyclosporin A, domperidone, digoxin and so on into the blood.

4.3 Blood-Cerebrospinal fluid barrier

A third barrier represented by the blood-Cerebrospinal fluid barrier also serves to prevent indiscriminate entry of substances in the CNS [41]. This barrier is made up of choroid plexus epithelial cells. The blood-Cerebrospinal fluid barrier is made up of choroid plexus epithelial cells, which have smaller tight junctions than the BBB endothelia. The blood-Cerebrospinal fluid barrier prevents the entry of macromolecules into the Cerebrospinal fluid. The active transport systems of the BBB actively remove therapeutic organic acids from the Cerebrospinal fluid [42].

5. Circumvention of the blood-brain barrier by NPs

Some of the ways by which NP can circumvent the blood brain barrier include the following (**Figure 1**):

- Transcellular diffusion—Low molecular weight solid lipid nanoparticles [43].
- Paracellular diffusion—this route is taken by silica and reduced graphene oxide NP [44, 45].
- Receptor-mediated transcytosis—Engineered nanomaterials with ligands such as transferrin, insulin, ApoE can avoid the BBB by this route [46].

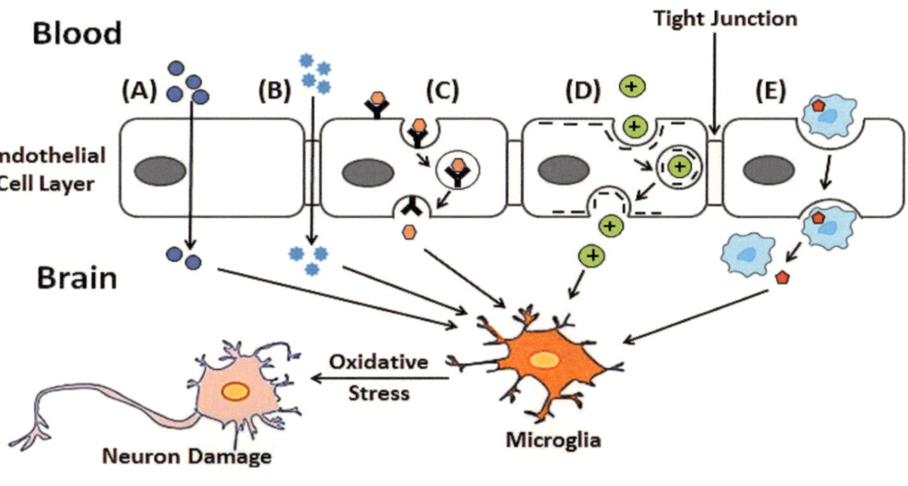

Figure 1.
Possible pathways through which nanoparticles cross the blood-brain barrier (BBB) and damage the neurons. Engineered nanomaterials with specific physicochemical properties can cross the BBB through various transport pathways such as (A) transcellular diffusion; (B) paracellular diffusion; (C) receptor-mediated transcytosis; (D) adsorptive-mediated transcytosis; and (E) cell mediated transcytosis. Nanoparticles interact directly with neuronal cells and cause neurotoxicity.

- Adsorptive-mediated transcytosis—Cationic albumin-conjugated pegylated NPs enter the brain by adsorptive-mediated transcytosis [47].

- Cell mediated transcytosis—Macrophages take up engineered nanomaterials and release them into the CNS [48].

6. Translocation of nanoparticles through the placenta

Exposure of pregnant mice to different NPs has been reported to induce pregnancy complications or damage to the fetus. Placenta is the maternal-fetal interface, which is formed of both maternal and fetal tissues that protects the embryo from harmful substances in the maternal blood. Placenta functions to exchange oxygen, nutrients, metabolic waste, and other molecules between the maternal and fetal bloodstream [49]. Factors that control the transfer of substances between maternal and fetal circulation include membrane surface area and thickness, blood flow, hydrostatic pressure in the intervillous chamber and the difference between fetal and maternal osmotic pressure [50]. Beside the placenta, amnion, chorion and parietal decidua also surround the fetus. These membranes are impervious to most of the xenobiotics in the maternal blood [51].

The brains from the fetuses of rats and mice have shown the presence of NP when the pregnant mothers were exposed to NP [52, 53]. Nano-silica and nano-TiO_2 have been reported to accumulate in the placenta, fetal liver, and fetal brain when injected to pregnant mice [54]. The extent of transfer of nanoparticle across the placenta depends on the characteristics and functionalization of the particles [55, 56]. NPs with diameters 1–100 nm have been shown to transverse the placental barrier and were detected in the brain of the offspring [57, 58]. Gestational age is an important factor affecting the toxicity of NP on the fetus [50]. Fennell et al. [59] have demonstrated that AgNP administered through oral and IV route on gestational day 18 resulted in placental accumulation after 48 h. Campagnolo et al. [60] demonstrated that inhalation of Ag NP during the first gestational day until the fifteenth gestational day in female rats caused fetal resorption. This was accompanied with an increased expression of pregnancy-relevant inflammatory cytokines in the placentas. Zhang et al. [19] have shown that maternal exposure of mice to TiO_2 NP decreased in angiogenesis in placental tissue and activated apoptotic pathways through caspase-3 in placental tissue.

Studies have demonstrated that various NPs can cross the BBB and placental barrier [61, 62]. Titanium dioxide nanomaterials ($nTiO_2$) have been reported to cross the placental barrier in pregnant mice and cause neurotoxicity in their offspring. Toxicity to the brain cells was reported to be caused due to necrosis (**Figure 2**) [63].

6.1 Mammalian embryonic model

Rodents, primarily mice and rats have been commonly used for gestational translocation of NPs [15]. Mice have been commonly used for mammalian embryo toxicity studies [64–66]. Although rabbits have been used in fewer studies, rabbit placentae bear closer resemblance to human placentae than that of other rodents. Therefore, rabbits should be the preferable animal model to study gestational particle exposure [15]. Other nonmammalian species like drosophila and zebrafish have also been used in *in vivo* studies [67].

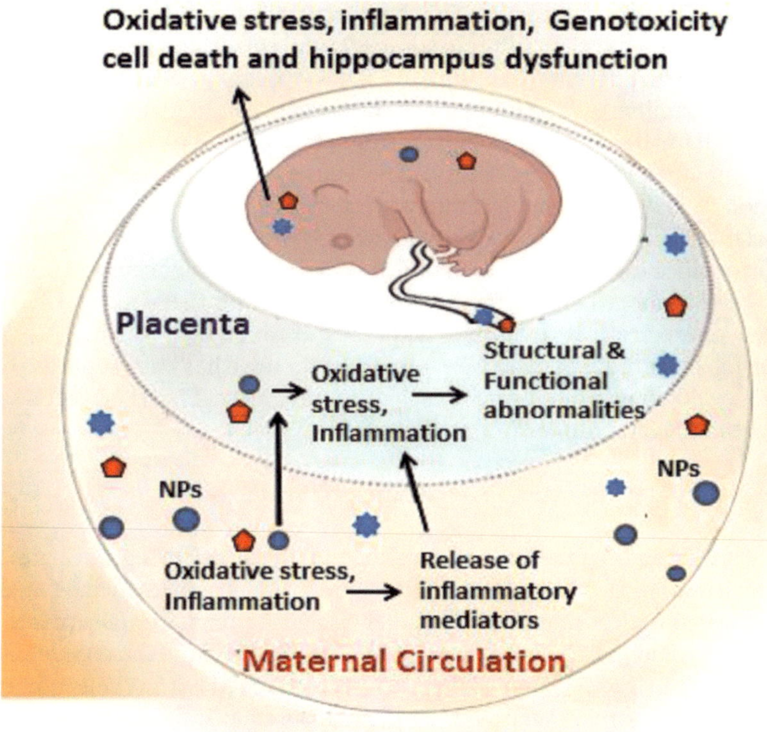

Figure 2.
Maternal exposure of nanoparticles (NPs) results in neural fetotoxicity and developmental abnormalities. Direct translocation of NPs from maternal circulation across the placental barrier into growing fetus has been recognized as the major factor involved in NP-induced fetotoxicity. Accumulation of NPs in the fetus can cause structural and functional abnormalities in various fetal tissues, including the central nervous system (CNS) which is the main target of metallic NPs. Oxidative stress, induction of inflammatory responses, alterations in gene expression, DNA damage, necrosis, and apoptosis are the mechanisms associated with NP-induced neural fetotoxicity.

6.2 Effects of nanoparticles on fetal brain

The developing brain is highly vulnerable to nanomaterials [18] due to the incomplete development of BBB in the fetus [68]. The CNS shows considerable plasticity in the early stages of development and therefore highly susceptible to the toxic effects of NP [69]. The placenta is a multifunctional organ forming a barrier between maternal and fetal tissues. In utero exposure to NPs is one of main routes of exposure during the development of the nervous system [70]. Neurodevelopmental studies have shown that both male and female offspring show differential phenotypes after prenatal insults by NPs [18].

Among various NPs, many studies have been reported on the neurotoxicity of TiO_2 NP. Injection of TiO_2 NP into pregnant mice resulted in altered expression of genes associated with brain development and function of the central nervous system in embryos [71]. The effects of TiO_2 seem to continue on the developing brain even during lactation [72]. The effects of titanium dioxide nanomaterials in pregnant mice include reduced size of the placenta and disrupted anatomical structure of the fetal brain and liver. Toxicity to the brain cells was reported to be caused due to necrosis [63]. One study showed that TiO_2 NPs administered subcutaneously to pregnant mice resulted in an increased number of apoptotic cells in the olfactory bulb of the brain and damage to cranial nerves [58]. A subsequent study showed that the mice fetuses that were exposed to TiO_2 NPs prenatally exhibited an increased level of dopamine and its metabolites in the prefrontal cortex and neostriatum. This demonstrates that prenatal exposure to TiO_2 NPs might affect the development of the central dopaminergic system in mouse offspring [73]. In utero exposure of mice to TiO_2, NP has been shown to cause changes in the genes associated with the brain development and functions of central nervous system in the embryo [71]. Accumulation of TiO_2 NP in the placenta may interfere with the development of nervous system of the fetus by impairing the transport of nutrients to the fetus [74].

Injection of silica (Si) NPs to pregnant mice resulted in their accumulation in the brain of the embryo [54]. Other studies have reported that ZnO and TiO_2 NPs causes neurotoxic effects in fetus after passing through the placenta [71, 75]. Injection of cobalt-chrome (CoCr) NPs into pregnant mice has been reported to cause neurodevelopmental abnormalities, like reactive astrogliosis and increased DNA damage in the fetal hippocampus [76].

6.3 Effects of prenatal exposure to NP on the offspring

Here, we briefly enumerate some of the effects of NPs in offspring associated with prenatal exposure. The effects of prenatal exposure to nanoparticles include neurobehavioral alterations in the offspring [77]. Other effects of prenatal exposure include accumulation of NP in the hippocampus [58, 78, 79]. These NPs in the fetal brain cause disturbances in the CNS homeostasis. The accumulated NP has been reported to cause psychiatric disorders such as autism, schizophrenia, and depression in offspring [80]. Exposure of pregnant mice to aluminum NP has been shown to induce neurodevelopmental changes which persisted during adulthood. This was accompanied by an anxiety-like behavior and impairment of cognitive function in offspring exposed to aluminum nanoparticles during in utero life [20]. Prenatal exposure to TiO_2 NPs has been shown to impair the antioxidant status, cause oxidative damage to nucleic acids and lipids in the brain of newborn pups and enhanced the depressive-like behaviors during adulthood. Prenatal exposure to TiO_2 NP has been associated with depressive behavior in adults [81]. In the case of ZnO NP, the depressive behavior has been attributed to their neurotoxic effects on neural development [82].

Pups from mice exposed to Al2O3 before and during pregnancy have been shown to have higher levels of Al accumulation in the hippocampus [20]. Similarly, in the case of Sprague Dawley rats the pups of dams exposed to silver NP showed the accumulation of silver in the brain, lung, liver, and kidneys [78]. Subcutaneous injection of TiO_2 NP to CD-1 pregnant mice caused the accumulation of TiO_2 NPs in the brain and testis of offspring [58]. However, exposure of Sprague Dawley rats to Zn NPs before mating and during lactation caused no accumulation of these NPs in the brain of offspring [83]. Prenatal exposure of mice to TiO_2 NPs causes anatomical alterations in cerebral cortex, olfactory bulb and regions associated with the dopamine systems in the offspring [84].

Studies of Mohammadipour et al. [85] and Gao et al. [72] showed that in pregnant rats treated with TiO_2 NPs significantly decreased hippocampal cell proliferation, impaired learning, and memory, and affected synaptic plasticity in the hippocampal dentate gyrus area in newborn rats. Similarly, the study of Zhou and his collogues [86] showed that maternal exposure to TiO_2 NP results in inhibition of hippocampal and dysfunction of the rho/NMDAR signaling pathway in offspring. Maternal CB-NP exposure induced the long-term activation of astrocytes resulting in reactive astrogliosis in the brains of young mice [87]. TiO_2 NP injection to pregnant mice has been reported to cause symptoms akin to autism spectrum disorder (ASD) and neurodevelopment disorders in neonates, without the detectable presence of NP in the placenta [88]. Another study indicated that nano-TiO_2 can cross the blood-fetal barrier and placental barrier, thereby delaying the development of fetal mice and inducing skeletal malformation [89].

7. Mechanisms of nanoparticle toxicity

Various hypothesizes have been proposed from time to time regarding the toxicity of NP. Nanoparticles can directly cross the placenta and cause damage to the fetus because of their high surface reactivity. Because of their small size, NPs can easily reach the brain and are taken up by the brain cells, such as neurons and glia. Mechanisms of NP uptake by cells include pinocytosis, endocytosis dependent on caveolae and lipid raft composition, clathrin-dependent endocytosis, and phagocytosis [90]. Due to their high surface reactivity, the nanoparticles can cause the generation of reactive oxygen species [91] and inflammation [92]. The metal ions of the NP have been proposed to contribute to their toxicity [93, 94]. The neurotoxic effects can either result in the direct alteration of the structure or activity of the neural system or lead to subsequent effects due to glial activations and glial-neuronal interactions [95]. The nanoparticles may also exert their toxic effects due to their limited elimination/excretion from the brain.

Oxidative stress has been implicated as one of the major mechanisms of NP toxicity. Consequences of oxidative stress include mitochondrial membrane damage and dysfunction, which in turn leads to cell death [96]. Inflammation caused by the production of cytokines appear to be a second mechanism by which the NP exerts their cytotoxic effects [97]. ZnO NPs have been shown to induce the production of pro-inflammatory cytokines in the brain of mice, accompanied by an impairment of cAMP/CREB signaling pathway. The degree of inflammation correlated with the age of the mice [56]. NPs interact with enzymes, potential apoptotic, or necrotic factors and induces inflammatory processes [12]. NP show properties similar to that of viruses and cause damage to DNA affecting cell proliferation [90]. NP can reduce mitochondrial function [98] and generate cellular morphological abnormalities [99] Cui et al. [81] postulated that prenatal exposure to NP resulted in an impairment of antioxidant capabilities in the brain of newborn pups.

Accumulation of NPs along the endosomal pathway may affect the morphology and functioning of the BBB. The interaction of the NP with biological macromolecules like DNA, lipids, and proteins may lead to the generation of oxidative stress, conformational changes in the macromolecules, mutations, alterations in membrane permeability, activation of various signaling pathways, alterations in the functions of enzymes, and exposure of new protein epitopes [100]. Genotoxic effects of NP include chromosomal aberrations, DNA strand breaks, oxidative DNA damage, DNA adducts, and micronucleus formation [101, 102]. Interactions of NP with microglia and astrocyte may activate NF-κB signaling and result in the release of mediators of inflammation and apoptosis [103]. On the other hand, oxidative stress induced mitochondrial DNA damage results in Nod-like receptor protein 3 (NLRP3) inflammasome activation, which subsequently regulates inflammatory responses by activating caspase-1 and interleukin-1β (IL-1β) release [104].

Most of the resulting damage of the nervous tissue is usually irreversible [18]. NPs have been reported to disrupt the cytoskeleton of cells of the CNS and thus cause cell death. NPs been shown to regulate the expression of neuronal channels and other proteins involved in excitability and neurotransmission [105]. Microglia, account for ~20% of the glial cells in the brain. They are a type of glial cells, which are the resident innate immune cells in the brain and regulate neuroinflammation [106]. Choi et al. [107] demonstrated that low levels of SiNPs can alter microglial function by changing the expression of proinflammatory genes and cytokine release. Excessively activated or uncontrollable microglia can cause nerve toxicity by inducing proinflammatory factors, such as interleukin-1β, tumor necrosis factor (TNF)-α, prostaglandin E2, and interferon-γ (**Figure 3**) [18].

Autophagy (autophagic flux) is a highly regulated cellular process which by eliminating long-lived proteins and damaged organelle components through the lysosomal mechanism maintains cellular homeostasis [18]. NPs have been demonstrated to be autophagic inducers [108]. Autophagy has been found to be correlated with increased DNA strand breaks and other defensive mechanisms [109]. NPs have been reported to induce autophagy through the generation of ROS and lysosomal-dependent mechanism [18]. Autophagy induced by NPs can have protective or detrimental effect on cells. During intracellular oxidative stress, imbalance and excessive ROS generation decline in autophagy-lysosome degradation function results in autophagic flux impairment, which leads to significant accumulation of the substrate of autophagy within the cell and may even trigger cell death through mitochondrial pathway [110].

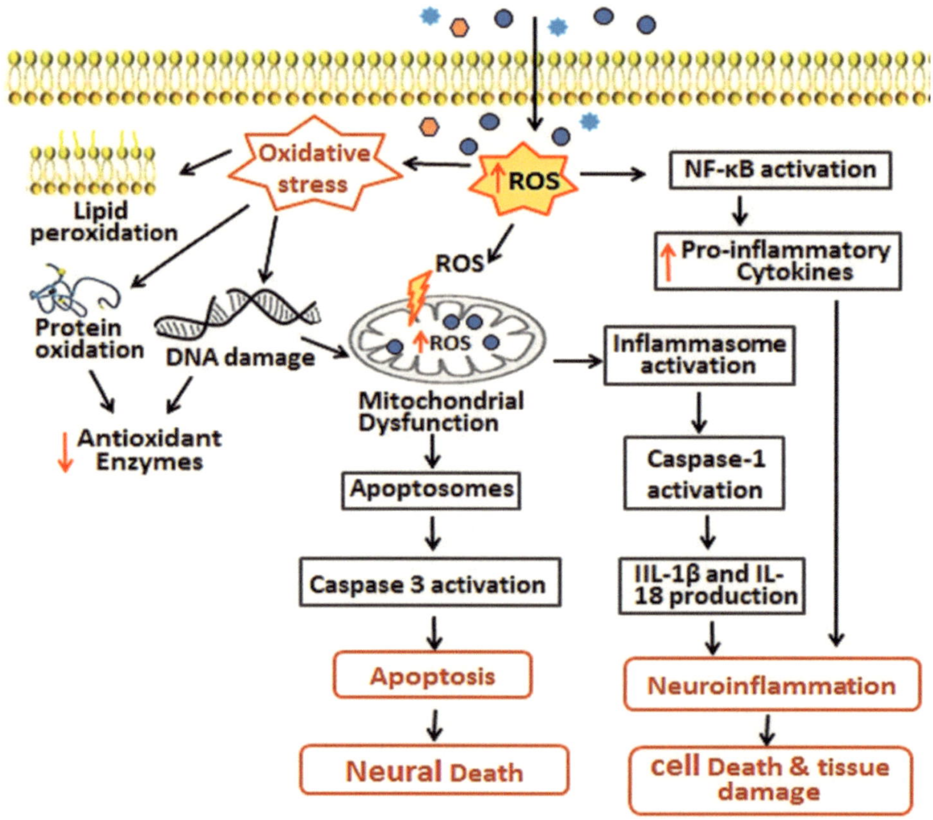

Figure 3.
Mechanism of nanoparticles (NPs)-induced neurotoxicity. Supraphysiological levels of reactive oxygen species (ROS) induce oxidative damage to the cellular macromolecules such as lipids, protein, and both mitochondrial and nuclear DNA. ROS-induced protein peroxidation may result in loss of catalytic activity of many enzymes including the antioxidant enzymes. NPs-mediated genotoxic stress in turn, can drive apoptosis mainly through the intrinsic mitochondrial apoptotic cell death pathway in neuronal cells. Mitochondrial dysfunction activates inflammasomes, which triggers the release of proinflammatory cytokines IL-1β and IL-18 via caspase-1 activation. Moreover, ROS-induced activation of nuclear factor kappa B (NF-κB) pathway may trigger proinflammatory responses, which is one of the key factors associated with NPs-induced neurological inflammation.

8. Conclusion

The brain has a limited capacity to excrete NPs [111]. Therefore, NPs that bypass the blood brain barrier and reach the fetal brain during embryonic development result in neurodevelopmental toxicity in growing fetus and psychiatric disorders in offspring. Compelling evidence from animal studies on nanotoxicity during pregnancy shows that cautions must be taken by pregnant women when using NP-based products or medicine. Deeper understanding of interaction of NPS with the biological system and the underlying mechanism on neurotoxicity will help in the development of safety guidelines on the use of engineered NPs in medicine and commercial products without health hazard. However, there is a need to study the effects of long-term exposure to NP with realistic routes and levels of exposure to identify the chronic effects of NP to fetal nervous system.

Acknowledgements

"The authors thank the Deanship of Scientific Research and RSSU at King Saud University for their technical support."

Author details

Nikhat J. Siddiqi[1]*, Sabiha Fatima[2], Bechan Sharma[3] and Mohamed Samir Elrobh[1]

1 Department of Biochemistry, College of Science, King Saud University, Riyadh, Saudi Arabia

2 Department of Clinical Laboratory Sciences, College of Applied Medical Sciences, King Saud University, Riyadh, Saudi Arabia

3 Department of Biochemistry, University of Allahabad, Allahabad, India

*Address all correspondence to: niksiddiqi@gmail.com

References

[1] Griffin S, Masood MI, Nasim MJ, Sarfraz M, Ebokaiwe AP, Schäfer KH, et al. Natural nanoparticles: A particular matter inspired by nature. Antioxidants (Basel). 2017;**7**(1):3. DOI: 10.3390/antiox7010003

[2] Lespes G, Faucher S, Slaveykova VI. Natural nanoparticles, anthropogenic nanoparticles, where is the frontier? Frontiers in Environmental Science. 2020;**8**(71). DOI: 10.3389/fenvs.2020.00071

[3] Hochella MF, Mogk DW, Ranville J, Allen IC, et al. Natural, incidental, and engineered nanomaterials and their impacts on the earth system. Science. 2019;**363**(6434):eaau8299. DOI: 10.1126/science.aau8299

[4] Sharma VK, Filip J, Zboril R, Varma RS. Natural inorganic nanoparticles—Formation, fate, and toxicity in the environment. Chemical Society Reviews. 2015;**44**(23):8410-8423. DOI: 10.1039/c5cs00236b

[5] Teleanu DM, Chircov C, Grumezescu AM, Teleanu RI. Neurotoxicity of nanomaterials: An up-to-date overview. Nanomaterials (Basel). 2019;**9**(1):96. DOI: 10.3390/nano9010096

[6] Asharani PV, Lian WY, Gong Z, Valiyaveettil S. Toxicity of silver nanoparticles in zebrafish models. Nanotechnology. 2008;**19**(25):255102. DOI: 10.1088/0957-4484/19/25/255102

[7] King-Heiden TC, Wiecinski PN, Mangham AN, Metz KM, Nesbit D, Pedersen JA, et al. Quantum dot nanotoxicity assessment using the zebrafish embryo. Environmental Science and Technology. 2009;**43**(5):1605-1611. DOI: 10.1021/es801925c

[8] Contado C. Nanomaterials in consumer products: A challenging analytical problem. Frontiers in Chemistry. 2015;**3**:48. DOI: 10.3389/fchem.2015.00048

[9] Smijs TG, Pavel S. Titanium dioxide and zinc oxide nanoparticles in sunscreens: Focus on their safety and effectiveness. Nanotechnology, Science and Applications. 2011;**4**:95-112. DOI: 10.2147/NSA.S19419

[10] Ghebretatios M, Schaly S, Prakash S. Nanoparticles in the food industry and their impact on human gut microbiome and diseases. International Journal of Molecular Sciences. 2021;**22**(4):1942. DOI: 10.3390/ijms22041942

[11] Gupta R, Xie H. Nanoparticles in daily life: Applications, toxicity and regulations. Journal of Environmental Pathology, Toxicology and Oncology. 2018;**37**(3):209-230. DOI: 10.1615/JEnviron Pathol Toxicol Oncol. 201802 6009

[12] Celá P, Veselá B, Matalová E, Večeřa Z, Buchtová M. Embryonic toxicity of nanoparticles. Cells, Tissues, Organs. 2014;**199**(1):1-23. DOI: 10.1159/000362163

[13] Sharma A, Muresanu DF, Patnaik R, Sharma HS. Size- and age-dependent neurotoxicity of engineered metal nanoparticles in rats. Molecular Neurobiology. 2013;**48**(2):386-396. DOI: 10.1007/s12035-013-8500-0

[14] Gratton SE, Ropp PA, Pohlhaus PD, Luft JC, Madden VJ, Napier ME, et al. The effect of particle design on cellular internalization pathways. Proceedings of the National Academy of Sciences of the United States of America. 2008;**105**(33):11613-11618. DOI: 10.1073/pnas.0801763105

[15] Bongaerts E, Nawrot TS, Van Pee T, Ameloot M, Bové H. Translocation of (ultra)fine particles and nanoparticles

across the placenta: A systematic review on the evidence of in vitro, ex vivo, and in vivo studies. Particle and Fibre Toxicology. 2020;**17**(1):56. DOI: 10.1186/s12989-020-00386-8

[16] Lao F, Chen L, Li W, Ge C, Qu Y, Sun Q, et al. Fullerene nanoparticles selectively enter oxidation-damaged cerebral microvessel endothelial cells and inhibit JNK-related apoptosis. ACS Nano. 2009;**3**(11):3358-3368. DOI: 10.1021/nn900912n

[17] Rogers NJ, Franklin NM, Apte SC, Batley GE. The importance of physical and chemical characterization in nanoparticle toxicity studies. Integrated Environmental Assessment and Management. 2007;**3**(2):303-304. DOI: 10.1002/ieam.5630030219

[18] Feng X, Chen A, Zhang Y, Wang J, Shao L, Wei L. Central nervous system toxicity of metallic nanoparticles. International Journal of Nanomedicine. 2015;**10**:4321-4340. DOI: 10.2147/IJN.S78308

[19] Zhang L, Xie X, Zhou Y, Yu D, Deng Y, Ouyang J, et al. Gestational exposure to titanium dioxide nanoparticles impairs the placentation through dysregulation of vascularization, proliferation and apoptosis in mice. International Journal of Nanomedicine. 2018;**13**:777-789. DOI: 10.2147/IJN.S152400

[20] Zhang Q, Ding Y, He K, Li H, Gao F, Moehling TJ, et al. Exposure to alumina nanoparticles in female mice during pregnancy induces neurodevelopmental toxicity in the offspring. Frontiers in Pharmacology. 2018;**9**:253. DOI: 10.3389/fphar.2018.00253

[21] Frank LA, Onzi GR, Morawski AS, Pohlmann AR, Guterres SS, Contri RV. Chitosan as a coating material for nanoparticles intended for biomedical applications. Reactive and Functional Polymers. 2020;**147**. DOI: org/10.1016/j.reactfunctpolym.2019.104459

[22] Oberdörster G, Maynard A, Donaldson K, Castranova V, Fitzpatrick J, Ausman K, et al. ILSI research foundation/risk science institute nanomaterial toxicity screening working group. Principles for characterizing the potential human health effects from exposure to nanomaterials: Elements of a screening strategy. Particle and Fibre Toxicology. 2005;**2**:8. DOI: 10.1186/1743-8977-2-8

[23] Oberdörster G, Sharp Z, Atudorei V, Elder A, Gelein R, Kreyling W, et al. Translocation of inhaled ultrafine particles to the brain. Inhalation Toxicology. 2004;**16**(6-7):437-445. DOI: 10.1080/08958370490439597

[24] Elder A, Gelein R, Silva V, Feikert T, Opanashuk L, Carter J, et al. Translocation of inhaled ultrafine manganese oxide particles to the central nervous system. Environmental Health Perspectives. 2006;**114**(8):1172-1178. DOI: 10.1289/ehp.9030

[25] Borm PJ, Robbins D, Haubold S, Kuhlbusch T, Fissan H, Donaldson K, et al. The potential risks of nanomaterials: A review carried out for ECETOC. Particle and Fibre Toxicology. 2006;**3**:11. DOI: 10.1186/1743-8977-3-11

[26] Geraets L, Oomen AG, Schroeter JD, Coleman VA, Cassee FR. Tissue distribution of inhaled micro- and nano-sized cerium oxide particles in rats: Results from a 28-day exposure study. Toxicological Sciences. 2012;**127**(2):463-473. DOI: 10.1093/toxsci/kfs113

[27] Wolak DJ, Thorne RG. Diffusion of macromolecules in the brain: Implications for drug delivery. Molecular Pharmaceutics. 2013;**10**(5):1492-1504. DOI: 10.1021/mp300495e

[28] Zlokovic BV. The blood-brain barrier in health and chronic neurodegenerative disorders. Neuron. 2008;**57**(2):178-201. DOI: 10.1016/j.neuron.2008.01.003

[29] Daneman R. The blood-brain barrier in health and disease. Annals of Neurology. 2012;**72**(5):648-672. DOI: 10.1002/ana.23648

[30] Daneman R, Prat A. The blood-brain barrier. Cold Spring Harbor Perspectives in Biology. 2015;7(1):a020412. DOI: 10.1101/cshperspect.a020412

[31] Sims DE. The pericyte—A review. Tissue and Cell. 1986;**18**(2):153-174. DOI: 10.1016/0040-8166(86)90026-1

[32] Abbott NJ, Rönnbäck L, Hansson E. Astrocyte-endothelial interactions at the blood-brain barrier. Nature Reviews Neuroscience. 2006;7(1):41-53. DOI: 10.1038/nrn1824

[33] O'Brown NM, Pfau SJ, Gu C. Bridging barriers: A comparative look at the blood-brain barrier across organisms. Genes and Development. 2018;**32**(7-8): 466-478. DOI: 10.1101/gad.309823.117

[34] Löscher W, Potschka H. Blood-brain barrier active efflux transporters: ATP-binding cassette gene family. NeuroRx. 2005;**2**(1):86-98. DOI: 10.1602/neurorx.2.1.86

[35] Mittapalli RK, Manda VK, Adkins CE, Geldenhuys WJ, Lockman PR. Exploiting nutrient transporters at the blood-brain barrier to improve brain distribution of small molecules. Therapeutic Delivery. 2010;**1**(6):775-784. DOI: 10.4155/tde.10.76

[36] Kluge MA, Fetterman JL, Vita JA. Mitochondria and endothelial function. Circulation Research. 2013;**112**(8):1171-1188. DOI: 10.1161/CIRCRESAHA.111.300233

[37] Wohlfart S, Gelperina S, Kreuter J. Transport of drugs across the blood-brain barrier by nanoparticles. Journal of Controlled Release. 2012;**161**(2):264-273. DOI: 10.1016/j.jconrel.2011.08.017

[38] Mc Carthy DJ, Malhotra M, O'Mahony AM, Cryan JF, O'Driscoll CM. Nanoparticles and the blood-brain barrier: Advancing from in-vitro models towards therapeutic significance. Pharmaceutical Research. 2015;**32**(4): 1161-1185. DOI: 10.1007/s11095-014-1545-6

[39] Persidsky Y, Ramirez SH, Haorah J, Kanmogne GD. Blood-brain barrier: Structural components and function under physiologic and pathologic conditions. Journal of Neuroimmune Pharmacology. 2006;**1**(3):223-236. DOI: 10.1007/s11481-006-9025-3

[40] Minn A, Ghersi-Egea JF, Perrin R, Leininger B, Siest G. Drug metabolizing enzymes in the brain and cerebral microvessels. Brain Research Reviews. 1991;**16**(1):65-82. DOI: 10.1016/0165-0173(91)90020-9

[41] Béduneau A, Saulnier P, Benoit JP. Active targeting of brain tumors using nanocarriers. Biomaterials. 2007;**28**(33): 4947-4967. DOI: 10.1016/j.biomaterials.2007.06.011

[42] Spector R. Nature and consequences of mammalian brain and Cerebrospinal fluid efflux transporters: Four decades of progress. Journal of Neurochemistry. 2010;**112**(1):13-23. DOI: 10.1111/j.1471-4159.2009.06451.x

[43] Neves AR, Queiroz JF, Lima SAC, Reis S. Apo E-functionalization of solid lipid nanoparticles enhances brain drug delivery: Uptake mechanism and transport pathways. Bioconjugate Chemistry. 2017;**28**(4):995-1004. DOI: 10.1021/acs.bioconjchem.6b00705

[44] Mendonça MC, Soares ES, de Jesus MB, Ceragioli HJ, Ferreira MS, Catharino RR, et al. Reduced graphene oxide induces transient blood-brain barrier opening: An in vivo study. Journal of Nanobiotechnology. 2015;**13**:78. DOI: 10.1186/s12951-015-0143-z

[45] Liu X, Sui B, Sun J. Blood-brain barrier dysfunction induced by silica

NPs in vitro and in vivo: Involvement of oxidative stress and Rho-kinase/JNK signaling pathways. Biomaterials. 2017;**121**:64-82. DOI: 10.1016/j.biomaterials.2017.01.006

[46] Kafa H, Wang JT, Rubio N, Klippstein R, Costa PM, Hassan HA, et al. Translocation of LRP1 targeted carbon nanotubes of different diameters across the blood-brain barrier in vitro and in vivo. Journal of Controlled Release. 2016;**225**:217-229. DOI: 10.1016/j.jconrel.2016.01.031

[47] Lu W, Sun Q, Wan J, She Z, Jiang XG. Cationic albumin-conjugated pegylated nanoparticles allow gene delivery into brain tumors via intravenous administration. Cancer Research. 2006;**66**(24):11878-11887. DOI: 10.1158/0008-5472.CAN-06-2354

[48] Ge D, Du Q, Ran B, Liu X, Wang X, Ma X, et al. The neurotoxicity induced by engineered nanomaterials. International Journal of Nanomedicine. 2019;**14**:4167-4186. DOI: 10.2147/IJN.S203352

[49] Maltepe E, Fisher SJ. Placenta: The forgotten organ. Annual Review of Cell and Developmental Biology. 2015;**31**:523-552. DOI: 10.1146/annurev-cellbio-100814-125620

[50] Pereira KV, Giacomeli R, Gomes de Gomes M, Haas SE. The challenge of using nanotherapy during pregnancy: Technological aspects and biomedical implications. Placenta. 2020;**100**(75-80). DOI: 10.1016/j.placenta.2020.08.005

[51] Menezes V, Malek A, Keelan JA. Nanoparticulate drug delivery in pregnancy: Placental passage and fetal exposure. Current Pharmaceutical Biotechnology. 2011;**12**(5):731-742. DOI: 10.2174/138920111795471010

[52] Di Bona KR, Xu Y, Ramirez PA, DeLaine J, Parker C, Bao Y, et al. Surface charge and dosage dependent potential developmental toxicity and biodistribution of iron oxide nanoparticles in pregnant CD-1 mice. Reproductive Toxicology. 2014;**50**:36-42. DOI: 10.1016/j.reprotox.2014.09.010

[53] Semmler-Behnke M, Lipka J, Wenk A, Hirn S, Schäffler M, Tian F, et al. Size dependent translocation and fetal accumulation of gold nanoparticles from maternal blood in the rat. Particle and Fibre Toxicology. 2014;**11**:33. DOI: 10.1186/s12989-014-0033-9

[54] Yamashita K, Yoshioka Y, Higashisaka K, Mimura K, Morishita Y, Nozaki M, et al. Silica and titanium dioxide nanoparticles cause pregnancy complications in mice. Nature Nanotechnology. 2011;**6**(5):321-328. DOI: 10.1038/nnano.2011.41

[55] Yang H, Sun C, Fan Z, Tian X, Yan L, Du L, et al. Effects of gestational age and surface modification on materno-fetal transfer of nanoparticles in murine pregnancy. Scientific Reports. 2012;**2**:847. DOI: 10.1038/srep00847

[56] Tian L, Lin B, Wu L, Li K, Liu H, Yan J, et al. Neurotoxicity induced by zinc oxide nanoparticles: Age-related differences and interaction. Scientific Reports. 2015;**5**:16117. DOI: 10.1038/srep16117

[57] Wick P, Malek A, Manser P, Meili D, Maeder-Althaus X, Diener L, et al. Barrier capacity of human placenta for nanosized materials. Environmental Health Perspectives. 2010;**118**(3):432-436. DOI: 10.1289/ehp.0901200

[58] Takeda K, Suzuki K, Ishihara A, Kubo-Irie M, Fujimoto R, Tabata M, et al. Nanoparticles transferred from pregnant mice to their offspring can damage the genital and cranial nerve systems. Journal of Health Science. 2009;**55**:95-102. DOI: 10.1248/jhs.55.95

[59] Fennell TR, Mortensen NP, Black SR, Snyder RW, Levine KE, Poitras E, et al. Disposition of

intravenously or orally administered silver nanoparticles in pregnant rats and the effect on the biochemical profile in urine. Journal of Applied Toxicology. 2017;**37**(5):530-544. DOI: 10.1002/jat.3387

[60] Campagnolo L, Massimiani M, Vecchione L, Piccirilli D, Toschi N, Magrini A, et al. Silver nanoparticles inhaled during pregnancy reach and affect the placenta and the foetus. Nanotoxicology. 2017;**11**(5):687-698. DOI: 10.1080/17435390.2017.1343875

[61] Keelan JA. Nanotoxicology: Nanoparticles versus the placenta. Nature Nanotechnology. 2011;**6**(5):263-264. DOI: 10.1038/nnano.2011.65

[62] Muoth C, Aengenheister L, Kucki M, Wick P, Buerki-Thurnherr T. Nanoparticle transport across the placental barrier: Pushing the field forward! Nanomedicine (London, England). 2016;**11**(8):941-957. DOI: 10.2217/nnm-2015-0012

[63] Naserzadeh P, Ghanbary F, Ashtari P, Seydi E, Ashtari K, Akbari M. Biocompatibility assessment of titanium dioxide nanoparticles in mice fetoplacental unit. Journal of Biomedical Materials Research. Part A. 2018;**106**(2): 580-589. DOI: 10.1002/jbm.a.36221

[64] Bailey GP, Wise LD, Buschmann J, Hurtt M, Fisher JE. Pre- and postnatal developmental toxicity study design for pharmaceuticals. Birth Defects Research. Part B, Developmental and Reproductive Toxicology. 2009;**86**(6):437-445. DOI: 10.1002/bdrb.20217

[65] Wise LD, Buschmann J, Feuston MH, Fisher JE, Hew KW, Hoberman AM, et al. Embryo-fetal developmental toxicity study design for pharmaceuticals. Birth Defects Research. Part B, Developmental and Reproductive Toxicology. 2009;**86**(6): 418-428. DOI: 10.1002/bdrb.20214

[66] Khan Z, Wolff HS, Fredrickson JR, Walker DL, Daftary GS, Morbeck DE. Mouse strain and quality control testing: Improved sensitivity of the mouse embryo assay with embryos from outbred mice. Fertility and Sterility. 2013;**99**(3):847-854. DOI: 10.1016/j.fertnstert.2012.10.046

[67] Haque E, Ward AC. Zebrafish as a model to evaluate nanoparticle toxicity. Nanomaterials (Basel). 2018;**8**(7):561. DOI: 10.3390/nano8070561

[68] Watson RE, Desesso JM, Hurtt ME, Cappon GD. Postnatal growth and morphological development of the brain: A species comparison. Birth Defects Research. Part B, Developmental and Reproductive Toxicology. 2006;**77**(5):471-484. DOI: 10.1002/bdrb.20090

[69] Siddiqui MA, Alhadlaq HA, Ahmad J, Al-Khedhairy AA, Musarrat J, Ahamed M. Copper oxide nanoparticles induced mitochondria mediated apoptosis in human hepatocarcinoma cells. PLoS One. 2013;**8**(8):e69534. DOI: 10.1371/journal.pone.0069534

[70] Rice D, Barone S Jr. Critical periods of vulnerability for the developing nervous system: Evidence from humans and animal models. Environmental Health Perspectives. 2000;**108**(Suppl. 3): 511-533. DOI: 10.1289/ehp.00108s3511

[71] Shimizu M, Tainaka H, Oba T, Mizuo K, Umezawa M, Takeda K. Maternal exposure to nanoparticulate titanium dioxide during the prenatal period alters gene expression related to brain development in the mouse. Particle and Fibre Toxicology. 2009;**6**:20. DOI: 10.1186/1743-8977-6-20

[72] Gao X, Yin S, Tang M, Chen J, Yang Z, Zhang W, et al. Effects of developmental exposure to TiO_2 nanoparticles on synaptic plasticity in hippocampal dentate gyrus area: An in vivo study in anesthetized rats. Biological Trace Element Research.

2011;**143**(3):1616-1628. DOI: 10.1007/s12011-011-8990-4

[73] Takahashi Y, Mizuo K, Shinkai Y, Oshio S, Takeda K. Prenatal exposure to titanium dioxide nanoparticles increases dopamine levels in the prefrontal cortex and neostriatum of mice. The Journal of Toxicological Sciences. 2010;**35**(5):749-756. DOI: 10.2131/jts.35.749

[74] Wu Y, Chen L, Chen F, Zou H, Wang Z. A key moment for TiO_2: Prenatal exposure to TiO_2 nanoparticles may inhibit the development of offspring. Ecotoxicology and Environmental Safety. 2020;**202**:110911. DOI: 10.1016/j.ecoenv.2020.110911

[75] Okada Y, Tachibana K, Yanagita S, Takeda K. Prenatal exposure to zinc oxide particles alters monoaminergic neurotransmitter levels in the brain of mouse offspring. The Journal of Toxicological Sciences. 2013;**38**(3):363-370. DOI: 10.2131/jts.38.363

[76] Hawkins SJ, Crompton LA, Sood A, Saunders M, Boyle NT, Buckley A, et al. Nanoparticle-induced neuronal toxicity across placental barriers is mediated by autophagy and dependent on astrocytes. Nature Nanotechnology. 2018;**13**(5):427-433. DOI: 10.1038/s41565-018-0085-3

[77] Hougaard KS, Jackson P, Jensen KA, Sloth JJ, Löschner K, Larsen EH, et al. Effects of prenatal exposure to surface-coated nanosized titanium dioxide (UV-Titan). A study in mice. Particle and Fibre Toxicology. 2010;**7**:16. DOI: 10.1186/1743-8977-7-16

[78] Lee Y, Choi J, Kim P, Choi K, Kim S, Shon W, et al. A transfer of silver nanoparticles from pregnant rat to offspring. Toxicology Research. 2012;**28**(3):139-141. DOI: 10.5487/TR.2012.28.3.139

[79] Zhang Y, Wu J, Feng X, Wang R, Chen A, Shao L. Current understanding of the toxicological risk posed to the fetus following maternal exposure to nanoparticles. Expert Opinion on Drug Metabolism and Toxicology. 2017;**13**(12):1251-1263. DOI: 10.1080/17425255.2018.1397131

[80] O'Connor MJ, Paley B. Psychiatric conditions associated with prenatal alcohol exposure. Developmental Disabilities Research Reviews. 2009;**15**(3):225-234. DOI: 10.1002/ddrr.74

[81] Cui Y, Chen X, Zhou Z, Lei Y, Ma M, Cao R, et al. Prenatal exposure to nanoparticulate titanium dioxide enhances depressive-like behaviors in adult rats. Chemosphere. 2014;**96**:99-104. DOI: 10.1016/j.chemosphere.2013.07.051

[82] Alimohammadi S, Hosseini MS, Behbood L. Prenatal exposure to zinc oxide nanoparticles can induce depressive-like behaviors in mice offspring. International Journal of Peptide Research and Therapeutics. 2019;**25**:401-409. DOI: 10.1007/s10989-018-9686-9

[83] Jo E, Seo G, Kwon JT, Lee M, Bc L, Eom I, et al. Exposure to zinc oxide nanoparticles affects reproductive development and biodistribution in offspring rats. The Journal of Toxicological Sciences. 2013;**38**(4):525-530. DOI: 10.2131/jts.38.525

[84] Umezawa M, Tainaka H, Kawashima N, Shimizu M, Takeda K. Effect of fetal exposure to titanium dioxide nanoparticle on brain development—Brain region information. The Journal of Toxicological Sciences. 2012;**37**(6):1247-1252. DOI: 10.2131/jts.37.1247

[85] Mohammadipour A, Fazel A, Haghir H, Motejaded F, Rafatpanah H, Zabihi H, et al. Maternal exposure to titanium dioxide nanoparticles during pregnancy; impaired memory and decreased hippocampal cell proliferation in rat offspring. Environmental Toxicology and Pharmacology. 2014;**37**(2):617-625. DOI: 10.1016/j.etap.2014.01.014

[86] Zhou Y, Ji J, Hong F, Zhuang J, Wang L. Maternal exposure to nanoparticulate titanium dioxide causes inhibition of hippocampal development involving dysfunction of the rho/NMDAR signaling pathway in offspring. Journal of Biomedical Nanotechnology. 2019;**15**(4):839-847. DOI: 10.1166/jbn.2019.2723

[87] Onoda A, Takeda K, Umezawa M. Dose-dependent induction of astrocyte activation and reactive astrogliosis in mouse brain following maternal exposure to carbon black nanoparticle. Particle and Fibre Toxicology. 2017;**14**(1):4. DOI: 10.1186/s12989-017-0184-6

[88] Notter T, Aengenheister L, Weber-Stadlbauer U, Naegeli H, Wick P, Meyer U, et al. Prenatal exposure to TiO_2 nanoparticles in mice causes behavioral deficits with relevance to autism spectrum disorder and beyond. Translational Psychiatry. 2018;**8**(1):193. DOI: 10.1038/s41398-018-0251-2

[89] Hong F, Zhou Y, Zhao X, Sheng L, Wang L. Maternal exposure to nanosized titanium dioxide suppresses embryonic development in mice. International Journal of Nanomedicine. 2017;**12**:6197-6204. DOI: 10.2147/IJN.S143598

[90] Asharani PV, Hande MP, Valiyaveettil S. Anti-proliferative activity of silver nanoparticles. BMC Cell Biology. 2009;**10**:65. DOI: 10.1186/1471-2121-10-65

[91] Fu PP, Xia Q, Hwang HM, Ray PC, Yu H. Mechanisms of nanotoxicity: Generation of reactive oxygen species. Journal of Food and Drug Analysis. 2014;**22**(1):64-75. DOI: 10.1016/j.jfda.2014.01.005

[92] Shirasuna K, Usui F, Karasawa T, Kimura H, Kawashima A, Mizukami H, et al. Nanosilica-induced placental inflammation and pregnancy complications: Different roles of the inflammasome components NLRP3 and ASC. Nanotoxicology. 2015;**9**(5):554-567. DOI: 10.3109/17435390.2014.956156

[93] Katsumiti A, Gilliland D, Arostegui I, Cajaraville MP. Mechanisms of toxicity of Ag nanoparticles in comparison to bulk and ionic ag on mussel hemocytes and gill cells. PLoS One. 2015;**10**(6):e0129039. DOI: 10.1371/journal.pone.0129039

[94] Xiao Y, Vijver MG, Chen G, Peijnenburg WJ. Toxicity and accumulation of Cu and ZnO nanoparticles in Daphnia magna. Environmental Science and Technology. 2015;**49**(7):4657-4664. DOI: 10.1021/acs.est.5b00538

[95] Li J, Martin FL. Chapter 4—Current perspective on nanomaterial-induced adverse effects: Neurotoxicity as a case example. In: Jiang X, Gao H, editors. Neurotoxicity of Nanomaterials and Nanomedicine. Cambridge, Massachusetts: Academic Press; 2017. pp. 75-98

[96] Sayes CM, Gobin AM, Ausman KD, Mendez J, West JL, Colvin VL. Nano-C60 cytotoxicity is due to lipid peroxidation. Biomaterials. 2005;**26**(36):7587-7595. DOI: 10.1016/j.biomaterials.2005.05.027

[97] Trickler WJ, Lantz SM, Murdock RC, Schrand AM, Robinson BL, Newport GD, et al. Silver nanoparticle induced blood-brain barrier inflammation and increased permeability in primary rat brain microvessel endothelial cells. Toxicological Sciences. 2010;**118**(1):160-170. DOI: 10.1093/toxsci/kfq244

[98] Chen X, Schluesener HJ. Nanosilver: A nanoproduct in medical application. Toxicology Letters. 2008;**176**(1):1-12. DOI: 10.1016/j.toxlet.2007.10.004

[99] Hussain SM, Hess KL, Gearhart JM, Geiss KT, Schlager JJ. In vitro toxicity of nanoparticles in BRL 3A rat liver cells. Toxicology in Vitro. 2005;**19**(7):975-983. DOI: 10.1016/j.tiv.2005.06.034

[100] Xia T, Li N, Nel AE. Potential health impact of nanoparticles. Annual Review of Public Health. 2009;**30**:137-150. DOI: 10.1146/annurev.publhealth.031308.100155

[101] Landsiedel R, Kapp MD, Schulz M, Wiench K, Oesch F. Genotoxicity investigations on nanomaterials: Methods, preparation and characterization of test material, potential artifacts and limitations—Many questions, some answers. Mutation Research. 2009;**681**(2-3):241-258. DOI: 10.1016/j.mrrev.2008.10.002

[102] Xie H, Mason MM, Wise JP Sr. Genotoxicity of metal nanoparticles. Reviews on Environmental Health. 2011;**26**(4):251-268. DOI: 10.1515/reveh.2011.033

[103] Albensi BC. What is nuclear factor kappa B (NF-κB) doing in and to the mitochondrion? Frontiers in Cell and Development Biology. 2019;7:154. DOI: 10.3389/fcell.2019.00154

[104] Gómez DM, Urcuqui-Inchima S, Hernandez JC. Silica nanoparticles induce NLRP3 inflammasome activation in human primary immune cells. Innate Immunity. 2017;**23**(8):697-708. DOI: 10.1177/1753425917738331

[105] Kang Y, Liu J, Song B, Feng X, Ou L, Wei L, et al. Potential links between cytoskeletal disturbances and electroneurophysiological dysfunctions induced in the central nervous system by inorganic nanoparticles. Cellular Physiology and Biochemistry. 2016; **40**(6):1487-1505. DOI: 10.1159/000453200

[106] Block ML, Elder A, Auten RL, Bilbo SD, Chen H, Chen JC, et al. The outdoor air pollution and brain health workshop. Neurotoxicology. 2012;**33**(5):972-984. DOI: 10.1016/j.neuro.2012.08.014

[107] Choi J, Zheng Q, Katz HE, Guilarte TR. Silica-based nanoparticle uptake and cellular response by primary microglia. Environmental Health Perspectives. 2010;**118**(5):589-595. DOI: 10.1289/ehp.0901534

[108] Podila R, Brown JM. Toxicity of engineered nanomaterials: A physicochemical perspective. Journal of Biochemical and Molecular Toxicology. 2013;**27**(1):50-55. DOI: 10.1002/jbt.21442

[109] Halamoda Kenzaoui B, Chapuis Bernasconi C, Guney-Ayra S, Juillerat-Jeanneret L. Induction of oxidative stress, lysosome activation and autophagy by nanoparticles in human brain-derived endothelial cells. The Biochemical Journal. 2012;**441**(3):813-821. DOI: 10.1042/BJ20111252

[110] Feng X, Zhang Y, Zhang C, Lai X, Zhang Y, Wu J, et al. Nanomaterial-mediated autophagy: Coexisting hazard and health benefits in biomedicine. Particle and Fibre Toxicology. 2020; **17**(1):53. DOI: 10.1186/s12989-020-00372-0

[111] Song B, Zhang Y, Liu J, Feng X, Zhou T, Shao L. Unraveling the neurotoxicity of titanium dioxide nanoparticles: focusing on molecular mechanisms. Beilstein Journals Nanotechnol. 2016 Apr **29**;7:645-654. DOI: 10.3762/bjnano.7.57. PMID: 27335754; PMCID: PMC4901937.

Chapter 2

Impact of Silver Nanoparticles on Neurodevelopment and Neurodegeneration

Yiling Hong

Abstract

Silver nanoparticles (AgNPs) are one of the most highly commercialized nanoparticles, having been used extensively as an antimicrobial agent in cosmetics, textiles, foods, and the treatment of diseases. However, the impact of AgNPs on human mental health has not yet been well characterized. Using the human pluripotent stem cell (hPSC) neuronal differentiation cellular model to assess AgNPs neurotoxicity has several benefits. First, hPSCs neuronal differentiation process can faithfully recapitulate stages of neural development from neuronal progenitors to mature neurons which can provide an excellent platform for neurodevelopment and neurodegeneration toxicity testing. Furthermore, it can limit the amount of animal use for toxicity studies. With this cellular model, we examined citrate-coated AgNPs (AgSCs) and Polyvinylpyrrolidone-coated (AgSP) mediated neurotoxicity. Our results suggested that AgNP induced neurotoxicity exhibited a coating and dose-dependent manner. AgSC had high neurotoxicity compared with AgSP. AgSC significantly up-graduated Metallothionein (1F, 1E, 2A) proteins, a metal-binding protein that plays an essential role in metal homeostasis, heavy metal detoxification, and cellular anti-oxidative defense. Transcriptome analysis indicated that AgSC inhibited neurogenesis and axon guidance, promoted gliogenesis and neuronal apoptosis through oxidative stress. Supplementation with ascorbic acid can act as an antioxidant to attenuate AgNP-mediated neurotoxicity.

Keywords: silver nanoparticles (AgNP), human pluripotent stem cell-derived neuronal network, transcriptome analysis, oxidative stress, neurogenesis and gliogenesis, neurodegeneration

1. Introduction

Engineered nanomaterials (ENMs) are ultra-fine materials (ranging from 1 to 100 nm in length or diameter) that are currently being developed for diverse applications due to their unique optical, electrical, and thermal properties [1–3]. Among them, silver nanoparticles (AgNPs) are one of the most widely used in medical and commercial products for their unique antibacterial functions [4–10]. The AgNP market is expected to reach USD 2.45 billion by 2022 (Globe Newswire, San Francisco, 2015). Furthermore, over the next decade, Nanotechnological approaches will continue to play a vital role in neuroscience, not just in the development of highly specific and sensitive imaging probes and biosensor interfaces, but also potential tools for treatment strategies [11, 12]. For example, molecules will be nano-engineered to cross the blood-brain barrier to target specific cell or signaling systems or act as vehicles for gene delivery [13, 14].

Although the translation of nanotechnology into the treatment of human neurological disorders is very promising, the biocompatibility of these materials is still a primary concern [8]. A wealth of data demonstrates that ENMs have the potential to induce inflammation, oxidative stress, and DNA damage, which point towards potential health risks for humans, including cardiovascular diseases, pulmonary diseases, impairment of brain function, and developmental toxicity [15–17]. Recently, researchers have begun to explore the potential neurotoxicity of ENMs such as AgNPs in cellular and animal models [18–21]. These studies showed that AgNPs can accumulate in the central nervous system (CNS) through the upper respiratory tract via the olfactory bulb or through crossing the blood-brain barrier, and thus induce neurodegeneration [10, 22, 23]. Furthermore, studies showed that AgNP exposure impairs neurodevelopment in PC12 cells and stem cell-derived neuronal networks and alters the expression of genes involved in neuronal function that are distinct from those of Ag^{+} alone, depending on size and coating [24–26].

So far, there has been limited information regarding the impact of AgNPs on neuronal development and neurodegeneration both in vivo and in vitro. hPSCs neuronal differentiation protocol evaluates the impact of AgNPs on multiple stages of differentiation ranging from neuronal progenitors to mature neuron and astrocyte networks [24, 25, 27]. This cellular model will help us to understand the mechanisms behind AgNP-mediated neuronal toxicity and identify the molecular markers to assess mental health risks associated with products containing EMNs. This book chapter is a summary of our recent studies regarding AgNP mediated neurotoxicity.

2. The impact of AgNP on neurogenesis

Neurogenesis is a series of developmental events leading to the formation of new neurons and astrocyte support cells. Neurogenesis is not only the most active process during the pre-natal stage but also happens in certain regions of the brain, such as the subgranular layer of the hippocampal dentate gyrus throughout life in mammals. Studies found that adult brains are more plasticity than previously thought. The process of neurogenesis is tightly regulated and influenced by both intrinsic genetic factors and extrinsic environmental factors. The process involves transitions from proliferation to differentiation, accompanied sequentially by the expression of the transcriptional factors such as Pax6, Tbr2, NeuroD, and Tbr1 [28]. If these gene expressions are altered, the neurogenesis events will be disrupted, which can lead to neuropsychiatric diseases such as anxiety, learning and memory, and Alzheimer's disease (AD) [29, 30].

Our study indicates that when citrate-coated AgNP (AgSC) were administered to the media during stem cell neuronal differentiation, neuronal progenitor rosettes were immunostained with neuronal progenitor markers: sex-determining region Y-box 2 (SOX2) and VI intermediate filament protein (Nestin). The results showed that AgSC exposure disrupted neuronal tube-like rosette formation and reduced neuronal progenitor population (**Figure 1A**). Quantification of SOX2 and Nestin relative fluorescence intensity showed that AgSC reduced SOX2 expression and increased Nestin expression in a concentration-dependent manner (**Figure 1B**). The alternation of the expression level of Sox2 and Nestin will change the neural progenitor fate. Furthermore, flow cytometric analysis for the population of neuronal progenitors with SOX2 and Nestin markers indicated that the percentage of $SOX2^{+}$ and $Nestin^{+}$ neuronal progenitors decreased from 54.3.3% to 20.9%, while $SOX2^{-}$ and $Nestin^{-}$ cells which would be unable to differentiate into neurons increased

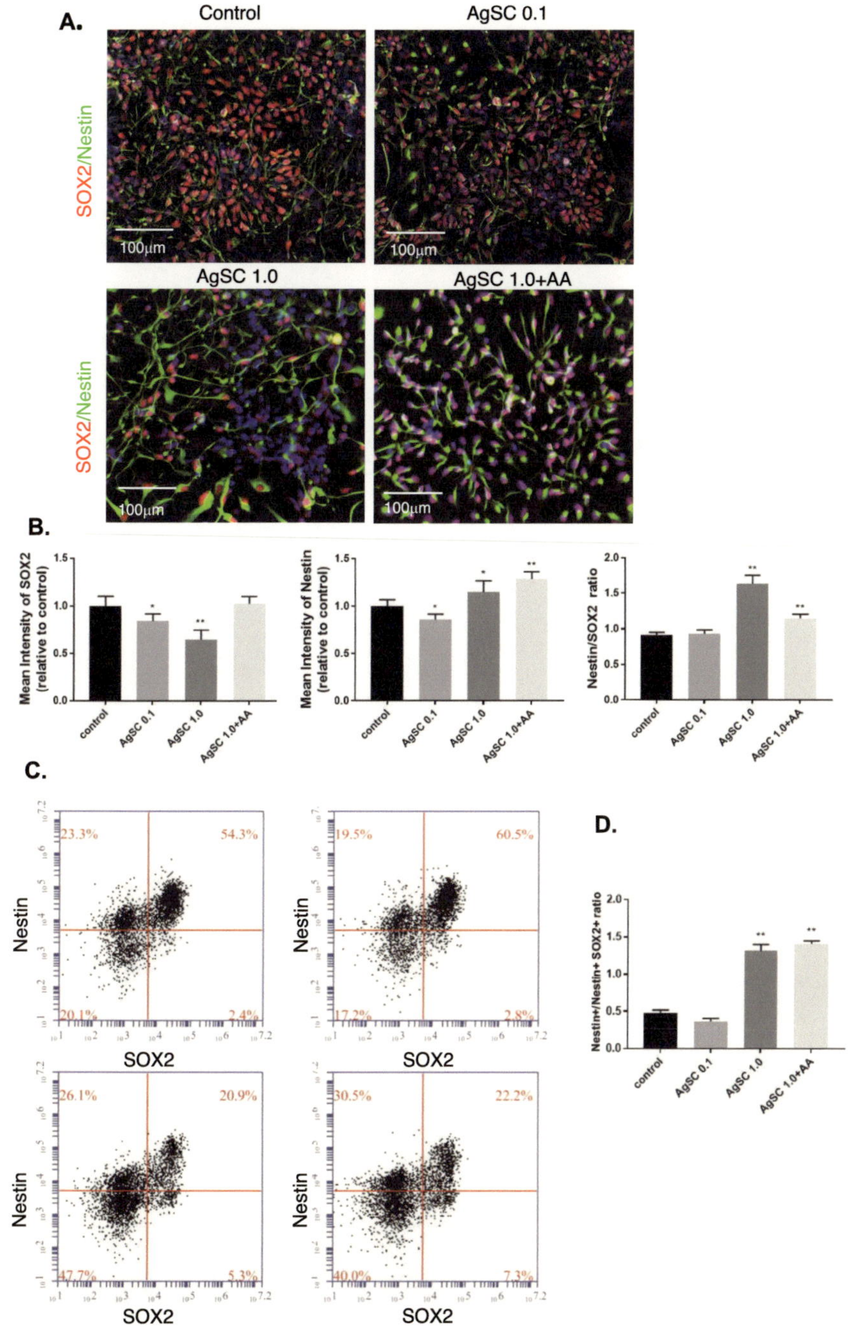

Figure 1.
*AgSC inhibited neurogenesis and promoted gliogenesis. A. AgSC inhibited neuronal rosette formation. Scale bar = 100 µm. B. Quantification of SOX2 and nestin relative intensities (fold of control), ratio of intensity between SOX2 and nestin from immunofluorescent staining images. C. BDAccuri C6 flow cytometer analysis the neuronal progenitor population. D. Ratio of nestin⁺/SOX2⁻ and nestin⁺ from flow cytometry result. Data is presented as mean ± SEM, *p < 0.05, or **p < 0.01 vs. control.*

from 20.19% to 47.7% at 1.0 µg/mL AgSC exposure compared to untreated sample. In contrast, $SOX2^-$ and $Nestin^+$ progenitors, which potentially could develop into astrocytes, increased from 23.3% to 26.1% with the same treatment (**Figure 2A**). The ratio of $Nestin^+/SOX2^-$ and $Nestin^+$ elevated to 1.45 at 1.0 µg/mL AgSC exposure, while the control group is 0.43. Those data support our hypothesis that AgSC

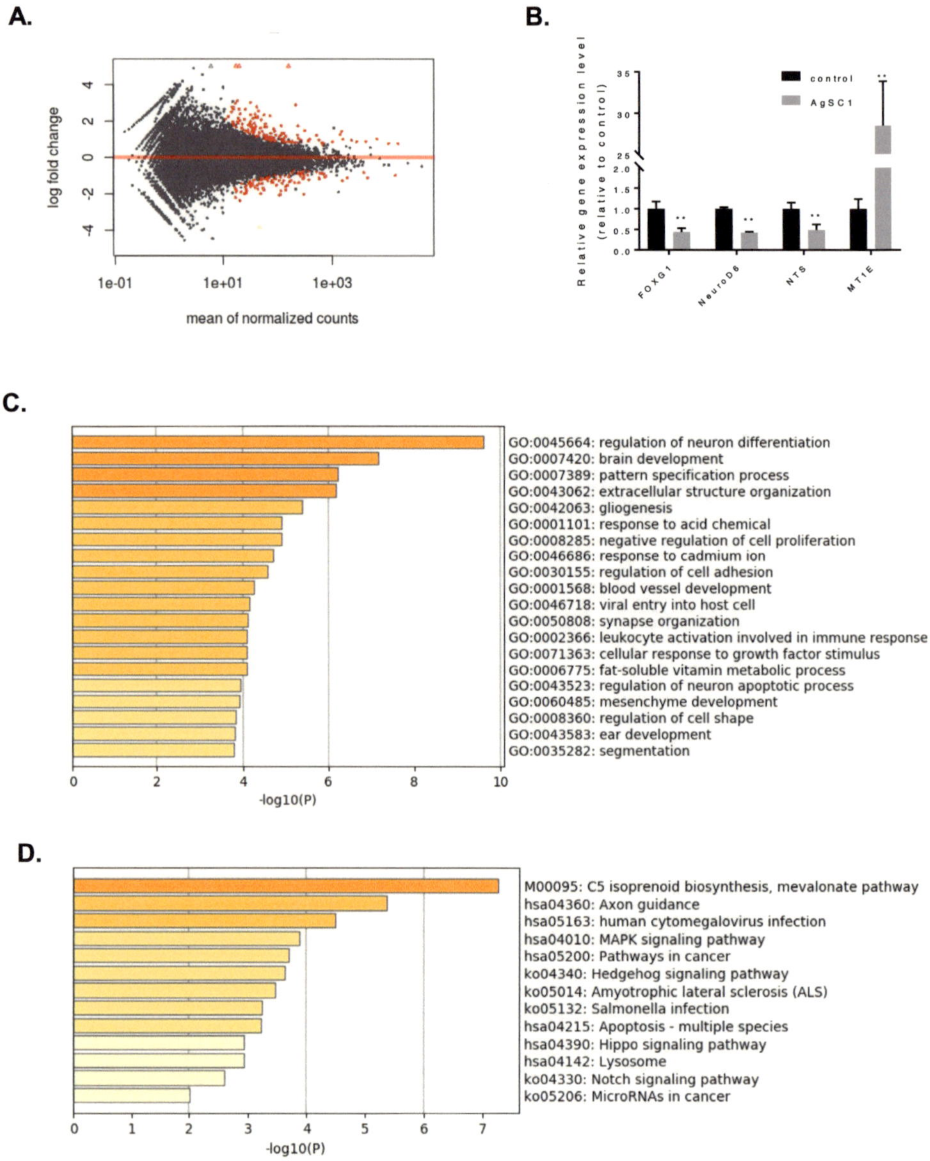

Figure 2.

*AgSC significantly altered gene expression A. Total DEGenes of 1.0 µg/mL AgSCs treated group compared with control group. The significant genes ($P \leq 0.05$) were labeled with red color. B. Quantitative real-time PCR to examine selected genes. FOXG1, NeuroD6 and NTS were significantly down-regulated. MT1E was significantly up-regulated. Data is presented as mean ± SEM, *$p < 0.05$, or **$p < 0.01$ vs. control. C. The clustered by GO biological processes. Result was shown as –log10(P) value. D. KEGG pathway and colored with –log10 (P) value. Min overlap ≥3, p-value ≤0.01 and min enrichment ≥1.5 were used for significant enrichments [25].*

inhibited neurogenesis and promoted gliagenesis. Lower concentrations of AgSC (0.1 µg/mL) slightly reduced SOX2 and Nestin expression, but the impact is insignificant. Supplements of AA partially reduced the effects (**Figure 1C**).

To further understand the molecular mechanisms of AgSC neuronal toxicity, a transcriptome analysis was performed., Total RNA was extracted from 3 replicates of 1.0 µg/ml AgSC exposure groups and untreated control groups to make libraries for sequencing. Significant differential expression (SDE) was cut off by padj <0.05 and |log2foldChange| > = 1. Among 322 SDE genes, 134 were up-regulated and 188 were down-regulated upon AgSC exposure (**Figure 2A**). The topmost up-regulated genes Metallothioneins 1F; Metallothioneins 1E; Metallothioneins 2A (45, 52, and 24 times), and frizzled class receptor 10 (FZD10) (**Table 1**). There are four main isoforms of cysteine-rich proteins Metallothioneins (MTs) which have the capacity to bind heavy metals such as zinc, copper, selenium, cadmium, mercury, silver, through the thiol group of its cysteine residues. MTs play important roles in metal homeostasis and protect against heavy metal toxicity, DNA damage, and oxidative stress. The other up-graduated gene is FZD10, a key regulator of the WNT signaling pathway. FZD10 plays acritical role in the neuronal pattern specification process, gliagenesis, and neurite outgrowth [31]. In addition, transcriptional factors NeuroD6, FOXG1, and NTS are among the top 20 significantly down-regulated genes (**Table 2**). Those genes play an important role in regulating neuronal differentiation, synaptogenesis, and axon extension during brain development [32]. The selected genes MT1E, NeuroD6, FOXG1, and NTS mRNA expression levels were examined with qPCR, respectively, and confirmed by RNA-seq data (**Figure 2B**).

These significantly differentially expressed genes were analyzed by metascape (http://metascape.org) for functional annotation clustering. Based on gene ontology analysis, in response to AgSC exposure, the most significant impact on the

Gene NAME	log2FoldChange
Metallothionein 1F (MT1F)	5.733703827
Frizzled class receptor 10 (FZD10)	5.63545845
Metallothionein 1E (MT1E)	5.55542047
Vestigial like family member 3 (VGLL3)	5.257650459
Pentraxin 3 (PTX3)	5.249022406
Metallothionein 2A (MT2A)	4.634538775
Cyclin O (CCNO)	4.614228599
FZD10 antisense RNA 1 (head to head) (FZD10-AS1)	3.906526795
Canopy FGF signaling regulator 1 (CNPY1)	3.102452269
NAD(P)H quinone dehydrogenase 1 (NQO1)	2.932494502
Sodium voltage-gated channel beta subunit 4 (SCN4B)	2.863730164
Transcription factor AP-2 beta (TFAP2B)	2.822828878
Zic family member 1 (ZIC1)	2.792907219
Actin, alpha 2, smooth muscle, aorta (ACTA2)	2.779703608
Actin, gamma 2, smooth muscle, enteric (ACTG2)	2.726196918
Alpha-2-macroglobulin (A2M)	2.584555887
Crumbs 2, cell polarity complex component (CRB2)	2.561792956
Zic family member 4 (ZIC4)	2.479236853
Neuronal pentraxin 2 (NPTX2)	2.443739583
Protein tyrosine kinase 2 beta (PTK2B)	2.421852257
Vasoactive intestinal peptide receptor 2 (VIPR2)	2.404813991
Collagen type I alpha 2 chain (COL1A2)	2.330235258
Zinc finger DHHC-type containing 22 (ZDHHC22)	2.286038754
Iroquois homeobox 1 (IRX1)	2.283963197
EF-hand and coiled-coil domain containing 1 (EFCC1)	2.280818988

Table 1.
AgSC mediated up-graduated differential expressed genes.

Gene name	log2FoldChange
CREBATF bZIPtranscription factor (CREBZF)	−3.554019527
LIM domain 7 (LMO7)	−3.064914689
SRSF protein kinase 2 (SRPK2)	−2.924926145
Myocyte enhancer factor 2C (MEF2C)	−2.81151306
Transmembrane protease, serine 13 (TMPRSS13)	−2.794313859
Neuritin1 (NRN1)	−2.770934839
Ring finger protein 175 (RNF175)	−2.724670035
G1 to S phase transition 2 (GSPT2)	−2.674801389
Methylsterol monooxygenase 1 (MSMO1)	−2.634382164
Coiled-coil domain containing 171 (CCDC171)	−2.583794397
Meis homeobox 2 (MEIS2)	−2.540498698
Gamma-aminobutyric acid type A receptor gamma2 subunit (GABRG2)	−2.503960528
Src-like-adaptor (SLA)	−2.478947195
calcium binding protein 1 (CABP1)	−2.341485603
semaphorin 3F (SEMA3F)	−2.336576641
fatty acid binding protein 6 (FABP6)	−2.333357057
B-cell CLLlymphoma 11A (BCL11A)	−2.268903493
neuronal differentiation 6 (NEUROD6)	−2.2525029
neurotensin (NTS)	−2.251646035
DLG associated protein 1 (DLGAP1)	−2.233930932
zinc finger CCCH-type containing 15 (ZC3H15)	−2.227494717
cerebellar degeneration related protein 1 (CDR1)	−2.217658748
neurotensinreceptor 1 (NTSR1)	−2.214928804
forkheadbox G1 (FOXG1)	−2.185129942
chromosome 12 open reading frame 65 (C12orf65)	−2.176721998

Table 2.
AgSC-mediated down-graduated differential expressed genes.

biological processes were regulation of neuron differentiation, brain development, synapse organization, pattern specification processes, gliogenesis, and cholesterol biosynthetic processes (**Figure 2B**). The KEGG analysis results showed that the affected genes were enriched in C5 isoprenoid biosynthesis, axon guidance, neuron apoptotic progress lysosomes, MAPK, WNT, Hedgehog, and Notch signaling pathways (**Figure 2D**). In conclusion, our data suggest that AgSCs interfere with metal homeostasis and cholesterol biosynthesis which induces oxidative stress, reduces neurogenesis and axon guidance and promotes gliogenesis and apoptosis.

3. Impact of AgNPs on neurodegeneration

Neurodegeneration is the progressive loss of structure or function of neurons due to aging, diseases, and environmental factors. Free radicals or oxidative stress may damage lipids, nucleic acids, and proteins. The brain is particularly vulnerable to oxidative stress because of its high level of protein and lipid content and low level of antioxidants [33]. Reactive oxygen species (ROS) such as superoxide (O_2^-) and hydrogen peroxide (H_2O_2) are typically categorized as neurotoxic molecules associated with decreased synaptic plasticity performances in cognitive function and cell death. ROS can initiate excitotoxicity effects by inducing an intracellular calcium influx that leads to the activation of glutamate receptors and apoptosis [24]. To investigate the molecular mechanisms underlying AgNP-induced neurodegeneration, mature glutamatergic neuronal networks containing astrocytes were generated from iPSC. ROS production were examined with 20 nm citrate-coated AgNPs (AgSCs) and polyvinylpyrrolidone-coated AgNPs (AgSPs) exposure. Our results showed AgNPs-induced ROS production was coating and dose-dependent (**Figure 3A**). AgSCs-treated neurons produced more ROS compared to the AgSPs-treated samples.

We examined our hypothesis, stating that AgNPs-induced ROS will promote astrocyte activation and neuronal cell death. Astrocytes are the most numerous neuroglial cells in the central nervous system (CNS). Astrocyte vital functions include blood-brain barrier formation, providing structural and metabolic support, and regulating synaptic transmission and water transport [34, 35]. Astrocytes are

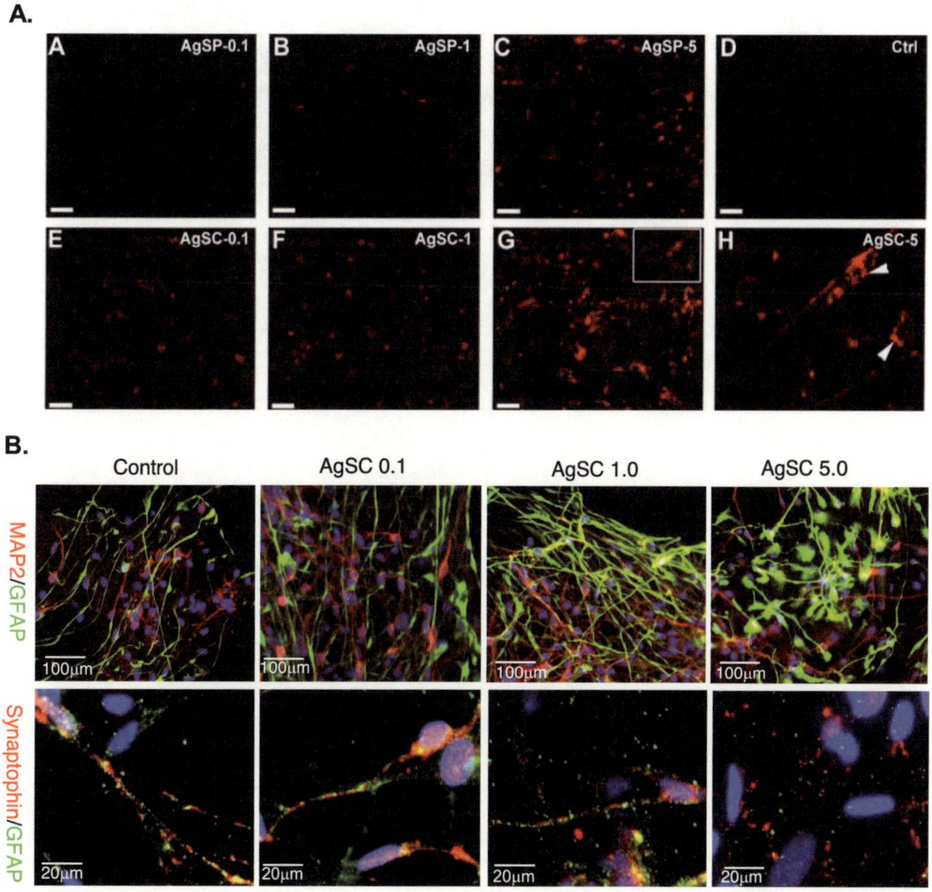

Figure 3.
AgNP promoted ROS production, induced astrocyte activation and synapse protein loss. A. ROS was generated in a dose-dependent manner in (A–C) AgSP-treated neurons. (E–G) AgSC-treated neurons produced a higher amount of ROS compared to (D) the untreated neurons (ctrl). (H) the inset image of hGNs treated with 5 mg/ml AgSC showed the interneuronal accumulation of ROS. Scale bar 100 mM. B. Immunofluorescent staining images showed AgSC promoted astrocyte activation. C. Effect of AgSC on the excitatory synaptic protein, vGlu1 and PSD95 expression. The co-localization of vGlut1(red) and PSD95 (green) in the controls. Exposure to AgSC (5 mg/ml) significantly diminished the vGlut1and PSD95 expression and co-localization [24, 27].

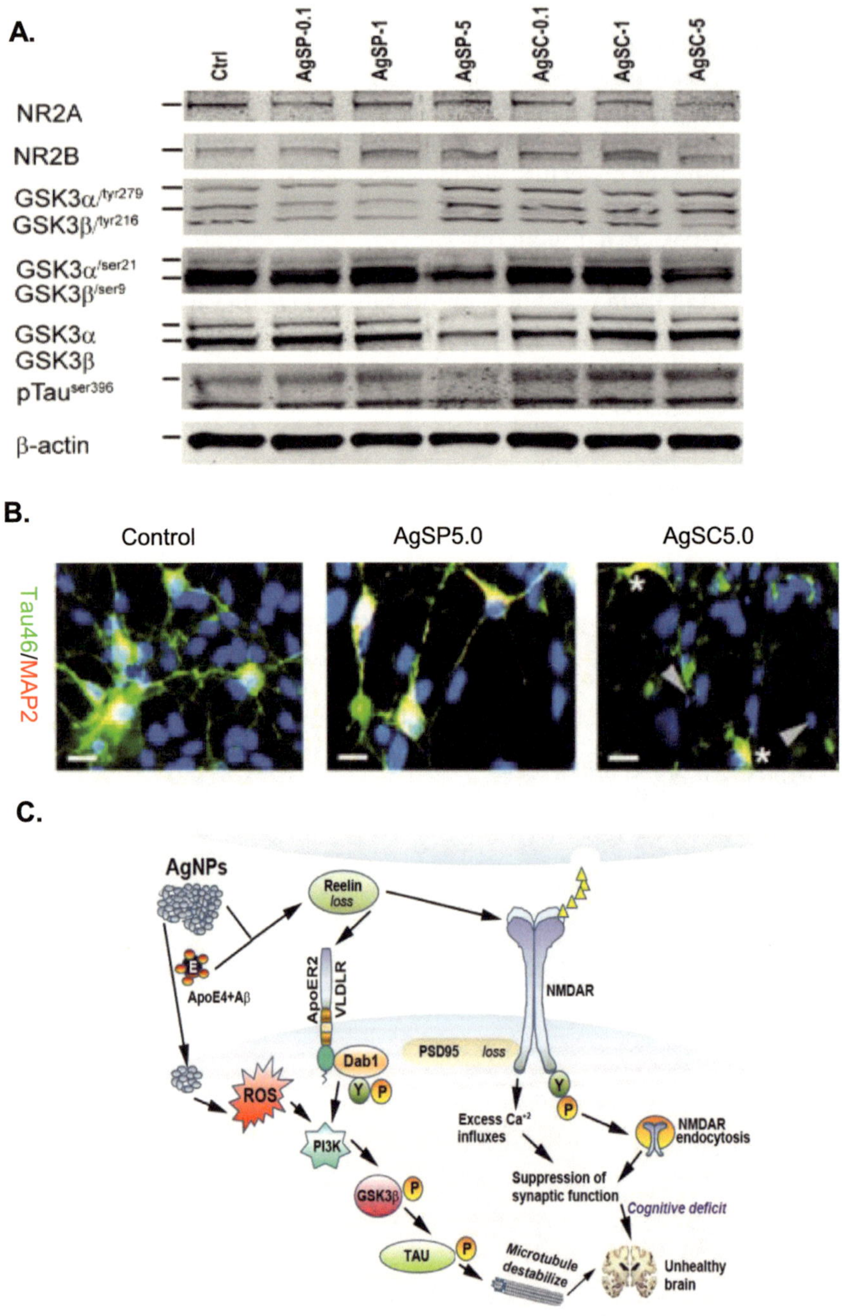

Figure 4.
The molecular mechanisms of the AgNP induced neurotoxicity. A. Immunoblotting of glutamate receptors NR2A/B, phosphorylated GSK-3α/β and Tau46 after espousing the AgNPs at three different concentrations for 72 h. β-Actin was used as a loading control. B. Immunostaining with Tau46/Map2 indicated that the effect of AgNPs on microtubule assembly proteins expression and axon outgrowth. C. Potential molecular mechanisms underlying AgNP induced neurotoxicity [24].

sensitive to environmental changes. Under the chronic stress condition, astrocytes will undergo significant structural remodeling which reduces process length, branching, and density length [36]. Our results indicated that 0.1 μg/ml dose AgSC exposure increased the number of GFAP positive astrocytes for neuronal protection. At high doses, 5.0 μg/ml AgSC exposure altered astrocyte morphology and induced astrocyte activation. Furthermore, we examined how AgSCs affect synaptic structural and functional components. Neurons were double-stained for the presynaptic vesicle membrane protein Synaptophin (Syn) and the postsynaptic marker PSD-95 (**Figure 3B**). Untreated control neurons showed extensive neuritis processes co-localized between Syn and PSD-95 (**Figure 3B**). Exposure with AgSCs at 1.0 and 5.0 μg/mL drastically reduced Syn and PSD-95 expression and their co-localization.

We further investigated the signaling cascade involved in AgNP mediated neurodegeneration with different coatings. Glutamate receptor *N*-methyl-D-aspartate receptor (NMDAR) plays a key role in synaptic plasticity, which is linked to a form of long-term depression (LTD) as well as neuron survival. The dysregulation of NMDAR in neurons will trigger an apoptosis-associated increase in caspase-3 activity. The immunoblotting results showed that AgSCs reduced the expression levels of the post-glutamate receptor subunits NR2A and NR2B and increased the phosphorylation of GSK3α/βTyr216/279, whereas AgSPs had similar effects, but only at a higher concentration (5 μg/ml) (**Figure 4A**). GSK3 α/β phosphorylation has been shown to be associated with neural apoptosis in many neurodegenerative disorders. An increase in GSK-3β activity via GSK3α/βTyr216/279 phosphorylation can lead to Tau phosphorylation (pTau) [37, 38]. Our immunoblotting results confirmed that the AgNPs can increase GSK3 α/β phosphorylation and increase Tau phosphorylation at serine 396 in a dose-dependent manner, whereas AgSPs had no effect on Tau phosphorylation (**Figure 4A**). Tau is involved in the loss of neuronal dendrites and the axonal network by disrupting microtubule assembly. The result of Tau46/MAP2 double immunostaining showed that AgSC treatment caused the reduction of both protein expression and axon outgrowth (**Figure 4B**). **Figure 4D** presents a model of molecular mechanisms for AgNPs induced neurodegeneration. We suggested that phosphorylation of GSK3a/bTyr216/279could be the potential biomarker for AgNPs neurotoxicity testing.

4. Conclusion

In our study, neuronal progenitors, mature glutamatergic neurons, and astrocytes were derived from hPSC which were used for testing AgNPs toxicity. The results indicated that citrate-coated AgSCs significantly affected neuronal progenitor proliferation, gliagenesis, neuronal neuritis outgrowth, and cell viability due to up-graduated Metallothionein (1F, 1E, 2A) gene expression and increased ROS production. AgSPs had similar effects but only exhibited the toxicities at higher concentration exposure. In this context, the proper coating can prevent or limit the neurotoxicity associated with the AgNPs exposure. Our study indicates that stem cell-derived neuronal differentiation is an excellent cellular platform for investigating the impact of AgNPs on neuronal development and neurodegeneration and identifying biomarkers for risky assessment. In addition, this cellular model could also be used for different types of nanoparticles such as carbon-based nanoparticles, ceramic nanoparticles, metal nanoparticles, semiconductor nanoparticles, and lipid-based nanoparticles neuronal toxicity assessment in the future.

Acknowledgements

This work was supported by the National Institutes of Environmental Health Sciences (1R15 ES019298-01A1). I would like to thank Aynun Begum, Hao Li, and Neza Repar who had worked on these projects and provided the data for this book chapter.

Conflict of interest statement

The authors report no conflicts of interest.

Author details

Yiling Hong
College of Veterinary Medicine, Western University of Health Sciences, Pomona, CA, USA

*Address all correspondence to: yhong@westernu.edu

References

[1] Bruchez M, Moronne M, Gin P, Weiss S, Alivisatos AP. Semiconductor nanocrystals as fluorescent biological labels. Science. 1998;**281**:2013-2016

[2] Chen X, Schluesener HJ. Nanosilver: a nanoproduct in medical application. Toxicology Letters. 2008;**176**(1):1-12

[3] Oberdorster G, Maynard A, Donaldson K, Castranova V, Fitzpatrick J, Ausman K, et al. Principles for characterizing the potential human health effects from exposure to nanomaterials: Elements of a screening strategy. Particle and Fibre Toxicology. 2005;**2**:8

[4] Choi O, Hu Z. Size dependent and reactive oxygen species related nanosilver toxicity to nitrifying bacteria. Environmental Science & Technology. 2008;**42**(12):4583-4588

[5] Domeradzka-Gajda KM, Nocun J, Roszak B, Janasik CD, Quarles W Jr, Wasowicz J, et al. A study on the in vitro percutaneous absorption of silver nanoparticles in combination with aluminum chloride, methyl paraben or di-n-butyl phthalate. Toxicology Letters. 2017;**272**:38-48. DOI: 10.1016/j.toxlet.2017.03.006

[6] Kim JS, Kuk E, Yu KN, Kim JH, Park SJ, Lee HJ. Antimicrobial effects of silver nanoparticles. Nanomedicine. 2007;**3**:95-101

[7] Westerband EI, Hicks AL. Nanosilver-enabled food storage container tradeoffs: Environmental impacts versus food savings benefit, informed by literature. Integrated Environmental Assessment and Management. 2018;**14**(6):769-776. DOI: 10.1002/ieam.4093

[8] Wang EC, Wang AZ. Nanoparticles and their applications in cell and molecular biology. Integrative Biology. 2014;**6**:9-26

[9] West J, Halas N. Applications of nanotechnology to biotechnology. Current Opinion in Biotechnology. 2000;**11**:215-217

[10] Ahamed M, Alsalhi MS, Siddiqui MK. Silver nanoparticle applications and human health. Clinica Chimica Acta. 2010;**411**(23-24):1841-1848. DOI: 10.1016/j.cca..08.016

[11] Samir TM, Mansour MM, Kazmierczak SC, Azzazy HM. Quantum dots: Heralding a brighter future for clinical diagnostics. Nanomedicine. 2012;7(11):1755-1769

[12] Silva J, Bowman DM. In: Hunter R, Preedy V, editors. The Regulation of Nanomedicine. Nanomedicine in Health and Disease. Boca Raton: Science Publishers; 2012. pp. 20-42

[13] Win-Shwe TT, Fujimaki H. Nanoparticles and neurotoxicity. International Journal of Molecular Sciences. 2011;**12**:6267-6280

[14] Etame AB, Diaz RJ, O'Reilly MA, Smith CA, Mainprize TG, Hynynen K, et al. Enhanced delivery of gold nanoparticles with therapeutic potential into the brain using MRI-guided focused ultrasound. Nanomedicine. 2012:**8**(7):1133-1142

[15] Colvin V. The potential environmental impacts of engineered nanomaterials. Nature Biotechnology. 2003;**21**:1166-1170

[16] Rajanahalli P, Stuck C, Hong Y. The effects of silver nanoparticles on cell cycle progression and cell viability in mouse embryonic stem cells. Toxicology Reports. 2015;**2**:758-765

[17] Zhu L, Dai L, Hong Y. DNA damage induced by multiwalled carbon nanotubes in mouse embryonic stem cells. Nano Letters. 2007;7(12):3592-3579

[18] Hadrup N, Loeschner K, Mortensen A, Sharma AK, Qvortrup K, Larsen EH, et al. The similar neurotoxic effects of nanoparticulate and ionic silver in vivo and in vitro. Neurotoxicology. 2012;**33**(3):416-423

[19] Rungby J, Danscher G. Localization of exogenous silver in brain and spinal cord of silver exposed rats. Acta Neuropathologica. 1983;**60**(1-2):92-98

[20] Rungby J, Danscher G. Neuronal accumulation of silver in brains of progeny from argyric rats. Acta Neuropathologica. 1983b;**61**(3-4):258-262

[21] Tang J, Xiong L, Wang S, Wang J, Liu L, Li J, et al. Distribution, translocation and accumulation of silver nanoparticles in rats. Journal of Nanoscience and Nanotechnology. 2009;**9**(8):4924-4932

[22] Hoet PH, Bruske-Hohlfeld I, Salata OV. Nanoparticles—Known and unknown health risks. Journal of Nanobiotechnology. 2004;**2**(1):12. DOI: 10.1186/1477-3155-2-12

[23] Yang Z, Liu ZW, Allaker RP, Reip P, Oxford J, Ahmad Z, et al. A review of nanoparticle functionality and toxicity on the central nervous system. Journal of the Royal Society, Interface. 2010; 7(Suppl. 4):S411-S422. DOI: 10.1098/rsif.2010.0158.focus

[24] Begum AN, Aguilar JS, Elias L, Hong Y. Silver nanoparticles exhibit coating and dose-dependent neurotoxicity in glutamatergic neurons derived from human embryonic stem cells. Neurotoxicology. 2016;**57**:45-53. DOI: 10.1016/j.neuro.2016.08.015

[25] Li H, Li QQ, Hong Y. Global gene expression signatures in response to citrate-coated silver nanoparticles exposure. Toxicology. 2021;**461**:152898. DOI: 10.1016/j.tox.2021.152898

[26] Power C, Badireddy AR, Ryde IT, Seidler FJ, Slotkin TA. Silver nanoparticles compromise neurodevelopment in PC12 Cells: critical contributions of silver ion, particle size, coating, and composition. Environmental Health Perspectives. 2011;**119**:37-44

[27] Repar N, Li H, Aguilar JS, Li QQ, Drobne D, Hong Y. Silver nanoparticles induce neurotoxicity in a human embryonic stem cell-derived neuron and astrocyte network. Nanotoxicology. 2018;**12**(2):104-116. DOI: 10.1080/17435390.2018.1425497

[28] Espósito MS, Piatti VC, Laplagne DA, Morgenstern NA, Ferrari CC, Pitossi FJ, et al. Neuronal differentiation in the adult hippocampus recapitulates embryonic development. The Journal of Neuroscience. 2005;**25**:10074-10086

[29] Hevner RF, Miyashita-Lin E, Rubenstein JL. Cortical and thalamic axon pathfinding defects in Tbr1, Gbx2, and Pax6 mutant mice: Evidence that cortical and thalamic axons interact and guide each other. The Journal of Comparative Neurology. 2002;**447**(1):8-17. DOI: 10.1002/cne.10219

[30] Martynoga B, Drechsel D, Guillemot F. Molecular control of neurogenesis: A view from the mammalian cerebral cortex. Cold Spring Harbor Perspectives in Biology. 2012;**4**:10. DOI: 10.1101/cshperspect.a008359

[31] Levy-Strumpf N, Culotti JG. Netrins and Wnts function redundantly to regulate antero-posterior and dorso-ventral guidance in *C. elegans*. PLoS Genetics. 2014;**10**(6):e1004381. DOI: 10.1371/journal.pgen.1004381

[32] Uittenbogaard M, Baxter KK, Chiaramello A. The neurogenic basic helix-loop-helix transcription factor NeuroD6 confers tolerance to oxidative stress by triggering an antioxidant response and sustaining the mitochondrial biomass. ASN Neuro. 2010;**2**(2):e00034. DOI: 10.1042/AN20100005

[33] Ermak G, Davies KJ. Calcium and oxidative stress: From cell signaling to cell death. Molecular Immunology. 2002;**38**:713-721

[34] Blanco-Suárez E, Caldwell AL, Allen NJ. Role of astrocyte-synapse interactions in CNS disorders. The Journal of Physiology. 2016;**595**(6):1903-1916. DOI: 10.1113/jp270988

[35] Hacimuftuoglu AA, Tatar D, Cetin N, Taspinar F, Saruhan U, Okkay H, et al. Astrocyte/neuron ratio and its importance on glutamate toxicity: An in vitro voltammetric study. Cytotechnology. 2016;**68**(4):1425-1433. DOI: 10.1007/s10616-015-9902-9

[36] Diniz DG, Oliveira MA, Lima CM, Fôro CA, Sosthenes MC, Bento-Torres J, et al. Age, environment, object recognition and morphological diversity of GFAP-immunolabeled astrocytes. Behavioral and Brain Functions. 2016;**12**(1):1-28. DOI: 10.1186/s12993-016-0111-2

[37] Elyaman W, Terro F, Wong NS, Hugon J. In vivo activation and nuclear translocation of phosphorylated glycogen synthase kinase-3beta in neuronal apoptosis: links to tau phosphorylation. The European Journal of Neuroscience. 2002;**15**:651-660

[38] Park CH, Lee BH, Ahn SG, Yoon JH, Oh SH. Serine 9 and tyrosine 216 phosphorylation of GSK-3beta differentially regulates autophagy in acquired cadmium resistance. Toxicological Sciences. 2013;**135**:380-389

Section 2

Neurotoxicity and Chemical Substances

Chapter 3

Neurotoxic Agents and Peripheral Neuropathy

Neslihan Eskut and Asli Koskderelioglu

Abstract

Neurotoxicity may develop with exposure to various substances such as antibiotics, chemotherapeutics, heavy metals, and solvents. Some plants and fungi are also known to be neurotoxic. Neurotoxicity can develop acutely within hours, or it can develop as a result of exposure for years. Neurotoxicity can be presented with central or peripheral nervous system findings such as neurobehavioral symptoms, extrapyramidal signs, peripheral neuropathy. Peripheral nerve fibers are affected in different ways by neurotoxicant injury. The pattern of injury depends on the target structure involved. The focus of this chapter includes signs, symptoms, pathophysiology, and treatment options of neurotoxicity.

Keywords: neurodegeneration, neuropathy, neurotoxic, mechanisms of neurotoxicity, chemicals

1. Introduction

The direct or indirect effects of chemical or physical agents that disrupt the function or structure of the nervous system of humans or animals are called neurotoxicants [1]. Neurotoxicity can be presented with central or peripheral nervous system findings such as neurobehavioral symptoms, extrapyramidal signs, and peripheral neuropathy. Peripheral nerve fibers are affected distinctly by neurotoxicant injury. Mild or severe polyneuropathy involves the peripheral nerves, affecting the myelinated, thinly myelinated, and unmyelinated fibers. A wide variety of etiological factors can cause polyneuropathy. In addition to frequent causes such as diabetes mellitus, alcohol abuse, the peripheral nervous system is vulnerable to several rare conditions [2]. Toxic peripheral neuropathies are caused by various chemicals, a basic form of acquired polyneuropathy [3]. Neurotoxicity may develop when exposed to heavy metals, solvents chemotherapeutics, monomers, gases and pesticides. The focus of this chapter includes signs, symptoms, pathophysiology, and treatment options of several neurotoxic agents that cause peripheral neuropathy.

2. Heavy metals

Heavy metals are naturally occurring elements with a high weight and a density at least five times greater than water [4]. In other words, any toxic metal can be defined as heavy metal, regardless of its atomic weight or density [5]. The industrial activities of the modern world have caused a massive rise in human exposure to heavy metals, and heavy metals have harmful effects on human health [6]. Heavy metals' contamination of water and air is an environmental threat, and hundreds of millions of people are being exposed worldwide. The concentration of heavy metals in water supplies, air, and food is evaluated in this respect [7, 8].

Heavy metals such as arsenic (As), lead (Pb), mercury (Hg), aluminum (Al), and cadmium (Cd) do not have any particular role in an organism and can be toxic even at low levels [9]. On the contrary, it has been reported that some of these heavy metals such as iron, magnesium, selenium, copper, zinc, cobalt, nickel, molybdenum, chromium, and manganese are essential nutrients that have functional roles for various diverse biochemical and physiological functions in the body [10]. However, in over adequate amounts, they may cause toxicities. Acute and chronic toxic effects of heavy metals have an impact on different organs of the human body. In addition to the nervous system disorders, gastrointestinal and kidney dysfunction, skin lesions, vascular damage, immune system dysfunction, birth malformations, and cancer are examples of the complications of heavy metals toxic effects [8, 11, 12].

2.1 Lead

Lead is a toxic heavy metal in different sources such as contaminated drinking water, battery manufacture, cosmetics, leaded gasoline, lead-based paint, cans, glazed ceramics, traditional herbal medicine products, water pipes, jewelry, tobacco smoke, and electronic cigarettes, and toys. Lead exposure can be considered a public health concern, especially in early childhood, because children have increased hand-to-mouth activity, so they are more at risk [13, 14]. While the half-life of Pb in the bloodstream is about 35 days, it is stored in bones for approximately 30 years [15, 16]. Oxidative stress, alterations in membrane biophysics, dysregulation of cell signaling, and the impairment of neurotransmission are considered the complex underlying mechanisms of lead-induced neurotoxicity [17].

One of the most critical endpoints of Pb toxication is neurological effects. Pb toxication frequently causes neuropathy in adults, while encephalopathy is mainly seen in children. Exposure to high Pb levels causes encephalopathy with signs such as hyperirritability, cerebellar findings, seizures, unconsciousness, and coma. It is reported that exposure to low Pb levels has been associated with impaired cognitive and intellectual function in children [18, 19]. In occupational exposure, it is reported that neurological signs and symptoms include weakness, forgetfulness, irritability, headache, impotence, decreased libido, vertiginous symptoms, and paresthesia in Pb exposure workers. Moreover, increased prevalence and severity of white matter lesions, changes in nerve conduction velocity, and alterations of somatosensory evoked potentials were documented [18, 19].

In lead toxicity, motor-predominant polyneuropathy, which causes the development of wrist-drop, may present. Additionally, because of secondary to autonomic nerve involvement, constipation may accompany [20]. After forbidden the usage of leaded gasoline, changes in lead mining practices, and the abandonment of lead-based paint, human exposure to the primary sources of Pb decreased. So the incidence of overt lead toxicity induced polyneuropathy decreased [21].

2.2 Arcenic (As)

Arsenic is an environmental toxin, and this heavy metal is widely distributed to the earth. Hundreds of millions of people consume inorganic contaminated tube well water [22, 23]. Burning the charcoal and metal foundry activities are known to cause atmospheric deposition of As. Excessive pesticides and fertilizers and mining use cause soil contamination with As [24, 25]. While As often exists in the world crust in the trivalent atomic state (inorganic) with other heavy metals such as Pd, iron, copper, it is generally oxidized to pentavalent form in the soil and water. It is reduced to in trivalent atomic state in low oxygen situations, such as deep seawater [26]. Inorganic As is more potent and has been implicated in neurotoxic effects. The inorganic form should be distinguished from the non-neurotoxic organic As found in some fish and shellfish [21].

It is reported that traditional folk medicines can be the other sources of As [27, 28]. Some herbal medicines commercially available have been reported to contain heavy metals such as lead, mercury, and arsenic. Using these products may cause heavy metal toxicity and secondary peripheral neuropathy [26]. As causes various adverse effects on human health such as carcinogenic and non-carcinogenic [26].

The exact metabolic pathways of As are yet to be proved. However, oxidative methylation and glutathione conjugation are the primary pathways suggested [29]. The primary mechanism in As-induced neurological pathologies has been suggested oxidative stress with Vitro and in vivo studies [9]. While exposure to high levels of As induces primarily central nervous system findings, exposure to low levels causes primarily peripheral nervous system findings [18].

Single high dose exposure to As may lead to severe gastrointestinal and systemic symptoms such as nausea, diarrhea, vomiting, pain, dehydration, and weakness. It is usually the result of suicide- homicide or accidental poisoning. If the patient survives acute poisoning with As, neurological symptoms such as light-headedness, weakness, delirium, encephalopathy, and peripheral neuropathy develop [30].

Chronic neurological symptoms of As exposure are delirium, encephalopathy, and also peripheral neuropathy. In neuropsychological tests, while psychomotor speed and attentive processes were mildly impaired, verbal learning and memory were severely impaired [31, 32]. It is known that peripheral neuropathy may last for several years or even life-long, but on the other hand, in severe cases, diffuse sensorimotor polyradiculoneuropathy may be seen, similar to the Guillan–Barré syndrome. At the same time, chronic As exposure can cause painless sensory-predominant peripheral neuropathy [32].

The diagnosis of arsenic toxicity can be made by demonstrating high urinary and increased arsenic levels in the nails and hairs. Serum arsenic level estimation is not recommended because of the rapid clearance of arsenic. There is no gold standard specific treatment for chronic arsenic toxicity. For acute arsenic toxicity treatment, chelating agents such as BAL, D-penicillamine, and meso-2,3-dimercap-tosuccinic acid are mainly used [33].

2.3 Mercury (Hg)

Mercury is heavy metal in the air, water, and soil in three chemical forms; metallic/elemental, inorganic, and organic Hg (methyl mercury and ethyl mercury). The elemental Hg is liquid at room temperature and can evaporate quickly. The vapor form of Hg is more dangerous and can is readily absorbed from the lungs (80%) and distributed throughout the body [8]. A wide variety of fields in that Hg have been used, such as gold mining, fluorescent light bulbs production, ingredients of antiaging creams, fungicides to protect plants against infections, and protection in multidose vials of vaccines [34, 35].

In the middle of the 1950s, around 200.000 people have affected by the consumption of organic Hg-contaminated fish in Minamata Bay, Japan. Because of chronic Hg toxicity, neurological signs and symptoms occurred, such as ataxia, weakness, numbness, disturbance in speech, chewing, and swallowing. Infants born with severe developmental disabilities from the poisoned pregnant women were reported. After that, the illness was called Minamata disease [36].

It is reported that organic mercury influences the dorsal root and trigeminal ganglia and causes paresthesia, usually just before causing widespread CNS dysfunction [20]. In nerve conduction studies, motor abnormalities were much more frequently reported than sensory abnormalities. Most frequently, findings were prolonged latencies and reduced amplitudes in both motor and sensory nerves. Nevertheless, interestingly, those abnormalities were shown more often in upper extremities, not lower extremities, a finding that differs from expectations [37]. Electromyography (EMG) was less frequently performed in the studies but reported results were always abnormal. The most frequently reported EMG findings (fibrillations, positive waves) were suggestive of active denervation and also reinnervation (prolonged motor unit potential duration, polyphasic motor unit potential durations) [38]. Electromyography (EMG) was less frequently performed in the studies but reported results were always abnormal. The most frequently reported EMG findings (fibrillations, positive waves) were suggestive of active denervation and also reinnervation (prolonged motor unit potential duration, polyphasic motor unit potential durations) [20].

2.4 Cadmium (Cd)

Cadmium is a highly toxic heavy metal. According to Agency for Toxic Substance and Disease Registry, Cd is the 7th most toxic heavy metal. The biological half-life of Cd is about 20–30 years in humans [39]. Cd exists naturally in unrefined rocks. Several sources of human exposure to Cd include mining works, contaminated groundwater use, commercial products (batteries, color pigments, several alloys, and Polyvinyl chloride, phosphate fertilizer) [40].

Exposure to Cd can be occurred by inhalation and also ingestion. It can accumulate into the lungs, olfactory bulb, and kidney [40]. Suggested mechanisms of Cd neurotoxicity include increased lipid peroxidation associated with oxidative stress and causing injury to the microvasculature of the brain. Experimental studies show that rats exposed to Cd, accumulation in choroid plexus, and Cadmium-related lipid peroxidation were demonstrated in brain areas such as the cerebellum and cerebral cortex [41, 42]. Cd neurotoxicity might be caused by defective neurogenesis, lead notably reduced neuronal differentiation and axonogenesis, leading to neuronal cell death [43].

Exposure to Cd causes very different neurological signs and symptoms of both the peripheral and central nervous systems. These are mental retardation, learning disabilities, behavioral pathologies [44]. Moreover, there is growing evidence about Cd-dependent neurotoxicity being one of the possible etiological factors of neurodegenerative diseases such as Alzheimer's, Parkinson's diseases, and sporadic amyotrophic lateral sclerosis [45, 46]. However, Little is known about the influence of cadmium on the peripheral nervous system. Experimental studies have shown that Cd can be a potent neurotoxicant for the peripheral nervous system. Viaene et al. investigated the influence of Cd on polyneuropathy in 13 retired, long-term Cd-exposed workers. They performed the neurological clinical examination, nerve conduction studies, and needle EMG were performed in the study. 54% of the retired Cd workers were diagnosed with polyneuropathy. The authors concluded that increased Cd body burden promotes PNP development at older age [47].

There is no consensus in the literature regarding the treatment of Cd toxicity. While clinical treatment protocols exist for the use of Ethylene Diamine Tetra Acetic Acid (EDTA), 2,3-Dimercapto-1-propane sulfonic acid (DMPS), and meso-2, 3-dimercaptosuccinic acid (DMSA), there are limited human studies. EDTA is the agent most widely accepted for clinical use. It should be noted that these chelation treatments applied during acute poisoning may aggravate damage to the renal tubules. EDTA, which has a long history of safe use, is approved by the FDA to chelation heavy metals. It should not be given faster than one gram per hour nor in dosage greater than three grams per session. Cd is also significantly present in sweat during sauna, which appears to be a moderately successful modality for reducing the body burden of Cd without risk of tubular damage [48–50].

2.5 Tallium (T.I.)

Thallium is one of the heavy metals found in the earth's crust. Tl is colorless, odorless, and tasteless, and it has been used as a pesticide and rodenticide. Although the use of T.I. in this field has been abandoned in most western countries, there are still countries where it continues to be used. Thallium has been used in a wide variety of industries fields such as electronics, lamps, jewelry, pigmentation [51].

Thallium can contaminate by skin contact, inhalation of contaminated air, or food consumption from contaminated soil or water. Suggested mechanisms of T.I. neurotoxicity include lipid peroxidation and lysosomal enzyme beta-galactosidase in brain regions [52].

Toxication of T.I. causes neurological and non-neurological disorders. Anorexia, vomiting, gastrointestinal bleeding, abdominal pain, alopecia, cardiac arrhythmias are the best-known disorders. In a dose-dependent manner, neuropsychiatric signs have been reported as following; coma, delirium, seizure, hallucination, fatigue, emotional changes, ataxia, and loss of sensation, cranial neuropathy, and polyneuropathy [51, 53, 54]. Thallium-related polyneuropathy can become evident within 1–2 days. It is reported that a painful sensory-motor polyneuropathy mimicking Guillain-Barre's syndrome occurs. In delayed admission, patients are more prone to severe polyneuropathy and other neurological disorders [51, 55].

Treatment for thallium intoxication consists of termination from exposure, supportive care, and enhanced elimination. Prussian blue is approved as an oral agent to prevent absorption of thallium. It is reported that hemodialysis combined with the usage of Prussian blue helps treat patients even delayed admission [51, 55, 56].

3. Solvents

Solvents used in industry as degreasing agents, adjuvants, thinners, and cleaners are widespread. N-Hexane, carbon disulfide, ethylene oxide are widely used solvents [57]. Adhesives containing n-hexane are also widely used in the manufacture of leather goods [58]. Repeated occupational exposure of solvents can be both inhalation and skin contact. While the hexane concentration limit of organ damage through prolonged or repeated exposure is suggested as 5%, the organic solvents used in the adhesives may contain a higher percentage of n-hexane [59]. The toxic effects of organic solvents can be considered a public health problem even though regulations have been made that reduce usage limits [60]. The organic solvent syndrome is the mildest form of chronic exposure. Irritability, fatigue, and reversible difficulty to concentrate are the related symptoms [61]. The neurotoxicity of solvents may occur in both the peripheral nervous system and central nervous system [62].

3.1 N-hexane

The molecular mechanisms of peripheral neuropathy induced by hexane exposure have been investigated in several studies. ɣ-diketone 2,5-hexanedione, which is a neurotoxin, is the metabolite of n-hexane. ɣ-diketone 2,5-hexanedione is the cause of sensory or sensory-motor peripheral neuropathy [63–66]. According to the suggested mechanism, the accused metabolite reacts with amino groups of proteins, including neuroproteins. Lysine-rich neuroproteins are especially vulnerable, including microtubule-associated proteins required for axonal transport. Disruption of axonal transport causes consecutive degenerative changes resulting in localized demyelination and remyelination, with initial changes in the most extensive and most prolonged axons in peripheral nerves and the spinal cord, with similar changes in shorter nerve fibers at a later stage. It results in distal symmetrical sensorimotor neuropathy supported by central-peripheral distal axonopathy [63].

Detailed neurological and neuropsychological examinations are recommended to confirming the clinical findings of central and peripheral nervous system dysfunctions in case of suspicion of toxication. Sensory abnormalities such as insensitivity to pinprick and touch, impaired two-point discrimination, changes in sensation to position, vibration, or temperature, diminished deep tendon reflexes are common neurological findings. Peripheral neuropathy is characterized by symmetrical progressive distal sensory and motor impairment [61, 62, 64]. Nerve conduction studies and electromyography should be performed to confirm peripheral neuropathy. It is reported that severe exposure and affected patients may develop muscle atrophy and foot drop [62]. Typical electrophysiological findings increase in distal latencies, slowing of nerve conduction velocities, conduction block with temporal dispersion, and the slowing down of transmission in electromyography in subjects with severe neuropathy [58, 62]. Neuroimaging Cranial magnetic resonance imaging (MRI) should be performed to detect the atrophic changes in the frontal lobes and cerebellum and white-matter lesions described after exposure to certain solvents [67, 68]. It is reported that acute, low-dose exposures might be related to specific changes in test performance, which improve after withdrawal from exposure. However, chronic exposure can also be associated with permanent cognitive changes [67].

3.2 Carbon disulfide

Carbon disulfide (CS2) is an organic solvent used for various industrial purposes, such as an insecticide, fresh fruit conservation, disinfectant against insects [69]. CS2 is a significant metabolite of the drug disulfiram used as a dissuasive for alcohol abuse. The occupational CS2 exposure can be by inhalation and skin contact. It is known that the highest degree of exposure is in the viscose rayon industry [70]. Exposure to carbon disulfide is likely to occur for the general population by inhaling contaminated ambient air, eating vegetables and fruits, or other food products containing carbon disulfide [69]. Since carbon disulfide has lipophilic nature, the distribution of C.S. 2 is easily in organs such as the brain and liver. C.S. 2 is metabolized to thiocarbamates in these organs, and it is considered that dithiocarbamates can take part in neurotoxic effects [71].

According to acute or sub-acute high-level exposures of CS2 can lead to unconsciousness, hallucinations, emotional lability, extrapyramidal signs, and polyneuropathy [69, 70]. It is reported that exposure of 200 to 500 ppm may cause death [69]. Peripheral neuropathy and extrapyramidal signs have been reported following chronic occupational low-level exposures. In low level (10 to 40 ppm) exposure, peripheral neuropathy may be asymptomatic and detected only electrophysiologically. As the concentration of CS 2 increases (20 to 60 ppm), a progressive sensorimotor distal asymmetrical polyneuropathy appears [72].

In neurological examination, findings include; paresthesia and dysesthesia tend to occur in a 'stocking and glove' distribution, loss of ankle and patellar reflexes, and diminished pain, touch, and vibration sensation in the distal lower limbs. In some cases, recovery may be slow and incomplete, possibly because of residual axonal damage [73].

There is no typical clinical profile and routine laboratory tests, including cerebrospinal fluid (CSF) examination. Nevertheless, CSF should be performed for differential diagnosis. Nerve conduction studies and electromyography should be performed to confirm peripheral neuropathy. It is reported that long-term exposure and a cumulative dose of CS2 exposure are related to electrophysiological findings [74]. In the electrophysiological examination, reduced motor and sensory amplitudes, slightly slowed motor conduction velocities prolonged distal latencies are reported in exposed patients with neuropathy symptoms. In the same patient group, needle EMG revealed chronic, length-dependent denervation with decreased recruitment, large motor units, and fibrillation potentials [75].

3.3 Ethylene oxide (EO)

Ethylene oxide is a powerful sterilizer for medical materials and antiseptic for furs and some foods. It is a gas at room temperature. The occupational EO exposure can be by inhalation. Since EO is a water-soluble substance, it can quickly spread to all organs shortly after inhalation exposure [72]. EO is a potent alkylating agent and can interact with all cellular components, including DNA [76].

The principal neurotoxicant effect of EO is polyneuropathy. EO-related distal symmetrical axonal polyneuropathy has been reported in several cases reports in the 1980s, and Ohnishi et al. established an experimental model of EO neuropathy [77–80]. Kuzuhara et al. showed axonal degeneration with mild changes of the myelin sheath in sural nerve biopsies [79]. Neurotoxic effects may develop in both intermittent high doses and chronic prolonged low-dose exposure [72]. Gross et al. reported four cases who had occupational EO exposure. One of the cases had encephalopathy syndrome, and three of them had polyneuropathy [80]. In clinically symptomatic cases, distal extremity numbness and weakness, diminished sensation in the feet and hands can be initial symptoms. However, some of the cases can be asymptomatic. The electrophysiological examination reported reduced motor and sensory amplitudes and mildly slowed motor and sensory nerve conduction velocities [80, 81]. Gradual improvement of neurotoxicant effects was found associated with withdrawal from exposure [81].

4. Medications and peripheral nervous system toxicity

Antineoplastic drugs' most frequent and sometimes serious complication is chemotherapy-induced peripheral neuropathy (CIPN). The estimated prevalence of CIPN is 19–85% [82]. Compared to other peripheral neuropathies, such as painful diabetic polyneuropathy, patients with CIPN are likely to develop more severe symptoms, suffering from pain affecting both feet and hands, with faster progression. The high prevalence of CIPN among patients with cancer poses a serious problem for both patients and doctors administering the treatment. Due to the CIPN and related symptoms, sometimes it may be necessary to interrupt, stop, or reduce the dose of drugs, limiting the treatment's efficacy [83].

Platinum analogs (Cisplatin, oxaliplatin), taxanes (Paclitaxel), vinca alkaloids, and proteasome inhibitors (bortezomib) are the most commonly preferred antineoplastic medications. These are successfully used as first-line treatment for several solid and blood cancers, such as breast, lung, colorectal, gastric cancers, and multiple myeloma [84]. Although these antineoplastic medications have different chemical structures and mechanisms, chemotherapy-induced peripheral neurotoxicity (CIPN) is one of their common side effects. The occurrence of CIPN varies according to the chemotherapeutic drugs, dose, duration of exposure, and method of assessment [85]. The highest rate of CIPN is reported in platinum analogs (70–100%), taxanes (11–87%), thalidomide, and its analogs (20–60%), and ixabepilone (60–65%) [86].

4.1 Platinum analogs; cisplatin, carboplatin, oxaliplatin

Platinum analogs interact with DNA, forming platinum-DNA compounds and cause apoptotic cell death. Most platinum analogs cause some degree of neurotoxicity. Dorsal root ganglion (Drg) is considered to be the primary target of neurotoxicity. It has been shown that platinum analogs cause apoptosis in dorsal root ganglia and morphological changes in the nucleus in-vitro [84]. Because of the lack of blood–brain barrier protection and be vascularized by fenestrated capillaries, the nuclei of Drg neurons are vulnerable to chemically-induced damages [87]. Platinum analogs induced peripheral neuropathy is a sensory neuronopathy caused by direct damage to Drg neurons, leading to an anterograde axonal degeneration. According to sensory neuronopathy, altered touch sensation, paresthesia in the distal extremities, tingling, altered touch sensation, proprioceptive loss, areflexia, and sensory ataxia occur. Patients frequently experience painful sensations, including spontaneous burning, electric shock-like pain, along with mechanical or thermal allodynia or hyperalgesia. Neuropathic pain symptoms have been reported, often even after treatment discontinuation [88, 89].

Since the 1980s, Cisplatin has been used to treat testicular, ovarian, and small cell lung cancers. Cisplatin administration induced severe toxicity, especially to the kidneys and nervous system [90]. Cisplatin causes primarily sensory neuropathy, characterized by distal parenthesis, progressing to proprioceptive loss, areflexia, and sensory ataxia [88]. Symptoms arise after cumulative doses above 300 mg/m2. Severe symptoms related to neuropathy have been reported to occur three to six months post-treatment cessation [91]. Electrophysiological studies have typically shown marked reduction in sensory action potential amplitudes with relative preservation of conduction velocity, indicative of axonal loss [84, 91]. Motor and autonomic symptoms and signs are infrequent but may occur in severe cases. Treatment with platinum analogs has been rarely associated with acute inflammatory demyelinating polyradiculoneuritis in patients with solid tumors [92].

Carboplatin is known to be less toxic, with neuropathy observed in 13–42% of patients. At the same time, carboplatin may induce mild neurotoxicity in quarter patients, with moderate to severe neurotoxicity in 5% of patients [93]. Peripheric neurotoxic side effects are common with high doses (800–1600 mg/m2) [94]. Electrophysiological studies reveal a reduction in compound sensory and motor amplitudes. Experimental studies have reported that at very high doses (10–15 mg/kg), carboplatin induces neurotoxicity and associated platinum deposition in the dorsal root ganglion, similar to Cisplatin [84].

Oxaliplatin has been effectively used as a first-line therapy against colorectal cancer. Its neurotoxicity may develop both acute and chronic. Acute and rapidly reversible peripheral neuropathy occurs in approximately 65–98% of patients within hours of drug infusion at a dose ranging 85–130 mg/m2 and may last up to one week. In 12 cycles of chemotherapy received, symptoms may persist up to 21 days or longer. Myelotoxicity and enteric and peripheral neuropathy may be induced by chemotherapy with oxaliplatin [95]. Cold-induced neuropathic symptoms are the most important difference in the clinical presentation between oxaliplatin and cisplatin-induced neuropathy [96]. Chronic peripheral neuropathy occurs in approximately 50–70% of patients, described as a pure sensory, axonal neuropathy [95]. Patients frequently experience distal paresthesia, sensory ataxia, jaw pain, leg cramps. Electrophysiological studies of oxaliplatin-induced peripheral neuropathy reduce the sensory action potentials with preserved motor amplitudes and conduction velocities. However, spontaneous activity can be obvious, suggesting an immediate effect of the drug on the axonal excitability rather than structural damage [84, 97].

4.2 Taxanes; paclitaxel

Paclitaxel, docetaxel, cabazitaxel are the class of taxanes that act on microtubules, interfering with the normal cycling of microtubule depolymerization and polymerization. The incidence of CIPN according to taxanes may be very high (11 to 87%), and the highest rates are reported for Paclitaxel [98]. Neuropathy caused by taxanes usually emerges as a dominant sensory neuropathy with the stocking-and-glove distribution. The manifestations are paresthesias, dysesthesias, numbness, altered proprioception, and loss of dexterity predominantly in the toes and fingers. Motor and autonomic involvement are infrequent [99]. Neurological symptoms and findings are dose-dependent and tend to improve after stopping the treatment. However, some patients experience symptoms up to 1–3 years and sometimes lifelong after the therapy [100]. Microtubule disruption, mitochondrial dysfunction, axonal degeneration, altered calcium homeostasis, altered expression and function of ion channels, production of pro-inflammatory cytokines are the suggested underlying mechanisms of CIPN [101, 102].

Paclitaxel is a microtubule-binding antineoplastic drug commonly used to treat various solid tumors like lung, breast, and ovarian cancer. Paclitaxel is highly potent against proliferating neoplastic cells, but neurons not dividing cells are vulnerable to Paclitaxel. The treatment with paclitaxel affects the peripheral nervous system and primarily causes sensory axonal polyneuropathy [103]. Peripheral nerves biopsies have revealed a pathology of axonal degeneration, secondary demyelination, and, in cases of severe neuropathy, nerve fiber loss has also been observed [104].

4.3 Vinca alkaloids; vincristine

Vinca Alkaloids are developed from the Madagascar periwinkle plant, including vincristine, vinblastine, vinorelbine, and vindesine. These drugs are commonly prescribed to treat various tumors, such as Hodgkin and non–Hodgkin lymphoma, testicular cancer, and non–small cell lung cancer [102]. Vinca alkaloids have well-documented effects on microtubules – including binding to tubulin and inhibiting microtubule Dynamics [105].

Vincristine was approved in July 1963 by the United States Food and Drug Administration (FDA). It is one of the most common anticancer drugs used in pediatrics oncology. However, its clinical use is accompanied by severe side effects, such as peripheral neuropathy and neuropathic pain leading to treatment discontinuation. Both sensory and motor dysfunctions characterize peripheral neuropathy related to vincristine [106]. The duration and therapeutic doses received by patients directly affect the severity of symptoms. Besides sensory symptoms, patients also experienced muscle weakness and cramping. Changes in axonal transport and dorsal root ganglia resulting in Wallerian degeneration, altered ion channels activity and hyperexcitability of peripheral neurons, production of pro-inflammatory cytokines are the suggested underlying mechanisms of vincristine-induced peripheral neuropathy [101].

Vincristine use in Charcot–Marie–Tooth disease (CMT) patients has a black box warning added by the FDA. The CMT patients with the ERG2 gene mutation and polymorphism in the CEP72 gene are associated with increased risk and severity of drug-induced neuropathy [107, 108].

There is no specific treatment for vinca alkaloid-induced peripheral neuropathy. Pyridoxine or pyridostigmine can be having a certain efficacy in vincristine-induced neuropathy. A topical capsaicin cream was demonstrated to give benefit in peripheral neuropathy. In neuropathic pain, carbamazepine, imipramine, or lignocaine can be used [101].

4.4 Proteasome inhibitors; bortezomib

Bortezomib is a reversible proteasome inhibitor antineoplastic drug that is successfully used against multiple myeloma and some types of solid tumors. It was first described as an inflammation inhibitor, but with its cytotoxic effects, it began to be used in cancer therapy. Bortezomib was approved in 2003 by FDA as a single agent against advanced myeloma but is now mostly used in combination therapies [109]. Although bortezomib is generally well tolerated, the most frequent limiting factor for its clinical use is a painful peripheral neuropathy side effect. Bortezomib-induced peripheral neuropathy is attributed to paresthesias, dysaesthesias, burning sensations, numbness, sensory loss, reduced proprioception, and vibratory sensation. Besides these symptoms and signs, demyelinating neuropathy may also be present. Deep tendon reflexes and autonomic innervation of the skin are reduced in patients treated with bortezomib [110]. Chronic, distal, and symmetrical sensory peripheral neuropathy is typical neuropathy induced by bortezomib.

Neuropathic pain symptoms have been reported to continue for weeks, months, or even years after treatment discontinuation.

Bortezomib-induced peripheral neuropathy is reported in approximately one-third of the patients [111]. Suggested mechanisms of bortezomib-induced peripheral neuropathy are increased sphingolipid metabolism in astrocytes, inflammation related to TNFa and IL-1, mitochondrial damage, reactive oxygen radical production, and alteration in Ca^{++} signaling [101].

5. Others

5.1 Acrylamide

Monomeric acrylamide is a potent neurotoxin used in different industrial and laboratory processes. Acrylamide is readily absorbed by inhalation, ingestion, or dermal contact. The acrylamide exposure affects the central nervous system (CNS) and peripheral nervous system (PNS). Chronic and high-level exposure to this water-soluble chemical mostly causes peripheral neuropathy. The peripheral neuropathy causes impairment in the arms and legs of exposed workers. Several studies reported that short-term occupational exposure to acrylamide resulted in weakness of lower extremities, loss of deep tendon reflexes and sensations in distal limbs, and numbness preceded by skin peeling from the hands [112–114]. Moreover, it has been shown that longer exposure involved more severe symptoms, including cerebellar dysfunction followed by peripheral neuropathy. Based on numerous investigations and risk assessments, acrylamide is generated in food preparation processes involving high temperatures [115, 116]. Different pathogenetic mechanisms were hypothesized; however, the exact mechanism of action is not completely elucidated. Like other toxic neuropathies, the prognosis of neuropathy is associated with the degree of central axonal degeneration. Three important hypotheses currently considering acrylamide neurotoxicity include inhibition of kinesin-based fast axonal transport, alteration of neurotransmitter levels, and direct inhibition of neurotransmission [117].

5.2 Styrene

Styrene is a colorless solvent found in paints, plastics, and resins. It is one of the essential monomers usually used in plastic production. This compound can cause intoxication when inhaled in high concentrations for longer periods. There are few case reports regarding styrene-induced peripheral neuropathies. Early studies demonstrated abnormal neurological findings in humans exposed to styrene in low doses [118]. Styrene-induced peripheral neuropathy is characterized by neuropathic symptoms that start within a few days after significant exposure to styrene. Goba et al. reported that two workers presented with styrene-induced neuropathy. The workers had sensory-motor peripheral neuropathy of a demyelinating type [119].

5.3 Organophosphates

Organophosphates (OP) are chemical substances involved in the main components of herbicides, pesticides, and insecticides. Acute or chronic exposure to organophosphates causes several toxic effects in humans and animals. The exposure to organophosphates might be accidental or intentional. The organophosphate intoxication may occur after exposure to pesticides, either through occupational contact or suicide attempts. Acute toxic effects and delayed toxic neuropathy are related to central and peripheral nervous system involvement. The main effect of OP exposure is poisoning; however, peripheral neuropathy has been linked to chronic exposure. Several recent cases were reported associated with organophosphate-induced delayed neuropathy (OPIDN) after ingestion of organophosphate insecticides. The peripheral neuropathy associated with organophosphate intoxication may be seen with mild exposure. The mechanism of OPIDN is explained by loss of function of both motor and sensory axons located distally and ascending and descending tracts of the spinal cord [120, 121]. Organophosphate-induced delayed neuropathy is an uncommon clinical condition characterized by a distal paresis in the lower limbs and sensory symptoms. Electrophysiological findings show motor axonal neuropathy. The delayed onset of peripheral neuropathy and axonal motor involvement without a progressive course is needed for the diagnosis. Organophosphates can irreversibly bind to acetylcholine esterase (AChE) and prevent the breakdown of acetylcholine (ACh). The liberation of ACh overstimulates the muscarinic and nicotinic receptors. The main mechanism of OPIDN development is related to the inhibition of neuropathy target esterase (NTE) via phosphorylation. Neuropathy target esterase is an essential integrated membrane protein in neurons that takes part in axonal maintenance [122]. Its activity plays a crucial role in axonal maintenance since it facilitates the transport of macromolecules to the end of axons [120].

The symptoms are attributed to the effects on sensory and motor nerves with a typical axonal length-associated pattern. Lower extremities are predominantly affected. However, upper extremities are affected at higher OP exposure. The prognosis of peripheral neuropathy varies due to clinical involvement. It is primarily associated with the age of the individual (a younger age is associated with mild neuropathy), type of organophosphate, the persistence of myelopathic features, pyramidal involvement, degree of CNS involvement to peripheral nerve dysfunction [120, 123, 124]. There is no treatment approved for OPIDN, and the recovery is slow and partial. Thivakaran et al. reported a 15-year-old female who developed OPIDN with a smaller dose of chlorpyrifos [124]. Akçay et al. reported a similar case diagnosed with organophosphate-induced delayed neuropathy (OPIDN) complicated with central nervous system findings. They observed partial improvement in muscle strength despite motor axonal polyneuropathy [125]. In addition, Moretto et al. reported electrophysiological findings in 11 patients with acute OP poisoning [126]. Three of these patients developed OPIDN, mainly sensory-motor polyneuropathy. The diagnostic approach should be made carefully in peripheral neuropathy patients, excluding other possible causes, especially those who did not display cholinergic toxicity before the onset of neuropathy. Early recognition of OP poisoning and a professional approach to intoxication can be life-saving.

6. Conclusion

Chemicals have toxic effects on the human body. Neurotoxicity demonstrates acute and chronic manifestations. A toxic chemical can produce an acute toxic response, besides prolonged exposure of a toxin may result in slowly developing chronic disease. In many cases, the putative neurotoxic damage present many years after initial exposure to the toxin. Therefore, the clinical signs elicited and symptoms expressed should be interpreted carefully. The neurotoxicity level and the circumstances of the exposure determine clinical presentation. The clinical signs and symptoms due to neurotoxicity may be expressed in central and peripheral nervous systems. Moreover, toxic agents disrupt cellular processes and result in epigenetic changes. While several heavy metals cause DNA damage which leads to carcinogenesis, the peripheral nervous system is also vulnerable to toxin-induced damage. A peripheral neuropathy may have its origin in the neurone, axon, myelin sheath or either Schwann cells. Patients may present with length-dependent sensorimotor peripheral neuropathy as well as mononeuropathy or radicular pathology. Organophosphates and acrylamide have been associated with severe damage to the motor nerve terminal. Many chemicals have the ability to cause axon damage including acrylamide, arsenic, carbon disulfide, n-hexane, lead, organic mercury, perhexilene, and thallium. Hexachlorophene and perhexilene have been involved in myelin disruption. Also, methyl mercury is well-known neurotoxin cause neuronopathy. Here, we discuss the peripheral nervous system manifestations of heavy metals, solvents, chemotherapeutics, monomers, gases and pesticides in detail.

Conflict of interest

The authors declare no conflict of interest.

Author details

Neslihan Eskut* and Asli Koskderelioglu
Department of Neurology, University of Health Sciences, Izmir Bozyaka Education and Research Hospital, Izmir, Turkey

*Address all correspondence to: nespur@hotmail.com

References

[1] Spencer PS, Lein PJ (2014). Neurotoxicity. *In Encyclopedia of Toxicology: Third Edition.* Elsevier. 2014.p:489-500 DOI:10.1016/B978-0-12-386454-3.00169-X

[2] Abraira VE, Ginty DD. The Sensory Neurons of Touch. Neuron 2013; 79: 618-639. DOI: 10.1016/j.neuron.2013.07.051

[3] Valentine WM. Toxic Peripheral Neuropathies: Agents and Mechanisms. Toxicol Pathol. 2020;48:152-173. DOI: 10.1177/0192623319854326.

[4] Chen YG, He XLS, Huang JH, et al. Impacts of heavy metals and medicinal crops on ecological systems, environmental pollution, cultivation, and production processes in China, Ecotoxicology and Environmental Safety 2021; 219:112336. DOI: 10.1016/j.ecoenv.2021.112336

[5] Singh MR. Impurities-heavy metals (2009): IR perspective Available from: http://www.usp.org/pdf/EN/meetings/asMeetingIndia/2008Session4track1.pdf

[6] Agnihotri SK, Kesari KK. Mechanistic Effect of Heavy Metals in Neurological Disorder and Brain Cancer. In: Kesari K. (eds) Networking of Mutagens in Environmental Toxicology. Environmental Science and Engineering. Springer, Cham. 2011. DOI:10.1007/978-3-319-96511-6_2

[7] Luo L, Wang B, Jiang J, et al. Heavy metal contaminations in herbal medicines: determination. comprehensive risk assessments. Front. Pharmacol 020;11:595335.DOI:10.3389/fphar.2020.595335

[8] Balali-Mood M, Naseri K, Tahergorabi Z, Khazdair MR and Sadeghi M (2021) Toxic Mechanisms of Five Heavy Metals: Mercury, Lead, Chromium, Cadmium, and Arsenic. Front. Pharmacol. 12:643972. DOI: 10.3389/fphar.2021.643972

[9] Andrade VM, Aschner M, Marreilha Dos Santos AP. Neurotoxicity of Metal Mixtures. Adv Neurobiol. 2017;18:227-265. DOI:10.1007/978-3-319-60189-2_12

[10] Bhattacharya PT, Misra SR, Hussain M. Nutritional Aspects of Essential Trace Elements in Oral Health and Disease: An Extensive Review. Scientifica (Cairo). 2016;2016:5464373. DOI: 10.1155/2016/5464373.

[11] Gazwi HSS, Yassien EE, Hassan H M. Mitigation of lead neurotoxicity by the ethanolic extract of Laurus leaf in rats. Ecotoxicol. Environ Safe 2020; 192: 110297. DOI:10.1016/j.ecoenv.2020.110297

[12] Costa M. Review of arsenic toxicity, speciation and polyadenylation of canonical histones. Toxicol. Appl. Pharmacol 2019; 375: 1-4. DOI:10.1016/j.taap.2019. 05.006

[13] Ramírez Ortega D, González Esquivel DF, Blanco Ayala T, et al. Cognitive Impairment Induced by Lead Exposure during Lifespan: Mechanisms of Lead Neurotoxicity. Toxics. 2021;9(2):23. DOI: 10.3390/toxics9020023.

[14] Sankhla MS, Sharma K, Kumar R. Heavy Metal Causing Neurotoxicity in Human Health. International Journal of Innovative Research in Science, Engineering and Technology 2017;6: 7721-7726. DOI:10.15680/IJIRSET.2017.0605054

[15] Papanikolaou NC, Hatzidaki EG, Belivanis S, et al. Lead toxicity update. A brief review. Med Sci Monit. 2005t;11(10):RA329-RA336.

[16] Hu H, Shih R, Rothenberg S, Schwartz BS. The epidemiology of lead

toxicity in adults: measuring dose and consideration of other methodologic issues. Environ Health Perspect. 2007;455-462. DOI: 10.1289/ehp.9783

[17] Khan DA, Qayyum S, Saleem S, Khan FA. Lead-induced oxidative stress adversely affects health of the occupational workers. Toxicol Ind Health. 2008;24:611-618. DOI: 10.1177/0748233708098127.

[18] Pohl HR, Roney N, Abadin HG. Metal ions affecting the neurological system. Met Ions Life Sci. 2011;8: 247-262.

[19] Bellinger DC. The protean toxicities of lead: new chapters in a familiar story. Int J Environ Res Public Health. 2011;8:2593-2628. DOI:10.3390/ ijerph8072593

[20] Jang DH, Hoffman RS. Heavy metal chelation in neurotoxic exposures. Neurol Clin. 2011;29:607-622. DOI: 10.1016/j.ncl.2011.05.002.

[21] Staff NP, Windebank AJ. Peripheral neuropathy due to vitamin deficiency, toxins, and medications. Continuum (Minneap Minn). 2014;20:1293-1306. DOI:10.1212/01.CON.0000455880. 06675.5a.

[22] World Health Organization (2017) Arsenic, fact sheet No 372. World Health Organization. http://www.who.int/ media centr e/facts heets/fs372 /en/. Accessed 25 Dec 2017

[23] Singh R, Singh S, Parihar P, et al. Arsenic contamination, consequences and remediation techniques: A review. Ecotoxicol. Environ. Saf 2015;112:247-270.DOI:10.1016/j.ecoenv.2014.10.009.

[24] O'Neil P. Heavy metals in soils. In: Alloway BJ, editor. Arsenic. London: Blackie Academic and Professional Arsenic; 1995. p. 105-121.

[25] Adriano DC. Trace elements in terrestrial environments. New York: Eds. Springer; 2001.p. 867.DOI:10.1007/ 978-0-387-21510-5

[26] Mochizuki H. Arsenic Neurotoxicity in Humans. Int J Mol Sci. 2019;11: 20(14):3418. DOI:10.3390/ijms 20143418.

[27] Refaz AD, Mohd S, Parvaiz HQ. Overview of medicinal plants spread and their uses in Asia. J.Phyto pharmacol. 2017;6:349-351

[28] Saper RB, Kales SN, Paquin J, et al. Heavy metal content of ayurvedic herbal medicine products. JAMA 2004; 292:2868-2873.DOI:10.1001/jama. 292.23.2868

[29] Hayakawa T, Kobayashi Y, Cui X, Hirano S. A new metabolic pathway of arsenite: Arsenic-glutathionecomplexes are substrates for human arsenic methyltransferase Cyt19. Arch. Toxicol. 2005;79:183-191. DOI: 10.1007/ s00204-004-0620-x

[30] Greenberg SA. Acute demyelinating polyneuropathy with arsenic ingestion. Muscle Nerve 1996; 19:1611-1613. DOI:10.1002/(SICI)1097-4598 (199612)19:12<1611::AID-MUS13> 3.0.CO;2-U

[31] Hall AH. Chronic arsenic poisoning. Toxicol Lett 2002; 128: 69-72. DOI: 10.1016/s0378-4274(01)00534-3

[32] Ratnaike RN. Acute and chronic arsenic toxicity. Postgrad Med J 2003;79(933):391Y396. DOI: 10.1136/ pmj.79.933.391

[33] Valappil AV, Mammen A. Subacute Arsenic Neuropathy: Clinical and Electrophysiological Observations. J Neurosci Rural Pract. 2019;10:529-532. DOI: 10.1055/s-0039-1695693.

[34] Chen J, Ye Y, Ran MLQ,et al. Inhibition of tyrosinase by mercury chloride: spectroscopic and docking studies. Front Pharmacol 2020;11; 81. DOI:10.3389/fphar.2020.00081

[35] Lohren H, Pieper I, Blagojevic L, et al. Neurotoxicity of organic and inorganic mercury species – effects on and transfer across the blood-cerebrospinal fluid barrier, cytotoxic effects in target cells. Perspect Sci. 2015;3:21-22

[36] Dos Santos AA, Chang LW, Liejun Guo G, Aschner M. Fetal Minamata disease: a human episode of congenital methylmercury poisoning. In Slikker W, Paule MG, Wang C, editors. Handbook of developmental neurotoxicology. 2nd Edn (Cambridge, MA: Academic Press), 399-406.

[37] Spencer PS, Schaumburg HH, Ludolph AC editors. Experimental and clinical neurotoxicology. 2nd ed New York: Oxford University Press;2000

[38] Feldman RG. Mercury. In: Feldman RG, editor. Occupational &environmental neurotoxicology. Philadelphia (PA): Lippincott-Raven; 1999. p.92-114.

[39] Agency for Toxic Substance and Disease Registry USA. Toxicological Profile for Cadmium. Department of Health and Humans Services, Public Health Service, Centers for Disease Control, Atlanta, GA, USA. 2017

[40] Branca JJV, Morucci G, Pacini A. Cadmium-induced neurotoxicity: still much ado. Neural Regen Res. 2018 Nov;13(11):1879-1882. DOI:10.4103/1673-5374.239434

[41] Nishimura N, Nishimura H, Ghaffar A, Tohyama C. Localizationof metallothionein in the brain of rat and mouse. J Histochem Cytochem. 1992;40:309-315. DOI: 10.1177/40.2.1552172

[42] Méndez-Armenta M, Villeda-Hernández J, Barroso-Moguel R, et al. Brain regional lipid peroxidation and metallothionein levels of developing rats exposed to cadmium and dexamethasone. Toxicol Lett. 2003;144:151-157. DOI: 10.1177/40.2.1552172

[43] Son J, Lee SE,Park BS, et al. Biomarker discovery and proteomic evaluation of cadmium toxicity on a collembolan species, Paronychiurus kimi (Lee). Proteomics 2011;11: 2294-2307. DOI: 10.1002/pmic.200900690

[44] Wang B, Du Y. Cadmium and its neurotoxic effects. Oxid Med Cell Longev. 2013;2013:898034.

[45] Chin-Chan M, Navarro-Yepes J, Quintanilla-Vega B. Environmental pollutants as risk factors for neurodegenerative disorders: Alzheimer and Parkinson diseases. Front Cell Neurosci. 2015;9:124. DOI: 10.3389/fncel.2015.00124

[46] Sheykhansari S, Kozielski K, Bill J, et al. Redox metals homeostasis in multiple sclerosis and amyotrophic lateral sclerosis: a review. Cell Death Dis. 2018;9:348. DOI: 10.1038/s41419-018-0379-2

[47] Viaene MK, Roels HA, Leenders J, et al. Cadmium: a possible etiological factor in peripheral polyneuropathy. Neurotoxicology. 1999;20(1):7-16.

[48] Rafati Rahimzadeh M, Rafati Rahimzadeh M, Kazemi S, Moghadamnia AA. Cadmium toxicity and treatment: An update. Caspian J Intern Med. 2017;8(3):135-145. DOI: 10.22088/cjim.8.3.135

[49] Smith SW. The role of chelation in the treatment of other metal poisonings. J Med Toxicol. 2013;9(4):355-369. DOI:10.1007/s13181-013-0343-6

[50] Bernhoft RA. Cadmium toxicity and treatment. ScientificWorldJournal. 2013 Jun 3;2013:394652. DOI: 10.1155/2013/394652

[51] Zhao G, Ding M, Zhang B, et al. Clinical manifestations and

management of acute thallium poisoning. Eur Neurol 2008;60(6): 292Y297. DOI: 10.1159/000157883

[52] Osorio Rico L, Santamaria A, Galvan Arzate S. Thallium toxicity: general issues, neurological symptoms, and neurotoxic mechanisms. Adv Neurobiol 2017; 18:345-353. DOI: 10.1007/978-3-319-60189-2_17

[53] Kalita J, Misra UK. Sequelae of thallium poisoning: Clinical and neurophysiological follow-up. Eur Neurol 2006;56:253-255. DOI: 10.1159/000096675

[54] Jha S, Kumar R, Kumar R. Thallium poisoning presenting as paresthesias, paresis, psychosis and pain in abdomen. J Assoc Physicians India 2006; 54:53-55.

[55] Lin G, Yuan L, Peng X, et al. Clinical characteristics and treatment of thallium poisoning in patients with delayed admission in China. Medicine (Baltimore). 2019;98(29):e16471. DOI: 10.1097/MD.0000000000016471.

[56] Ghannoum M, Nolin TD, Goldfarb DS, et al. Extracorporeal treatment for thallium poisoning: recommendations from the EXTRIP Workgroup. Clin J Am Soc Nephrol 2012;7:1682-1690. DOI: 10.2215/CJN.01940212

[57] Dick FD. Solvent neurotoxicity. Occup Environ Med 2006;63:221-226. DOI: 10.1136/oem.2005.022400

[58] Wang C, Chen SJ, Wang ZT. Electrophysiological follow-up of patients with chronic peripheral neuropathy induced by occupational intoxication with *n*-hexane. CellBiochem Biophys 2014;70:579-585. DOI: 10.1007/s12013-014-9959-7

[59] Zhang X, Tong Y, Lu Y. Peripheral nerve injury in patients exposed to *n*-hexane: an analysis of eight cases. J Zhejiang Univ Sci B. 2021;15;22: 248-252. DOI: 10.1631/jzus.B2000601

[60] Public Health England, 2016. n-Hexane incident management. https://assets.publishing.service.gov.uk/government/uploads/system/uploads/attachment_data/file/566787/n-hexane_incident_management.pdf [Accessed on June. 25, 2021]

[61] Pan JH, Peng CY, Lo CT, Dai CY, Wang CL, Chuang HY. n-Hexane intoxication in a Chinese medicine pharmaceutical plant: a case report. J Med Case Rep. 2017;11(1):120. DOI: 10.1186/s13256-017-1280-9.

[62] Huang CC. Polyneuropathy induced by n-hexane intoxication in Taiwan. Acta Neurol. Taiwan 2008;17(1): 3-10.

[63] Spencer PS, Chen X. The Role of Protein Adduction in Toxic Neuropathies of Exogenous and Endogenous Origin. Toxics 2021; 9(5):98. DOI:10.3390/toxics9050098

[64] Misirli H, Domac FM, Somay G, Araal O, Ozer B, Adigüzel T. N-hexane induced polyneuropathy: a clinical and electrophysiological follow up. Electromyogr Clin Neurophysiol. 2008;48(2):103-108

[65] Puri V, Chaudhry N, Tatke M. N-hexane neuropathy in screen printers. Electromyogr Clin Neurophysiol. 2007;47(3):145-152

[66] Kutlu G, Gomceli YB, Sonmez T, Inan LE. Peripheral neuropathy and visual evoked potential changes in workers exposed to n-hexane. J Clin Neurosci. 2009t;16(10):1296-1269. DOI: 10.1016/j.jocn.2008.12.021.

[67] White RF, Proctor SP. Solvents and neurotoxicity. Lancet. 1997 Apr 26;349(9060):1239-1243. DOI:10.1016/S0140-6736(96)07218-2.

[68] Visser I, Lavini C, Booij J, et al. Cerebral impairment in chronic

solvent-induced encephalopathy. Ann Neurol 2008;63:572-580. DOI: 10.1002/ana.21364

[69] Abdollahi M, Hosseini A. Carbon Disulfide. In: Wexler, P. editors. Encyclopedia of Toxicology, 3rd edition vol 1. Elsevier Inc Academic Press, 2014; p.678-681. DOI:10.1016/B978-0-12-386454-3.00475-9

[70] Liu CH, Huang CY, Huang CC. Occupational neurotoxic diseases in Taiwan. Saf Health Work 2012;3(4): 257-267.

[71] Johnson DJ, Graham D G, Amarnath V, et al. Release of carbon disulfide is a contributing mechanism in the axonopathy produced by N,N-diethyldithiocarbamate. Toxicology and Applied Pharmacology 1998;148: 288-296. DOI: 10.1006/taap.1997.8344

[72] Berger AR, Schaumburg H H. Human Toxic Neuropathy Caused by Industrial Agents. In: *Peripheral Neuropathy.* Elsevier Inc; 2005.p. 2505-2525. DOI:10.1016/B978-0-7216-9491-7.50115-0

[73] Albers JW, Wald JJ. Industrial and environmental toxic neuropathy. In: WF Brown, CF Bolton, MJ Aminoff, editors. Clinical Neurophysiology and Neuromuscular Diseases,WB Saunders, Philadelphia, 2002; p. 1143-1168

[74] Albers JW. Industrial and environmental agents. In: JW Albers, S Berent, editors. Neurobehavioral Toxicology. Neurological and Neuropsychological Perspectives.Vol. II. Peripheral Nervous System, Taylor & Francis,London, 2005;pp. 329-427

[75] Chu CC, Huang CC, Chu NS et al. Carbon disulfide induced polyneuropathy: sural nerve pathology, electrophysiology,and clinical correlation. Acta Neurol Scand 1996; 94: 258-263. DOI: 10.1111/j.1600-0404.1996.tb07062.x

[76] Shore RE, Gardner M J, Pannett B. Ethylene oxide: an assessment of the epidemiologic evidence on carcinogenicity. Br J Ind Med 1993; 50:971-997. DOI:10.1136/oem.50.11.971

[77] Zampollo A, Zacchetti O, Pisati G. On ethylene oxide neurotoxicity: report of two cases of peripheral neuropathy. Ital J Neurol Sci. 1984;5(1):59-62. DOI:10.1007/BF02043971

[78] Ohnishi A, Murai Y. Polyneuropathy due to ethylene oxide, propylene oxide, and butylene oxide. Environ Res. 1993;60(2):242-247. DOI:10.1006/enrs.1993.1032

[79] Kuzuhara S, Kanazawa I, Nakanishi T, Egashira T. Ethylene oxide polyneuropathy. Neurology. 1983;33(3):377-280. DOI: 10.1212/wnl.33.3.377

[80] Gross JA, Haas ML, Swift TR. Ethylene oxide neurotoxicity: report of four cases and review of the literature. Neurology. 1979;29(7):978-983. DOI: 10.1212/wnl.29.7.978.

[81] Ohnishi A. Ethylene oxide. In Spencer, P. S., and Schaumburg, H. H. (eds.): Experimental and Clinical Neurotoxicology. New York, Oxford University Press, p. 563, 2000

[82] Glare PA, Davies PS, Finlay E, et al. Pain in cancer survivors. J Clin Oncol. 2014;32(16):1739-1747. DOI: 10.1200/JCO.2013.52.4629

[83] Bonhof CS, Mols F, Vos MC, et al. Course of chemotherapy induced peripheral neuropathy and its impact on health-related quality of life among ovarian cancer patients: a longitudinal study. Gynecol Oncol 2018;149(3):455-463. DOI: 10.1016/j.ygyno.2018.03.052

[84] Park SB, Krishnan AV, Lin CS, et al. Mechanisms underlying chemotherapy-induced neurotoxicity and the potential for neuroprotective strategies. Curr Med

Chem. 2008;15(29):3081-3094. DOI: 10.2174/092986708786848569

[85] Mols F, Beijers T, Vreugdenhil G, van de Poll-Franse L. Chemotherapy-induced peripheral neuropathy and its association with quality of life: a systematic review. Support Care Cancer 2014; 22(8):2261. DOI: 10.1007/s00520-014-2255-7

[86] Banach M, Juranek JK, Zygulska AL. Chemotherapy-induced neuropathies-a growing problem for patients and health care providers. Brain Behav. 2016;7(1):e00558. DOI: 10.1002/brb3.558

[87] McDonald ES, Windebank AJ. Cisplatin-induced apoptosis of DRG neuronsinvolves bax redistribution and cytochrome c release but not fas receptorsignalling. Neurobiol Dis. 2002;9(2):220-233. DOI: 10.1006/nbdi.2001.0468

[88] Carozzi VA, Canta A, Chiorazzi A. Chemotherapy-induced peripheral neuropathy: What do we know about mechanisms? Neurosci Lett. 2015;596:90-107. DOI: 10.1016/j.neulet.2014.10.014

[89] Bernhardson BM, Tishelman C, Rutqvist LE. Chemosensory changes experienced by patients undergoing cancer chemotherapy: A qualitative interview study. J Pain Symptom Manag. 2007;34(4): 403-412. DOI: 10.1016/j.jpainsymman.2006.12.010

[90] Lebwohl D, Canetta R. Eur. J. Cancer 1998;34(10):1522-1534. DOI: 10.1016/s0959-8049(98)00224-x

[91] Krarup-Hansen A. Helweg-Larsen S. Schmalbruch H, et al. Brain, 2007;130(4): 1076-1088. DOI: 10.1093/brain/awl356

[92] Yoon JY, Nam TS, Kim MK, et al. Acute inflammatory demyelinating polyradiculoneuropathy in a patient receiving oxaliplatin-based chemotherapy. Asia Pac J Clin Oncol 2012;8(2):201-204. DOI: 10.1111/j.1743-7563.2011.01515.x

[93] Hausheer FH, Schilsky RL, Bain S, et al. Diagnosis, management, and evaluation of chemotherapy-induced peripheral neuropathy. Semin Oncol 2006;33(1):15-49. DOI: 10.1053/j.seminoncol.2005.12.010

[94] Pfisterer J, Vergote I, Du Bois A, et al. Combination therapy with gemcitabine and carboplatin in recurrent ovarian cancerInt J GynecolCancer 2005;15(1):36-41. DOI: 10.1111/j.1525-1438.2005.15355.x

[95] Gebremedhn EG, Shortland PJ, Mahns DA. The incidence of acute oxaliplatin-induced neuropathy and its impact on treatment in the first cycle: A systematic review. BMC Cancer 2018;18(1): 410. DOI: 10.1186/s12885-018-4185-0

[96] Deuis JR, Zimmermann K, Romanovsky AA, et al. An animal model of oxaliplatin-induced cold allodynia reveals a crucial role for NaV1.6 in peripheral pain pathways. Pain 2013;154(9):1749-1757. DOI: 10.1016/j.pain.2013.05.032

[97] Pietrangeli A, Leandri M, Terzoli E, Jandolo B, Garufi C. Persistence of high-dose oxaliplatin-induced neuropathy at long-term follow-up. Eur Neurol. 2006;56(1):13-16. DOI: 10.1159/000094376

[98] Yared JA, Tkaczuk KH. Update on taxane development: New analogs and new formulations. Drug DesDev Ther 2012; 6:371-384. DOI: 10.2147/DDDT.S28997

[99] De Iuliis F, Taglieri L,Salerno G, et al. Taxane induced neuropathy in patients affected by breast cancer: Literature review. Crit Rev

Oncol/Hematol 2015; 96(1): 34-45. DOI: 10.1016/j.critrevonc.2015.04.011

[100] Eckhoff AS, Knoop MB, Jensen M, et al. Persistence of docetaxel-induced neuropathy and impacton quality of life among breast cancer survivors. Eur J Cancer 2015;51(3): 292-300. DOI: 10.1016/j.ejca.2014.11.024

[101] Laforgia M, Laface C, Calabrò C, et al. Peripheral Neuropathy under Oncologic Therapies: A Literature Review on Pathogenetic Mechanisms. Int J Mol Sci. 2021;17;22(4):1980. DOI: 10.3390/ijms22041980

[102] Zajączkowska R, Kocot-Kępska M, Leppert W, et al. Mechanisms of Chemotherapy-Induced Peripheral Neuropathy. Int J Mol Sci. 2019; 22;20(6):1451. DOI: 10.3390/ijms200 61451

[103] M Jordan, L Wilson. Microtubules as a target for anticancer drugs. Nat RevCancer 2004;4(4):253-265. DOI: 10.1038/nrc1317

[104] Sahenk Z, Barohn R, New P, et al. Taxol neuropathy, electrodiagnosticand sural nerve biopsy findings, Arch Neurol 1994;51:726-729. DOI: 10.1001/archneur.1994.00540190110024

[105] Raffa RB, Pergolizzi JV. Cancer Chemotherapy–Induced Neuropathic Pain. The Underlying Peripheral Neuropathy. In Chemotherapy Induced Neuropathic Pain; Raffa RB, Langford R, Pergolizzi JV, et al. Eds.; CRC Press, Taylor & Francis Group: Boca Raton, FL, USA, 2013; 113-135.

[106] Postma TJ, Benard BA, Huijgens PC, Ossenkoppele GJ, Heimans JJ. Long-term effects of vincristine on the peripheral nervous system. J Neurooncol. 1993;15(1):23-27. DOI: 10.1007/BF01050259

[107] Nakamura T, Hashiguchi A, Suzuki S, et al. Vincristine exacerbates asymptomatic Charcot–Marie–Tooth disease with a novel EGR2 mutation. Neurogenetics 2012;13(1):77-82. DOI: 10.1007/s10048-012-0313-1

[108] Diouf B, Crews KR, Lew G, et al. Association of an inherited genetic variant with vincristine-related peripheral neuropathy in children with acute lymphoblastic leukemia. JAMA 2015;313(8):815-823. DOI: 10.1001/jama.2015.0894

[109] Kouroukis CT, Baldassarre FG, Haynes AE, Imrie K, Reece DE, Cheung MC; Cancer Care Ontario Hematology Disease Site Group. Bortezomib in multiple myeloma: a practice guideline. Clin Oncol (R Coll Radiol) 2014; 26(2):110-119. DOI: 10.1016/j.clon.2013.11.022

[110] Argyriou AA, Iconomou G, Kalofonos HP. Bortezomib-induced peripheral neuropathy in multiple myeloma: a comprehensive review of the literature. Blood. 2008 Sep 1;112(5):1593-1599. DOI: 10.1182/blood-2008-04-149385

[111] Peng L, Ye X, Zhou Y, Zhang J, Zhao Q. Meta-analysis of incidence and risk of peripheral neuropathy associated with intravenous bortezomib. Support Care Cancer 2015;23(9):2813-2824. DOI: 10.1007/s00520-015-2648-2

[112] Myers JE, Macun I. Acrylamide neuropathy in a South African factory: An epidemiologic investigation. Am J Ind Med 1991;19(4):487-493. DOI: 10.1002/ajim.4700190406

[113] He FS, Zhang SL, Wang HL, et al. Neurological and electroneuro myographic assessment of the adverse effects of acrylamide on occupationally exposed workers. Scand J Work Environ Health 1989;15(2):125-129.

[114] Loeb AL, Anderson RJ. Antagonism of acrylamide neurotoxicity by supplementation with vitamin B6. Neurotoxicology 1981;2(4):625-633.

[115] Xu Y, Cui B, Ran R, et al. Risk assessment, formation, and mitigation of dietary acrylamide: Current status and future prospects. Food Chem Toxicol 2014; 69: 1-12. DOI: 10.1016/j.fct.2014.03.037

[116] Mucci LA, Wilson, KM. Acrylamide intake through diet and human cancer risk. J. Agric. Food Chem 2008;56(15): 6013-6019. DOI: 10.1021/jf703747b

[117] Sickles DW, Stone JD, Friedman MA. Fast axonal transport: A site of acrylamide neurotoxicity? Neurotoxicology 2002;23(2):223-251. DOI: 10.1016/s0161-813x(02)00025-6

[118] Stewart RD, Dodd HC, Baretta ED, et al. Human exposure to styrene vapor. Arch Environ Health 1968;16(5): 565-662. DOI: 10.1080/00039896.1968.10665124

[119] Gobba F, Cavelleri F, Bontadi D, Torri P, Dainese R. Peripheral neuropathy in styrene exposed workers. Scand J 1work Environ Health 1995; 21(6):517-520. DOI: 10.5271/sjweh.69

[120] Jokanović M, Kosanović M, Brkić D, Vukomanović P. Organophosphate induced delayed polyneuropathy in man: an overview. Clin Neurol Neurosurg 2011;113(1):7-10. DOI: 10.1016/j.clineuro.2010.08.015

[121] Jokanovic M, Kozanovic M and Stukalov PV. Organophosphate Induced Delayed Polyneuropathy. Medicinal Chemistry reviews Online 2004;1(6): 123-131.

[122] Li Y, Dinsdale D, Glynn P. Protein domains, catalytic activity, and subcellular distribution of neuropathy target esterase in Mammalian cells. J Biol Chem 2003;278(10):8820-8825. DOI: 10.1074/jbc.M210743200

[123] Lotti M. The pathogenesis of organophosphate polyneuropathy. Crit Rev Toxicol 1991;21:465-487. DOI: 10.3109/10408449209089884

[124] Thivakaran. Thivakaran T, Gamage R, Gunarathne KS, Gooneratne IK. Chlorpyrifos-induced delayed myelopathy and pure motor neuropathy: a case report. Neurologist 2012;18:226-228. DOI: 10.1097/NRL.0b013e318261035b

[125] Akçay Yalbuzdağ S, Ince, AG Karatepe, I Sengul, T Kaya. Organophosphate induced delayed neuropathy: a case report. Turkish Journal of Physical Medicine & Rehabilitation 2017;63(1):88-91. DOI: 10.5606/tftrd.2017.13549

[126] Moretto A, Lotti M.Poisoning by organophosphorus insecticides and sensory neuropathy.Journal of Neurology, Neurosurgery & Psychiatry 1998;64(4):463-468. DOI: 10.1136/jnnp.64.4.463

Chapter 4

Neurotoxic Effects of Insecticides Chlorpyrifos, Carbaryl, Imidacloprid, in Different Animal Species

Alejandra Mora-Gutiérrez, Carmen Rubio, Ángel Alonso Romero-López and Moisés Rubio-Osornio

Abstract

Insecticides are pesticides used to control insects in agriculture, ornamental gardens, homes, and veterinary medicine. Although the toxic effects on the environment and the health of living beings are not fully understood, these pesticides have become the first options for crop protection in agriculture. After herbicides, insecticides are the most extensively used pesticides in agriculture, with large quantities consumed on every continent, primarily in America. Chlorpyrifos, carbaryl, and imidacloprid are among the top ten most used insecticides. Amidst organophosphates, chlorpyrifos has been reported to be used in over fifty food crops. Carbaryl is a carbamate employed as an insecticide, fungicide, herbicide, and nematicide. Similarly, neonicotinoids are the most used insecticide on a global scale. Neonicotinoids include imidacloprid, the second most frequently used pesticide, surpassed only by glyphosate. It is used because it is less toxic to humans. However, insects appear to be less resistant to its compounds. Evidence suggests that these insecticides persist in soils for a long time and have neurotoxic effects in animal species not intended to receive its consequences. Thus, this chapter's aim is to describe these three pesticides effects and contrast them with the most recent findings regarding their neurotoxic effects in various animal species.

Keywords: insecticides, chlorpyrifos, carbaryl, imidacloprid, neurotoxicity

1. Introduction

Pesticides are substances that exist in our daily lives. Their most widespread use is in agriculture, where they are used to protect crops from pests caused by plants and animals. They are also used to prevent diseases caused by ectoparasites in farm animals and pets. These substances are used in gardening and brought into our homes to protect us from mosquitoes and other insects. Pesticides come into intimate touch with all forms of life through drinking water and eating food. However, the use of these substances is so widespread and poorly controlled that environmental contamination is inevitable.

Pesticide exposure occurs in a variety of ways. Not all living organisms are exposed to the same periods or the same dose, or not even to a single type of pesticide or to the same mixtures. The above may have yet unknown, synergistic, or potentiating effects on organisms.

Insecticides are a class of pesticides used to kill or control insects. It is not only used in agriculture, but also in ornamental gardens, homes, and veterinary medicine. Although the hazardous effects on the environment and the health of living beings are not yet fully understood, they have become one of the primary solutions for crop protection in agriculture. Regardless of the fact that pesticides come in a wide variety of families, the major goal of this chapter is to highlight the effects of imidacloprid (neonicotinoid), chlorpyrifos (organophosphate), and carbaryl (carbamate), insecticides widely used in agriculture, despite recent findings of their neurotoxic effects on several animal species.

2. Worldwide use of insecticides

After herbicides, insecticides are the most extensively used pesticides in agriculture [1]. The principal insecticide consumers by continent were America (44.9%), Asia (29%), Europe (16%), Africa (6.4), and Oceania (3.7%), with the United States being the country with the highest insecticide consumption worldwide (**Figure 1**) [2]. Recently collected data, dating from 1998 to 2014, indicates that chlorpyrifos was the third most used organophosphate pesticide in the United States, only for corn cultivation, with a total of 1,122kg/ha. In the same country, the most widely used carbamate was carbaryl with a total of 1,024 kg/ha; while imidacloprid was the most used neonicotinoid, with 0.057 kg/ha. During the same time period, chlorpyrifos, carbaryl, and imidacloprid were among the top 10 most widely used insecticides in the United States [3]. Currently, these same pesticides are used in agriculture and are included among the principal insecticides for each insecticide family aforementioned [4–6].

Furthermore, organophosphate insecticides account for roughly half of all insecticides used worldwide, and chlorpyrifos is one of the most widely used. This insecticide is approved for use on more than 50 food crops in both developed and

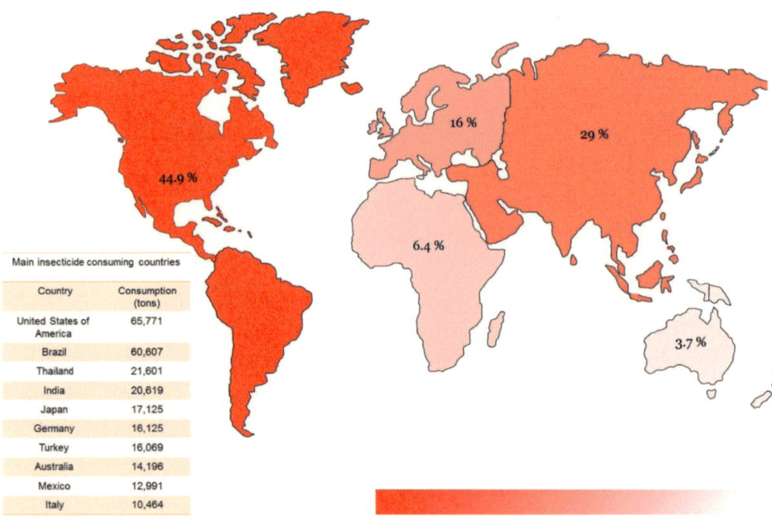

Country	Consumption (tons)
United States of America	65,771
Brazil	60,607
Thailand	21,601
India	20,619
Japan	17,125
Germany	16,125
Turkey	16,069
Australia	14,196
Mexico	12,991
Italy	10,464

Figure 1.
Highest to lowest insecticide use by continent.

developing countries [7]. About 50 chemicals belong to the carbamate family, which are utilized as fungicides, herbicides, and nematicides in addition to having insecticidal properties. Carbaryl was the first carbamate to be commercialized, and it is now more widely used than all other carbamates combined [8]. Neonicotinoids, on the other hand, appear to be the most widely employed insecticides worldwide, according to the literature. In fact, imidacloprid is the world's second most widely used pesticide, after only the controversial herbicide glyphosate [9, 10]. Neonicotinoids have largely replaced carbamates and organophosphates because they are considered less toxic to humans and insects, and they appear to be less resistant to neonicotinoids compared to other conventional insecticide classes [11].

3. Of the molecule, its structure, and mechanism of action

3.1 Chlorpyrifos

Organophosphates are compounds of organic nature that contain phosphorus. Chlorpyrifos (O, O-diethyl-O-3,5,6-trichloropyridin-2-yl phosphorothioate) is an organic thiophosphate of the chloropyridine class [12]. The latter is one of the most widely used organophosphate insecticides in agriculture, primarily used on corn, soy, fruit trees, walnut trees, brussels sprouts, blueberries, broccoli, and cauliflower, among others. This pesticide is also used on golf courses, on ornamental plants, for treating wood, and in homes to combat mosquitoes, cockroaches, and ants [13]. Chlorpyrifos act by irreversibly inhibiting the acetylcholinesterase enzyme activity, which causes acetylcholine accumulation in the synaptic cleft, causing overstimulation of postsynaptic receptors and the consequent signs of intoxication [14].

3.2 Imidacloprid

Imidacloprid [1-[(6-chloropyridin-3-yl) methyl] imidazolidin-2-ylidene] nitramide is a neonicotinoid of the chloropyridinyl class [15], which like the insecticides of the same family, acts as an agonist of nicotinic cholinergic receptors (nAChRs) of insects and mammals [16, 17]. IImidacloprid is used in agriculture for corn, cotton, soybean, potato, wheat, and some vegetable seeds, as well as for soil treatment and foliar application on crops like orange, potato, and cotton. It is also utilized in the treatment of decorative plants and residential areas, industrial vegetation and forestry management [18]. Additionally, it is used as veterinary medicine in presentations such as pipettes or collars for direct application on dogs and cats to prevent infestations by internal and external parasites [19].

3.3 Carbaryl

Carbaryl (1-naphthyl methylcarbamate) is a carbamate-based pesticide. It's a carbamate ester made up of 1-naphthol and methylcarbamic acid. On plants, this pesticide is insecticidal, acaricidal, and even growth retardant when used in plants. It is currently used to treat corn, soybean, cotton, nuts, fruit, and vegetable crops in agriculture [20]. It is mostly used on apple, nut, and soybean crops in the United States. However, it is found in more than 40 crops around the world, including asparagus, squash, and potatoes. Its non-agricultural uses include ornamental plants, lawns, grass, roads, and buildings [21]. Carbaryl acts by inhibiting acetylcholinesterase. Nevertheless, unlike organophosphates, carbamates do it reversibly [22].

4. Persistence in soil and water

When pesticides are manually or aerially sprayed on seeds, soil, or even directly on plants, they can last for days, months, or even years. They might also filter through the soil into surface and deep waterways, polluting food and water sources for living beings by coming into contact with animal and plant life. **Table 1** illustrates the soil-water partition coefficients (Koc) and octanol–water partition coefficients (Kow), which are used to characterize the mobility and bioaccumulation properties of pesticides, respectively. While these coefficients are not the only indicators used to determine pesticide behavior in the environment and in organisms, they do serve as referents for pesticide toxicity.

The Koc is a coefficient that is used to determine the pesticide concentration "attached" to soil particles as well as the phase present in the solution, i.e., dissolved in the same soil's water. As a result, the lower the temperature, the higher the Koc of the pesticide in solution, and the greater the likelihood of it leaching into groundwater. The Kow is a coefficient that is used to calculate pesticide concentrations in octanol and water. Pesticides having a high Kow, which are more soluble in octanol and less soluble in water, have been found to accumulate in organisms [23]. Chlorpyrifos accumulates greater in organisms than carbaryl and imidacloprid, as shown in **Table 1**. It does, however, have a lesser tendency to leak into the soil as compared to them. In this sense, imidacloprid would pose a greater risk as a groundwater pollutant.

To estimate a substance's environmental fate in diverse environments, scientists must first determine its degradation half-life, or DT_{50}, which is the time it takes for

	Chlorpyrifos	**Carbaryl**	**Imidacloprid**
Structural formula	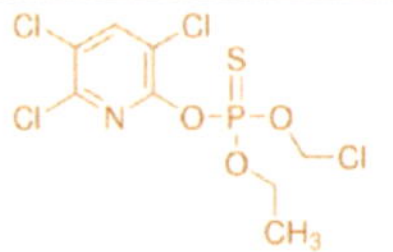	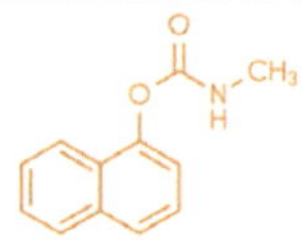	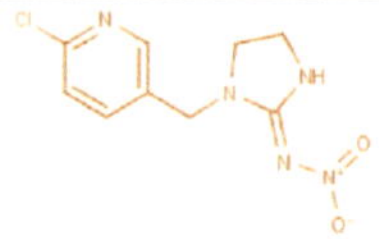
Chemical name	O, O-dietil-O-3,5,6-trichloropyridin-2-il fosforotioato	1-naphthyl methylcarbamate	1-[(6-chloropyridin-3-yl) methyl]imidazolidin-2-ylidene]nitramide
Color and form	White granular crystals	Colorless to light tan crystals	Colorless crystals
Odor	Mild mercaptan	Odorless	Slight characteristic odor
Melting Point	42 °C	145°C	144°C
Boiling Point	Decomposes before boiling	Decomposes before boiling	Decomposes before boiling
Molecular Weight	350.6	201.22	255.7
Water solubility (mg/L)	1.4	110 (at 22°C)	610 (at 20 °C)
Vapor pressure	2.49×10^{-3} mmHg at 25°C	$1{,}36 \times 10^{-6}$ mmHg at 25° C	3.99×10^{-10} mmHg at 20°C
Octagonal-water coefficient (K_{ow})	4.7	1.59 at 2.3	0.57 at 21°C
Soil sorption coefficient (K_{oc})	360 at 31000	290	249 at 336

Table 1.
Crucial physicochemical characteristics for insecticides are chlorpyrifos, carbaryl, and imidacloprid.

50% of a chemical to degrade or disappear from water or soil [7]. For the purposes of this review, the three pesticides DT_{50} examined will be provided below, depending on their average persistence in soil and water,

Chlorpyrifos can have a long persistence even in arctic regions, where its presence has been assessed in samples of ice, snow, a microcosm of water, sediments, air, and flora. The persistence of this pesticide (due to its high resistance to hydrolysis) has been reported to be greater in aquatic habitats than in soil. However, the LD_{50} in soil, has a wide range of values as reported in the literature, ranging from a few days to four years. It is also suggested to be more stable in low-pH soils, dark settings, and cold environments [7]. Chlorpyrifos DT_{50} has been found to last from 1 to 120days in the field and up to 180 days in the soil in the absence of light. It is worth noting that in organic soils, the half-life is longer than in mineral soils. A DT_{50} of 150 to 200 days has been documented in anaerobic pond sediments, while 106 + 54 days has been reported in experimental circumstances of wetland and anaerobic sediments. Chlorpyrifos has a DT_{50} of 18.7 days in freshwater and 49.4 days in seawater at 10°C, which decreases with increasing temperature [24].

In the case of carbaryl, its DT_{50} in the soil ranges from 17 to 28 days. It is considered to have low persistence, where it is degraded mainly by the action of light and bacteria. In sandy soil conditions, its half-life is 7 to 14 days, while in clay soil it ranges from 14 to 28 days, hydrolyzing itself rapidly in alkaline soils. The DT_{50} in water is highly variable, increased in acidic conditions; for example, in acidic water with a pH of 5, degradation is slow and can persist for up to 1500 days [23]. The DT_{50} of carbaryl in soil has recently been reported to be 16 days, while it can reach 12 and 5.8 days in water and sediments, respectively [25].

Neonicotinoids have a high DT_{50}, which means they can last a long time in the soil, with values in the range from 6.7 to 1230 days, while imidacloprid has the highest DT_{50}, with a value of 35.9 to 1230 days. Though it should be noted that the degradation of neonicotinoids and other pesticides in soil is dependent on pH, temperature, humidity, chemical concentration, and even the presence of microorganisms [26]. As evidence, imidacloprid has been found to remain for 42 to 129 days in vegetated soils and more than 180 days in soils free of vegetation [27]. The data on this insecticide's water persistence is varied, with half-lives ranging from 1 to 3 hours, 48 hours, and even 31 to 43 days [28].

5. Neurotoxic effects in different animal species

The lethal dose 50 or LD_{50}, is a measure that in toxicology is used to estimate the dose of a test substance that produces 50% of death in a certain animal species. It is used as a reference to determine how toxic it is to humans [29]. The LC_{50} or lethal concentration 50, corresponds to the concentration of a chemical substance in the

Class		LD_{50} for rat (mg / kg body weigth)	
		Oral	Dermal
Ia	Extremely dangerous	<5	<50
Ib	Highly dangerous	5–50	5–200
II	Moderately dangerous	50–2000	200–2000
III	Slightly dangerous	>2000	>2000
U	Acute hazard unlikely	5000 or more	

Table 2.
Toxicological classification for pesticides with moderate toxic effects.

Insecticide	Class	Nerve target	LD_{50} or LC_{50} in different species				Toxicological classification (WHO)
			Rat	Honey bee	Fish	Bird	
			Acute oral LD_{50} (mg/kg)	Acute contact LD_{50} (mg/bee)	Acute exposure LC_{50} (mg/L)	Acute oral LD_{50} (mg/kg)	
Chlorpyrifos	Organophosphate	AChE	182	0.072	108	27.36	Ia
Carbaryl	Carbamate	AChE	230	0.84	3470	1870.5	II
Imidacloprid	Neonicotinoid	nAChR	439.8	0.061	229,100	35.36	II

Table 3.
Effect of LD_{50} or LC_{50}: chlorpyrifos, carbaryl, and imidacloprid in different animal species.

air or in the water that causes half of the exposed animals to die [30]. According to the WHO toxicological classification for pesticides (**Table 2**) [31], both imidacloprid and carbaryl are in class II, which includes those pesticides with moderate toxic effects, while chlorpyrifos is located in class 1b since its LD_{50} is below 200 mg. Therefore, it is considered highly dangerous. In **Table 3**, the LD_{50} or LC_{50} for chlorpyrifos, carbaryl, and imidacloprid in different animal species are illustrated.

6. Neurotoxic effects of chlorpyrifos, carbaryl, and imidacloprid

Although insecticides are substances designed to kill some kinds of insects that cause pests, for decades it has been documented that they can also kill insects that should not be the target of their toxic effects and that overall, are essential for life on planet Earth. The most documented case is the decrease in pollinator populations and its possible association with insecticides utilization. In recent reviews, information supporting that insecticides can interfere with localization capacity, alteration of foraging and motor behavior, olfactory learning, and flight ability has been gathered. Additionally, they negatively impact the immune system and increase the death rate, among other toxic effects in bees [32–35], bumblebees [36–38], butterflies and moths [39–42], ants [43, 44], earthworms [39, 45] and various aquatic invertebrates [46–48]. They have also been associated with neuronal and colony performance alterations in bumblebees [32]. Insecticides such as dichlorvos, imidacloprid, and malathion, among others, can harm butterfly populations, resulting in decreased survival and changes in feeding and oviposition patterns [49].

Therefore, the effects on non-target insects have received special attention. According to studies on these species, an environmental emergency has been declared due to the decline in their populations. It is worth noting that insecticides have effects not confined to insects, which exacerbates the existing problem because all living beings are exposed to varying degrees of insecticides, making humans vulnerable to their toxic effects. Following, there is a brief overview of the effects identified in the last five years for each of the insecticides that have been the subject of this chapter, grouped into three different types of effects: behavioral, neurochemical, and cellular (**Tables 4–6**). However, for more detailed information, consider the present bibliography.

6.1 Chlorpyrifos

The recent literature regarding chlorpyrifos toxic effects in different species is extensive. However, this chapter has focused on those that are associated with effects

Behavioral effects			
	Chlorpyrifos	**Carbaryl**	**Imidacloprid**
Insects	Alters caste differentiation in *Plebeia droryana* bees [50]. Alters the formation and recovery of olfactory memories in bees [51]. It alters the locomotor activity of the cockroach *Nauphoeta cinerea* [52]. Alteration of olfactory learning and memory retention in *Apis mellifera* and *Apis cerana* bees [53]. Impaired locomotor performance manifested with altered swimming activity in Diamesa zernyi larvae [54].	It causes alterations in the percentage of copulations in adults of *Rhynchophorus palmarum* (Coleoptera: Curculionidae) [55]. No more recent studies for the review period in the literature.	Paralysis, tremors, prostration, and death in *Scaptotrigona postica* Latreille bees [56]. Decreased food consumption, digging, and foraging behavior in the red ant *Solenopsis Invicta* [57]. Alterations in sexual behavior and search for hosts in parasitic wasps Nasonia vitripennis [58]. It affects the queen selection behavior of the stingless bee *Plebeia droryana* [59]. Reduced visual movement and deterioration in-flight behavior in the migratory locust Locusta [60]. Disruption of copulation in adults of *Rhynchophorus palmarum* (Coleoptera: Curculionidae) [55].
Aquatic organisms	Alterations in the straightening of the gastropod *Gibbula umbilicalis* [61]. Irregular hatching patterns in shrimp *Artemia salina* [62]. Alteration of swimming activity, such as hypoactivity and spasms in the *Physalaemus gracilis* tadpole [63] Alterations in the swimming pattern in the catfish *Heteropneustes fossilis* [64].	General hypoactivity, decrease in escape swim, and feeding behavior in tadpoles of the terrestrial Anaxyrus toad [65]. Decrease in hatching speed of shrimp *Artemia salina* [62]. Delay in the ocular peduncle retraction speed in the blue crab *Callinectes sapidus* [66]. Hypoactivity, alterations in exploratory, social and feeding behavior in zebrafish exposed during embryonic life [67]. Decreased shell closing time and increased mucus secretion from the gills in the *Unio pictorum* mussel [68]. Decreased startle behavior and habituation in zebrafish larvae [69].	It decreases exploratory behavior, swimming activity and increases the sensorimotor response to startling stimuli in zebrafish [70]. It alters the swimming behavior and avoidance behavior of the predators of the tadpole Limnodynastes tasmaniensisy [71]. Decreased response to predators in the *Lithobates sylvaticus* frog [72]. Alterations in swimming and feeding behavior in the *Farfantepenaeus aztecus* shrimp [73]. Locomotor alterations and decreased aggressive behavior in the *Procambarus clarkii*es crab [74]. Hypoactivity in the zebrafish *Danio rerio* [75]. Lethargy is followed by hyperactivity and spasms in the tadpole *Leptodactylus latrans* [76].

Behavioral effects			
	Chlorpyrifos	**Carbaryl**	**Imidacloprid**
Birds	Salivation, tearing, panting, frequent defecation, tremors, and seizures in broilers [77]. Alteration in migratory orientation in the white-crowned sparrow *Zonotrichia leucophrys* [78].	Difficulty walking, weak legs, dizziness, frequent defecation, less food consumption, decrease in aggressive behavior [79].	Alteration in migratory orientation in the white-crowned sparrow *Zonotrichia leucophrys* [78]. Hypoactivity, decreased flight behavior, spasms, drooping wings, ataxia, prostration in the pigeon *Zenaida auriculata* [80]. Decrease in food consumption and delay in migration in the white-crowned sparrow *Zonotrichia leucophrys* [81]. Muscle tremors, ataxia, and depression in domestic chickens *Gallus gallus* domesticus [82].
Non-human vertebrates	Anxiety affects exposure in fetal life in male Wistar rats [83]. Alterations in social behavior and recognition memory in C57Bl6 / J mice [84]. Decreased locomotor activity and muscle strength in Sprague–Dawley rats [85] Alteration of the reference memory; Anxious behavior in male Wistar rats [86]. Catalytic behavior decreased motor coordination and gait disturbances in Swiss mice [87]. Piloerection, tremors, seizures, hypoactivity, among other neurological signs after administration in mice [88]. Impairment of social behavior and sensorimotor reflexes in PON 1/1 mice [89].	Memory and learning deficits. As well as habituation behavior alterations in NMRI mice [90]. Hypoactivity in Norwegian gray rats [91]. Hypersalivation, miotic pupils, lethargy, coma in bats *Eidolon helvum* [92].	Hypoactivity increased grooming behavior and behaviors associated with anxiety and depression in male Sprague–Dawley rats [93]. Decreased exploratory behavior, a deficit in sensorimotor functions, and depression in male Sprague–Dawley rats [94]. It alters the vocal, auditory, orientation, and memory systems in bats *Hipposideros armiger terasensis* [95].
Humans	Arm tremors in prenatally exposed children [96]. Alterations in the social and motor function of 3-year-old children are exposed postnatally [97]. Neurobehavioral deficits in exposed Egyptian workers [98].	Semi-conscious state due to acute intoxication [99].	Coma, dyspnea, and sweating in acute poisonings [100]. Drowsiness, confusion, incoherence, lack of orientation, and unconsciousness after acute poisoning [101]. Somnolence, Glasgow Coma Scale with a score of 10/15 and Miotic pupils after acute poisoning [102].

Table 4.
Behavioral effects of chlorpyrifos, carbaryl and imidacloprid on five animal species.

Neurochemical effects			
	Chlorpyrifos	**Carbaryl**	**Imidacloprid**
Insects	Decreased acetylcholinesterase activity and oxidative stress in *Nauphoeta cinerea* cockroaches' heads [52]. Lipid peroxidation and protein carbonylation in Diamesa zernyi larvae [54]. Increased levels of acetylcholinesterase in *Apis mellifera* bees' heads [103].	Inhibition of carbonic anhydrase in the bee *Apis mellifera* [104]. Decreased levels of acetylcholinesterase in the head of the bee *Apis mellifera* [103].	Increased levels of acetylcholinesterase in the heads of the bee *Apis mellifera* [103]. It decreases the activity of acetylcholinesterase and 8-hydroxy-2-deoxyguanosine, increases the levels of antioxidant enzymes in the brain tissue of the rainbow trout *Oncorhynchus mykiss* [105].
Aquatics organisms	Cholinesterase inhibition in the protobrain of shrimp *Artemia salina* [62]. Inhibition of acetylcholinesterase in the gastropod *Gibbula umbilicalis* [83]. Oxidative stress and acetylcholinesterase inhibition in common carp *Cyprinus carpio* brain tissue [106]. Decreased acetylcholinesterase activity and oxidative stress in *Physalaemus gracilis* tadpoles [63]. Cholinesterase inhibition in Chilina gibbosa [107].	Decreased levels of acetylcholine, GABA, choline, tryptophan, and phenylalanine in *Danio rerio* zebrafish larvae [108]. Cholinesterase inhibition in the protobrain of shrimp *Artemia salina* [62]. Inhibits acetylcholinesterase activity in the brain of tropical fish Phalloceros harpagos, *Pterygoplichthys pardalis*, and *Astyanax altiparanae* [109]. Inhibition of cholinesterase and carboxylesterase in Chilina gibbosa [107].	It increases acetylcholinesterase activity and causes oxidative stress in *Gobiocypris rarus* fish brain tissue [110]. Inhibition of brachial acetylcholinesterase in Sydney rock oyster [111]. Oxidative stress and acetylcholinesterase inhibition in zebrafish *Danio rerio* [75]. Inhibition of acetylcholinesterase in the muscle of *Astyanax altiparanae* fish [112].
Birds	Decreased acetylcholinesterase activity in blood, serum, and plasma of broilers [77]. Inhibition of acetylcholinesterase and butyrylcholinesterase; oxidative stress in the brain of the Coturnix japanica quail [113].	Inhibition of plasma acetylcholinesterase in the vulture *Gyps fulvus* [114].	It increases the levels of monoamines in the cerebral cortex of the *Coturnix coturnix* quail [115]. Alteration of acetylcholinesterase and glutathione-S-transferase activity in the muscle and brain of the gray bay-wing bird Agelaioides baduis [116].

Neurochemical effects			
	Chlorpyrifos	**Carbaryl**	**Imidacloprid**
Non-human vertebrates	Decreased activity of acetylcholinesterase; down-regulation of genes related to Parkinson's disease, synaptic transmission, plasticity, and dopaminergic and GABAergic signaling [117]. Acetylcholinesterase increased activity; increased levels of nitric oxide and reactive oxygen species in the amygdala and hippocampus of male Wistar rats [86]. Decreased acetylcholinesterase activity in the brain and cerebellum of Sprague Dawley rats [85]. Decreased dopamine levels and acetylcholinesterase activity in the striatum of Swiss mice [87]. Decreased brain levels of dopamine, serotonin and the activity of monoamine oxidase, acetylcholinesterase, and sodium-potassium ATPase in rats [118].	Acetylcholinesterase inhibition in Norwegian gray rats [91].	Increased acetylcholinesterase activity and calcium levels in the hypothalamus and pituitary of the Wistar rat [119]. Increased levels of epinephrine, norepinephrine, and cortisone in the serum of male Sprague–Dawley rats [93]. Reduction of serotonin, GABA, and dopamine levels, as well as oxidative stress in the brain of male Sprague–Dawley rats [94]. Reduction of GABA and glutathione levels, as well as a decrease in SDH in the albino rat brain [120].
Humans	Humans Decreased intracellular ATP levels and mitochondrial dysfunction in induced pluripotent stem cells [121].	Binding to human melatonin receptors [122]. Inhibition of plasma acetylcholinesterase after acute poisoning [99].	Increases intracellular calcium levels in LUHMES and SH-SY5Y neurons [123].

Table 5.
Neurochemical effects of chlorpyrifos, carbaryl and imidacloprid on five animal species.

Effects on the cellular level			
	Chlorpyrifos	**Carbaryl**	**Imidacloprid**
Insects	No recent studies for the review period in the literature.	No recent studies for the review period in the literature.	Induction of apoptosis by increased levels of caspase-3 and caspase-1 mRNA in the bee *Apis mellifera* [124]. Apoptosis and autophagy in neurons of the brain of the bee *Apis mellifera* [124]. Decreased density of synaptic units in the fungal bodies of the bee *Apis mellifera* [125]. Decreased driving speed in locusta migratoria [60].
Aquatics organisms	Increased expression of BNDF and c-fos in brain tissues of the zebrafish *Danio rerio* [126]. Degeneration and vacuolization in neurons of the dorsal pars medialis in the catfish *Heteropneustes fossilis* [64].	No recent studies for the review period in the literature.	Increased expression of BDNF and c-fos in brain tissues of the zebrafish *Danio rerio* [126].
Birds	Necrosis and degeneration in the brain of broilers [77]. Neurodegeneration, infiltration of mononuclear cells in the brain, and congestion of blood vessels of the meninges of broilers [127]. Neurodegeneration, liquefactive necrosis, vacuolar degeneration, glia cell enlargement, and satellitosis in the broiler brain [128].	No recent studies for the review period in the literature.	Pyknosis, karyolysis, perineuronal edema, reactive astrocytosis, among other histopathological findings in the white Leghorn hen embryos cerebellum [129]. Neurodegeneration, axonal degeneration with demyelination, congestion, perivascular edema, neuronal vacuolization in the *Columba livia* domestica pigeon [130].
No humans vertebrates	Histological alterations in the brain and cerebellum of Sprague Dawley rats [85]. Lewy body formation and neurodegeneration in the substantia nigra of Swiss albino mice [131]. Gliosis and Purkinje cell degeneration in male Wistar rats [132].	Alterations in normal brain development due to changes in important protein levels during neonatal exposure in NMRI mice [90]. Alterations in the electroencephalogram of the visual and frontal cortex of the male Long Evans rat [133]. Neuroinflammation in the hippocampus of male Wistar rats exposed during pregnancy and lactation [134].	Neurodegeneration and increased GFAP expression in the brain of male Sprague–Dawley rats [94]. Absence of the cellular band of the hippocampal formation in mice [135]. Decreased proteins related to echolocation in different brain regions of the bat *Hipposideros armiger terasensis* [95]. DNA damage of male Wistar rat brain cells [136].

Effects on the cellular level			
	Chlorpyrifos	**Carbaryl**	**Imidacloprid**
Humans	Inhibition of voltage-gated calcium channels in human PC12 cells [137]. Inhibition of neurite length, number of neurites, and branch points per neuron in human neural progenitor cells [138]. Apoptotic cell death in human neural stem cells [139]. Alterations in the morphology of different brain regions in exposed children [140].	Associated with meningiomas in people involved in agriculture [141].	Brain edema after acute poisoning [101]. Cell death in neurons of SH-SY5Y human neuroblastoma [142].

Table 6.
Effects on the cellular level of chlorpyrifos, carbaryl and imidacloprid on five animal species.

on the nervous system. For example, in non-target insects, such as bees, it has been observed that it can have adverse effects on caste differentiation [50], as well as on olfactory learning and memory retention [51, 53]; in cockroaches [52] and mosquito larvae [54] has been associated with locomotor alterations (**Table 4**) [143]. It has also been documented that chlorpyrifos can cause alterations in acetylcholinesterase activity and induce oxidative stress in different insects [52, 54, 103] and annelids (**Table 5**). On the other hand, in aquatic organisms such as mollusks, crustaceans, amphibians, and fish, it has been reported that it can cause alterations in locomotor activity [61, 63, 64, 144], inhibit acolinesterase in shrimp [62, 144], copepods [145], common carp [106], tadpoles [63] and snails [61, 107], as well as causing neuronal degeneration in catfish [64]. In toxicity studies carried out in broilers, it has been described that it can cause nervous signs such as salivation, tearing, panting, frequent defecation, tremors, and seizures [77], in sparrows, it can alter the migratory orientation [78] and inhibit acetylcholinesterase activity in broilers [77] and quail (**Tables 4** and **5**) [113]. Regarding its cellular effects, in repeated studies, chlorpyrifos has been reported to be associated with neurodegeneration in broilers [127, 128]. The neurotoxic effects of chlorpyrifos scale to small mammal species. In fact, in rodents under experimental conditions, it has been seen that it can have anxiogenic effects [83, 86] and cause alterations in the memory of recognition [84] and reference [86] in locomotor activity [85, 87], in social behavior (**Table 4**) [84, 89].

While, acute poisonings are associated with signs of piloerection, tremors, seizures, and hypoactivity, among other neurological manifestations [88]. Regarding brain neurochemistry in experimental rodents, it has been reported that chlorpyrifos can alter the activity of acetylcholinesterase. It participates in the downregulation of genes related to Parkinson's disease, causes oxidative stress and decreases dopamine and serotonin levels [86, 87, 117, 118]. Overall, it has also been associated with neurodegeneration in rodents for experimentation [85, 131, 132]. In humans, it has been reported that chlorpyrifos can alter social and motor function in children (**Table 5**) [96, 97]. As well as having fallout related to neurobehavioral deficits in workers exposed to the insecticide [98]. At the neurochemical level, in an in vitro study with human cells, it was shown that it can decrease intracellular levels of ATP and cause mitochondrial dysfunction [121]. Finally, at the cellular level, it has been reported to cause inhibition of activated calcium channels by voltage [137], alter morphology [138], and induce apoptosis in vitro [139]. In human cells exposed to chlorpyrifos, a recently published study reported that it may be associated with alterations in the morphology of different brain regions in children exposed to the substance (**Table 6**) [140].

6.2 Carbaryl

Recent studies on the neurotoxic effects associated with carbaryl are scarce. However, it has been reported that in bees, it can inhibit carbonic anhydrase [104] and decrease acetylcholinesterase levels [103], as well as its negative effect on isopod growth and survival (**Table 5**) [146]. In aquatic organisms, it has been discovered that carbaryl can cause embryonic deformities and growth inhibition in crustaceans [147], affect hatching speed in shrimp [62], locomotives alterations in blue crabs [66], mussels [68], and zebrafish [69]. Besides, in this same species, it has been associated with alterations in exploratory, social, and feeding behavior [67]. Likewise, in tadpoles, it causes hypoactivity, reduction in escape swimming, and feeding behavior (**Table 4**) [65]. Regarding the effects on brain chemistry, it has been reported that carbaryl may be related to the decrease in the levels of acetylcholine, GABA, choline, tryptophan, and phenylalanine in zebrafish [108]. Additionally, it inhibits acetylcholinesterase in shrimp [62], in some species of tropical fish [109], and also in mollusks (**Table 5**) [107]. On the other hand, it has been documented that in broilers, acute poisoning can cause walking difficulty, weakness in the legs, dizziness, frequent defecation, less food consumption, and a decrease in aggressive behavior (**Table 4**) [79]. Overall, acetylcholinesterase inhibition has been reported, particularly in the vulture [114]. Simultaneously, in experimental rodents, it has been associated with deficits in memory and learning. As well as alterations in habitual behavior [90] and hypoactivity [91]. Furthermore, in a supposed carbaryl poisoning in bats, signs such as hypersalivation, miotic pupils, lethargy, and coma were reported [92]. This substance can also inhibit acetylcholinesterase in Norwegian gray rats [91] and in experimental rodents. The above has been related to neurodevelopmental alterations [90], as depicted in the visual and frontal cortex electroencephalogram [133] and hippocampal neuroinflammation [134]. In humans, it has been linked to a semi-conscious state and acetylcholinesterase inhibition after acute poisoning in a 3-year-old child, without further details on other associated neurological signs (**Table 4**) [99]. Moreover, in an in vitro study, it was observed that carbaryl could bind to human melatonin receptors [122]. Carbaryl was recently associated with meningiomas in people agriculturally involved in an epidemiological investigation [141].

While, acute poisonings are associated with signs of piloerection, tremors, seizures, and hypoactivity, among other neurological manifestations [88]. Regarding brain neurochemistry in experimental rodents, it has been reported that chlorpyrifos can alter the activity of acetylcholinesterase [86, 87, 117, 118]. It participates in the downregulation of genes related to Parkinson's disease [117], causes oxidative stress [86] and decreases dopamine and serotonin levels [87, 118]. Overall, it has also been associated with neurodegeneration in rodents for experimentation [131, 132]. In humans, it has been reported that chlorpyrifos can alter social and motor function in children [96, 97]. As well as having fallout related to neurobehavioral deficits in workers exposed to the insecticide [98]. At the neurochemical level, in an in vitro study with human cells, it was shown that it can decrease intracellular levels of ATP and cause mitochondrial dysfunction [121]. Finally, at the cellular level, it has been reported to cause inhibition of activated calcium channels by voltage [137], alter morphology [138], and induce apoptosis in vitro [139]. In human cells exposed to chlorpyrifos, a recently published study reported that it may be associated with alterations in the morphology of different brain regions in children exposed to the substance (**Table 6**) [140].

6.3 Imidacloprid

Despite being considered harmless for most living organisms, neonicotinoid insecticide have been the focus of extensive investigation, as their toxicity has been proven to extend beyond insects [148], to humans. Imidacloprid poisoning in bees has been associated to neurological symptoms such as paralysis and tremors [56], and fire ant exposure has been linked to decreased consumption, foraging, and digging behavior, as well as parasitic wasps with alterations in host-seeking behavior (**Table 4**) [57, 58]. Reduced visual mobility and degradation in in-flight behavior in lobsters, in addition to influencing queen selection behavior in stingless bees have been other reported consequences of the exposure to this insecticide [59, 60]. Imidacloprid has been linked to a decrease in the density of synaptic units in fungiform bodies [125] and a decrease in driving speed in lobsters [103]. It can also increase acetylcholinesterase levels [103] and induce apoptosis and neuronal autophagy [60, 124]. In edaphic invertebrates, imidacloprid causes diverse effects on the survival, growth, and reproduction of earthworms, springtails, mites, and isopods based on LC_{50}, EC_{50}, and EC_{20} toxicity tests [149]. In aquatic organisms, a decrease in acetylcholinesterase levels in mollusks has been reported [150], as well as varied effects on exploratory behavior, swimming activity, and sensorimotor response to startling stimuli in zebrafish (**Tables 4** and **5**) [70].

Moreover, exposure to imidacloprid has been associated with alterations in swimming behavior in tadpoles [71] and shrimp [73], decreased response to predators in frogs [72], and locomotor alterations in crabs [74], zebrafish [75] and tadpoles (**Table 4**) [76]. At the neurochemical level, it has been proposed that imidacloprid can alter acetylcholinesterase activity and cause oxidative stress in fish [75, 105, 110]. It also inhibits brachial acetylcholinesterase in oysters [111] and in fish muscles (**Table 5**) [112]. At the cellular level, it has been documented that the above may be associated with increased expression of BNDF and c-fos in the brain tissues of zebrafish (**Table 6**) [126]. In birds, it has been reported that exposure to imidacloprid can cause hypoactivity, decreased flight behavior, spasms, drooping wings, ataxia, and prostration in pigeons [80]. It has also been stated that it can alter the migratory orientation and delay the time of starting migration in the white-crowned sparrow [151]. In one of the most recently published studies, it was reported that in chickens, it can generate neurological signs such as muscle tremors, ataxia and depression (**Table 4**) [82]; in quail, it can increase monoamine levels in the cerebral cortex [115] and alter the activity of acetylcholinesterase in the muscles and brain of the gray laurel wing bird (**Table 5**) [116]. At the cellular level, it has been associated with neurodegeneration in chicken embryos' cerebellum [129] and pigeons [130]. In experimentation rodents, it has been associated with hypoactivity, increased grooming behavior, and conduct associated with anxiety and depression [93, 94]. While in bats, it may be associated with alterations in the vocal, auditory, orientation, and memory systems (**Table 4**) [95]. Also, in rodents, it can increase acetylcholinesterase activity [119], adrenaline, norepinephrine, and cortisone levels [93], and reduce serotonin, GABA, dopamine, and glutathione (**Table 5**) [120, 152]. Regarding the cellular effects, exposure to imidacloprid can also cause neurodegeneration, an increase in the expression of GFAP [152], and DNA damage in neurons [136]. In bats, it has been related to a decrease in proteins related to echolocation in different brain regions [95]. Moreover, in humans, acute imidacloprid poisonings have been associated with neurological signs such as dyspnea, coma, sweating, drowsiness, confusion, incoherence, lack of orientation, and miotic pupils, among others [100–102].

In an in vitro study with LUHMES and SH-SY5Y cells, an increase in intracellular calcium levels was found [123] (**Table 5**) On the other hand, after acute poisoning, cerebral edema has been reported as a necropsy finding [101], while in an in vitro study it was revealed that it can cause the death of SH-SY5Y cells [135].

On the other hand, acute poisonings are linked to piloerection, tremors, seizures, and hypoactivity, among other neurological manifestations. Regarding brain neurochemistry in experimental rodents, it has been reported that chlorpyrifos can alter the activity of acetylcholinesterase [86, 87, 117, 118]. It participates in the downregulation of genes related to Parkinson's disease [117], causes oxidative stress [86] and decreases dopamine and serotonin levels [87, 118]. Overall, it has also been associated with neurodegeneration in rodents for experimentation [85, 132]. In humans, it has been reported that chlorpyrifos can alter social and motor function in children [96, 97]. As well as having fallout related to neurobehavioral deficits in workers exposed to the insecticide [98]. At the neurochemical level, in an in vitro study with human cells, it was shown that it can decrease intracellular levels of ATP and cause mitochondrial dysfunction [121]. Finally, at the cellular level, it has been reported to cause inhibition of activated calcium channels by voltage [137], alter morphology [138], and induce apoptosis in vitro [139]. In human cells exposed to chlorpyrifos, a recently published study reported that it may be associated with alterations in the morphology of different brain regions in children exposed to the substance [140].

7. Conclusions and perspectives

Insecticides are pesticides commonly associated with neurotoxic effects [153] and although the general population is exposed on a daily basis to low doses through water and food [154–156] the highest risk is presented by agricultural workers, their families and people who live in the areas surrounding the fields, unfortunately, these people are the most exposed and also the least informed about the toxic effects, which leads to bad practices of use, handling and disposal of these substances, which put wildlife and the environment at risk. Since the effects that cause the greatest impact are usually those that directly affect human health, in conclusion some neurotoxic effects associated with the use of insecticides are revealed. In epidemiological studies in humans, organophosphates have been linked to effects such as cholinergic syndrome, polyneuropathy and neuropsychiatric disorders such as cognitive deficits, anxiety, depression, peripheral neuropathy, extrapyramidal symptoms such as dystonia, tremor at rest, bradykinesia, postural instability and rigidity of facial muscles, among others, and have even been associated with neurodegenerative diseases such as Parkinson's and Alzheimer's disease [157, 158]; neonicotinoids have been linked to developmental diseases such as autism and anencephaly and in acute poisonings with neurological signs such as memory loss, finger tremors, muscle spasms, coma and dilated pupils [159–161]; On the other hand, with regard to epidemiological studies on neurotoxicity of carbamates in humans, the literature is limited, however, in the most recently published article, it has been reported that after acute poisoning, these pesticides can cause signs such as coma, drowsiness, seizures, disorientation, tremors and fasciculations, among others [157]. However, although there are epidemiological studies in which the possible relationship between exposure to pesticides and neurological disorders has been determined, to date they remain limited and in fact most of the toxic effects of many pesticides used in the field are unknown. agriculture and therefore it is difficult to determine how we can protect ourselves from them, although there are studies in which the neuroprotective effect of various substances has been experimentally demonstrated, which could counteract the neurotoxic effects of pesticides, for example in the case of pesticides.

Organophosphates it has been documented that the flavonoid kaempferol may have protective effects on chlorpyrifos-induced neurotoxicity [162] and that crocin and citric acid may also have the same effect on malathion-induced toxicity [163, 164]; in the case of neonicotinoids, reduced glutathione, curcumin, resveratrol, ascorbic acid, and aqueous ginger extract have been shown to act as neuroprotectors against imidacloprid-induced toxicity [165–168], as well as curcumin and N-acetylcysteine can protect against acetamiprid-induced neurotoxicity [169, 170]; In the case of carbamates, it has been described that naringenin can combat oxidative stress induced by exposure to carbaryl [171]. Previous studies offer alternatives as possible neuroprotectors, therefore, it is necessary to continue investigating the mechanisms of toxicity and target species of pesticides that exist on the market, before thinking of creating new, more powerful and, of course, more toxic pesticides ; In addition to banning those that pose a high risk to living beings and the environment and making strict policies to control their distribution and sale, since it is clear that it is difficult to live without pesticides, however, it is our duty to use them responsibly.

Acknowledgements

The present work has been possible thanks to Grant from Consejo Nacional de Ciencias y Tecnología (CONACYT) México, registry number 287959.

Conflict of interest

The authors declare no conflict of interest.

Author details

Alejandra Mora-Gutiérrez[1], Carmen Rubio[2], Ángel Alonso Romero-López[3] and Moisés Rubio-Osornio[1*]

1 Department of Neurochemistry, National Institute of Neurology and Neurosurgery, M.V.S., Mexico City, Mexico

2 Department of Neurophysiology, National Institute of Neurology and Neurosurgery, M.V.S., Mexico City, Mexico

3 Faculty of Biological Sciences, Benemerita Autonomous University of Puebla, Puebla, Mexico

*Address all correspondence to: ruomon@gmail.com.mx

References

[1] Sharma A, Kumar V, Shahzad B. Worldwide pesticide usage and its impacts on ecosystem. SN Appl. Sci. 2019;**1**:1446. DOI: 10.1007/s42452-019-1485-1

[2] FAO (Food and Agriculture Organization of the United Nations). FAOSTAT. Pesticides Use, 2021. Available from: http://www.fao.org/faostat/en/#data/RP

[3] Perry ED, Moschini G. Neonicotinoids in US maize: insecticide substitution effects and environmental risk. Journal of Environmental Economics and Management. 2020;**102**:102320. DOI: 10.1016/j.jeem.2020.102320

[4] Borsuah JF, Messer TL, Snow DD, Comfort SD, Mittelstet AR. Literature review: global neonicotinoid insecticide occurrence in aquatic environments. Water. 2020;**12**(12):3388. DOI: 10.3390/w12123388

[5] Adeyinka A, Muco E, Pierre L. Organophosphates. In: StatPearls [Internet]. Treasure Island (FL): StatPearls Publishing; 2021. Jan-. Available from: https://www.ncbi.nlm.nih.gov/books/NBK499860/

[6] Silberman J, Taylor A. Carbamate ToxicityIn: StatPearls [Internet]. Treasure Island (FL): StatPearls Publishing; 2021. Jan-. Available from: https://www.ncbi.nlm.nih.gov/books/NBK482183/

[7] ur Rahman HU, Asghar W, Nazir W, Sandhu MA, Ahmed A, Khalid N. A comprehensive review on chlorpyrifos toxicity with special reference to endocrine disruption: Evidence of mechanisms, exposures and mitigation strategies. Science of the Total Environment. 142649. DOI. 2020. DOI: 10.1016/j.scitotenv.2020.142649

[8] Struger J, Grabuski J, Cagampan S, Sverko E, Marvin C. Occurrence and distribution of carbamate pesticides and metalaxyl in southern Ontario surface waters 2007-2010. Bulletin of environmental contamination and toxicology. 2016;**96**(4):423-431. DOI: 10.1007/s00128-015-1719-x

[9] Simon-Celso N, Amaral-Rogers V, Belzunces LP, Nonmatin JM, Chagnon M, Downs C, et al. Systemic insecticides (neonicotinoids and fipronil): trends, uses, mode of action and metabolites. Environmental Science snd Pollution Research. 2015;**22**(1):5-34 https://doi.org/10.1007/s11356-014-3470-y

[10] Kundoo AA, Dar S, Mushtaq M, Bashir Z, Dar M, Gul S, et al. Role of neonicotinoids in insect pest management: A review. Journal of Entomology and Zoology Studies. 2018;6(1):333-9. Available online: https://www.entomoljournal.com/archives/2018/vol6issue1/PartE/5-5-303-183.pdf

[11] Craddock HA, Huang D, Turner PC, Quirós-Alcalá L, Payne-Sturges DC. Trends in neonicotinoid pesticide residues in food and water in the United States, 1999-2015. Environmental Health. 2019;**18**(1):1-16. DOI: 10.1186/s12940-018-0441-7

[12] National Center for Biotechnology Information PubChem Compound Summary for CID 2730, Chlorpyrifos. 2021. Retrieved July 11. Available from: https://pubchem.ncbi.nlm.nih.gov/compound/Chlorpyrifos.

[13] US EPA (United States Environmental Protection Agency). Chlorpyrifos. 2020. Available from: https://www.epa.gov/ingredients-used-pesticide-products/chlorpyrifos#:~:text=

[14] Hinojosa MG, Prieto AI, Gutiérrez-Praena D, Moreno FJ,

Caméan AM, Jos A. In vitro assessment of the combination of cylindrospermopsin and the organophosphate chlorpyrifos on the human neuroblastoma SH-SY5Y cell line. Ecotoxicology and environmental safety. 2020;**191**:110222. DOI: 10.1016/j.ecoenv.2020.110222

[15] Pang S, Lin Z, Zhang W, Mishra S, Bhatt P, Chen S. Insights into the microbial degradation and biochemical mechanisms of neonicotinoids. Frontiers in microbiology. 2020;**11**:868. DOI: 10.3389/fmicb.2020.00868

[16] Tomizawa M, Casida JE. Neonicotinoid insecticide toxicology: mechanisms of selective action. Annu. Rev. Pharmacol. Toxicol. 2005;**45**:247-268. DOI: 10.1146/annurev.pharmtox.45.120403.095930

[17] Matsuda K, Ihara M, Sattelle DB. Neonicotinoid insecticides: molecular targets, resistance, and toxicity. Annual review of pharmacology and toxicology. 2020;**60**:241-255. DOI: 10.1146/annurev-pharmtox-010818-021747

[18] US Environmental Protection Agency. Imidacloprid Proposed Interim Registration Review Decision Case Number 7605. Washington, DC. 2020. Available online: https://www.regulations.gov/document?D=EPAHQ-OPP-2008-0844-1619.

[19] Anthe M, Valles-Ebeling B, Achtenhagen J, Arenz-Leufen M, Atkinson J, Starp M, et al. Development of an aquatic exposure assessment model for Imidacloprid in sewage treatment plant discharges arising from use of veterinary medicinal products. Environmental Sciences Europe. 2020;**32**(1):1-21. DOI: 10.1186/s12302-020-00424-4

[20] National Center for Biotechnology Information. PubChem Compound Summary for CID 6129, Carbaryl. Retrieved July 11, 2021. From https://pubchem.ncbi.nlm.nih.gov/compound/Carbaryl.

[21] US EPA (United States Environmental Protection). APPENDIX 1-4. Usage Data for Carbaryl–SUUM. 2020. Available from: Agency https://www3.epa.gov/pesticides/nas/carbaryl/appendix-1-4.pdf.

[22] Ahn S, Lee JY, Kim B. Accurate Determination of Carbaryl, Carbofuran and Carbendazim in Vegetables by Isotope Dilution Liquid Chromatography/Tandem Mass Spectrometry. Chromatographia. 2021;**84**(1):27-35. DOI: 10.1007/s10337-020-03976-y

[23] Food and Agriculture Organization of the United Nations. FAO pesticide disposal series 8. Assessing soil contamination. A reference manual. 2002. Available online: http://www.fao.org/fileadmin/templates/agphome/documents/Pests.

[24] Watts M. Chlorpyrifos as a possible global POP. Pesticide Action Network North America, Oakland, CA. 2012. https://www.pan-europe.info/old/News/PR/121009 Chlorpyrifos_as_POP_final.pdf.

[25] Guarda PM, Pontes AM, Domiciano R, Gualberto LB, Mendes DA, Guarda E, da Silva JE. Determination of carbamates and thiocarbamates in water, soil and sediment of the Formoso River, TO, Brazil. Chemistry & biodiversity. 2020;17(4):e1900717. DOI: 10.1002/cbdv.201900717.

[26] Pietrzak D, Kania J, Kmiecik E, Malina G, Wątor K. Fate of selected neonicotinoid insecticides in soil–water systems: Current state of the art and knowledge gaps. Chemosphere. 2020;**255**:126981. DOI: 10.1016/j.chemosphere.2020.126981

[27] Romeh AA. Synergistic use of *Plantago major* and effective

microorganisms, EM1 to clean up the soil polluted with imidacloprid under laboratory and field condition. International Journal of Phytoremediation. 2020;**22**(14):1515-1523. DOI: 10.1080/15226514.2020.1785388

[28] Tišler T, Jemec A, Mozetič B, Trebše P. Hazard identification of imidacloprid to aquatic environment. Chemosphere. 2009;**76**(7):907-914. DOI: 10.1016/j.chemosphere.2009.05.002

[29] Erhirhie EO, Ihekwereme CP, Ilodigwe EE. Advances in acute toxicity testing: strengths, weaknesses and regulatory acceptance. Interdisciplinary Toxicology. 2018;**11**(1):5-12. DOI: 10.2478/intox-2018-0001

[30] Canadian Centre for Occupational Health & Safety. What is a LD50 and LC50? 2021. Available online: https://www.ccohs.ca/oshanswers/chemicals/ld50.html.

[31] World Health Organization. The WHO recommended classification of pesticides by hazard and guidelines to classification 2019. World Health Organization. 2020. Available online: https://apps.who.int/iris/bitstream/handle/10665/332193/9789240005662-eng.pdf.

[32] Godfray HCJ, Blacquiere T, Field LM, Hails RS, Potts SG, Raine NE, et al. A restatement of recent advances in the natural science evidence base concerning neonicotinoid insecticides and insect pollinators. Proceedings of the Royal Society B: Biological Sciences. 2015;**282**:20151821. DOI: 10.1098/rspb.2015.1821

[33] Kumar S, Joshi PC, Nath P, Singh VK. Impacts of insecticides on pollinators of different food plants. Entomol Ornithol Herpetol. 2018;**7**(2):7. DOI: 10.4172/2161-0983.1000211

[34] Siviter H, Muth F. Do novel insecticides pose a threat to beneficial insects? Proceedings of the Royal Society B. 2020;**287**(1935):20201265. DOI: 10.1098/rspb.2020.1265

[35] Gomes IN, Vieira KIC, Gontijo LM, Resende HC. Honeybee survival and flight capacity are compromised by insecticides used for controlling melon pests in Brazil. Ecotoxicology. 2020;**29**(1):97-107. DOI: 10.1007/s10646-019-02145-8

[36] Spurgeon D, Hesketh H, Lahive E, Svendsen C, Baas J, Robinson A, et al. Chronic oral lethal and sublethal toxicities of different binary mixtures of pesticides and contaminants in bees (*Apis mellifera*, *Osmia bicornis* and *Bombus terrestris*). EFSA supporting publication. 2016. DOI: 10.2903/sp.efsa.2016.EN-1076

[37] Sterk G, Peters B, Gao Z, Zumkier U. Large-scale monitoring of effects of clothianidin-dressed OSR seeds on pollinating insects in northern Germany: effects on large earth bumble bees (*Bombus terrestris*). Ecotoxicology. 2016;**25**:1666-1678. DOI: 10.1007/s10646-016-1730-y

[38] Switzer CM, Combes SA. The neonicotinoid pesticide, imidacloprid, affects *Bombus impatiens* (bumblebee) sonication behavior when consumed at doses below the LD_{50}. Ecotoxicology. 2016;**25**:1150-1159. DOI: 10.1007/s10646-016-1669-z

[39] Pisa LW, Amaral-Rogers V, Belzunces LP. Effects of neonicotinoids and fipronil on non-target invertebrates. Environ. Sci. Pollut. Res. 2015;**22**:68-102. DOI: 10.1007/s11356-014-3471-x

[40] Pecenka JR, Lundgren JG. Non-target effects of clothianidin on monarch butterflies. Sc. Nat. 2015;**102**:19. DOI: 10.1007/s00114-015-1270-y

[41] Yu RX, Wang YH, Hu XQ, Wu SG, Cai LM, Zhao XP. Individual and joint

acute toxicities of selected insecticides against *Bombyx mori* (Lepidoptera: Bombycidae). J. Econ. Entomol. 2015;**109**:327-333. DOI: 10.1093/jee/tov316

[42] Botías C, David A, Hill E, Goulson D. Contamination of wild plants near neonicotinoid seed-treated crops, and implications for non-target insects. Sci. Total. Environ. 2016;**566**:269-278. DOI: 10.1016/j.scitotenv.2016.05.065

[43] Wang L, Zeng L, Chen J. Sublethal effect of imidacloprid on *Solenopsis invicta* (Hymenoptera: Formicidae) feeding, digging, and foraging behaviour. Environ. Entomol. 2015a;**44**:1544-1552. DOI: 10.1093/ee/nvv127

[44] Wang L, Zeng L, Chen J. Impact of imidacloprid on new Queens of imported fire ants, *Solenopsis invicta* (Hymenoptera: Formicidae). Sci. Rep. 2015b;**5**:17938. DOI: 10.1038/srep17938

[45] Douglas MR, Rohr JR, Tooker JF. Neonicotinoid insecticide travels through a soil food chain, disrupting biological control of non-target pests and decreasing soya bean yield. J. Appl. Ecol. 2015;**52**:250-260. DOI: 10.1111/1365-2664.12372

[46] Morrissey CA, Mineau P, Devries JH, Sánchex-Bayo F, Liess M, Cavallaro MC, et al. Neonicotinoid contamination of global surfacewaters and associated risk to aquatic invertebrates: a review. Environ. Int. 2015;**74**:291-303. DOI: 10.1016/j.envint.2014.10.024

[47] de Perre C, Murphy TM, Lydy MJ. Fate and effects of clothianidin in fields using conservation practices. Environ. Toxicol. Chem. 2015;**34**:258-265. DOI: 10.1002/etc.2800

[48] Kunce W, Josefsson S, Örberg J, Johansson F. Combination effects of pyrethroids and neonicotinoids on development and survival of *Chironomus riparius*. Ecotoxicol Environ Saf. 2015;**122**:426-431. DOI: 10.1016/j.ecoenv.2015.09.008

[49] Mulé R, Sabella G, Robba L, Manachini B. Systematic review of the effects of chemical insecticides on four common butterfly families. Frontiers in Environmental Science, 2017;5:32. DOI. https://doi.org/10.3389/fenvs.2017.00032

[50] Dos Santos CF, Acosta AL, Dorneles AL, Dos Santos PD, Blochtein B. Queens become workers: pesticides alter caste differentiation in bees. Scientific Reports. 2016;6(1): 1-9. DOI. https://doi.org/10.1038/srep31605

[51] Urlacher E, Monchanin C, Rivière C, Richard FJ, Lombardi C, Michelsen-Heath S, et al. Measurements of chlorpyrifos levels in forager bees and comparison with levels that disrupt honey bee odor-mediated learning under laboratory conditions. Journal of Chemical Ecology. 2016;42(2):127-138. DOI. https://doi.org/10.1007/s10886-016-0672-4

[52] Adedara IA, Rosemberg DB, de Souza D, Farombi EO, Aschner M, Souza DO, et al. Neurobehavioral and biochemical changes in *Nauphoeta cinerea* following dietary exposure to chlorpyrifos. Pesticide Biochemistry and Physiology. 2016;**130**:22-30. DOI: 10.1016/j.pestbp.2015.12.004

[53] Li Z, Li M, Huang J, Ma C, Xiao L, Huang Q, Su S. Effects of sublethal concentrations of chlorpyrifos on olfactory learning and memory performances in two bee species, *Apis mellifera* and *Apis cerana*. Sociobiology. 2017;64:174-181. DOI: 10.13102/sociobiology.v64i2.1385

[54] Di Nica V, González ABM, Lencioni V, Villa S. Behavioural and

biochemical alterations by chlorpyrifos in aquatic insects: an emerging environmental concern for pristine Alpine habitats. Environmental Science and Pollution Research. 2020;**27**(25):30918-30926. DOI: 10.1007/s11356-019-06467-2

[55] Martínez LC, Plata-Rueda A, Rodríguez-Dimaté FA. Exposure to insecticides reduces populations of *Rhynchophorus palmarum* in oil palm plantations with bud rot disease. Insects. 2019;**10**:111. DOI: 10.3390/insects10040111

[56] Soares HM, Jacob CRO, Carvalho SM, Nocelli RCF, Malaspina O. Toxicity of imidacloprid to the stingless bee *Scaptotrigona postica* Latreille, 1807 (Hymenoptera: Apidae). Bulletin of Environmental Contamination and Toxicology. 2015;**94**(6):675-680. DOI: 10.1007/s00128-015-1488-6

[57] Wang L, Zeng L, Chen J. Sublethal effect of imidacloprid on *Solenopsis invicta* (Hymenoptera: Formicidae) feeding, digging, and foraging behavior. Environmental Entomology. 2015;**44**(6):1544-1552. DOI: 10.1093/ee/nvv127

[58] Tappert L, Pokorny T, Hofferberth J, Ruther J. Sublethal doses of imidacloprid disrupt sexual communication and host finding in a parasitoid wasp. Scientific Reports. 2017;**7**(1):1-9. DOI: 10.1038/srep42756

[59] Otesbelgue A, Dos Santos CF, Blochtein B. Queen bee acceptance under threat: Neurotoxic insecticides provoke deep damage in queen-worker relationships. Ecotoxicology and Environmental Safety. 2018;**166**:42-47. DOI: 10.1016/j.ecoenv.2018.09.048

[60] Parkinson RH, Gray JR. Neural conduction, visual motion detection, and insect flight behaviour are disrupted by low doses of imidacloprid and its metabolites. Neurotoxicology. 2019;**72**:107-113. DOI: 10.1016/j.neuro.2019.02.012

[61] Silva CO, Novais SC, Alves LM, Soares AM, Barata C, Lemos MF. Linking cholinesterase inhibition with behavioural changes in the sea snail *Gibbula umbilicalis*: Effects of the organophosphate pesticide chlorpyrifos. Comparative Biochemistry and Physiology Part C: Toxicology & Pharmacology. 2019;**225**:108570. DOI: 10.1016/j.cbpc.2019.108570

[62] Gambardella C, Nichino D, Iacometti C, Ferrando S, Falugi C, Faimali M. Long term exposure to low dose neurotoxic pesticides affects hatching, viability and cholinesterase activity of Artemia sp. Aquatic Toxicology. 2018;**196**:79-89. DOI: 10.1016/j.aquatox.2018.01.006

[63] Rutkoski CF, Macagnan N, Folador A, Skovronski VJ, do Amaral AM, Leitemperger J, Hartmann MT. Morphological and biochemical traits and mortality in *Physalaemus gracilis* (Anura: Leptodactylidae) tadpoles exposed to the insecticide chlorpyrifos. Chemosphere. 2020;250:126162. DOI: 10.1016/j.chemosphere.2020.126162.

[64] Mishra AK, Gopesh A, Singh KP. Acute toxic effects of chlorpyrifos and indoxacarb on dorsal pars medialis of telencephalon and swimming behavior of a catfish, *Heteropneustes fossilis*. Journal of Applied Biology & Biotechnology. 2021;9(03):137-143. DOI. https://doi.org/10.7324/JABB.2021.9317

[65] Wood L, Welch AM. Assessment of interactive effects of elevated salinity and three pesticides on life history and behavior of southern toad (*Anaxyrus terrestris*) tadpoles. Environmental Toxicology and Chemistry. 2015;**34**(3):667-676. DOI: 10.1002/etc.2861

[66] Schroeder-Spain K, Fisher LL, Smee DL. Uncoordinated: effects of

sublethal malathion and carbaryl exposures on juvenile and adult blue crabs (*Callinectes sapidus*). Journal of Experimental Marine Biology and Ecology. 2018;**504**:1-9. DOI: 10.1016/j.jembe.2018.03.005

[67] Correia D, Almeida AR, Santos J, Machado AL, Ucun OK, Žlábek V, et al. Behavioral effects in adult zebrafish after developmental exposure to carbaryl. Chemosphere. 2019;**235**:1022-1029. DOI: 10.1016/j.chemosphere.2019.07.029

[68] Khudhur SM, Shekha YA. Histopathological and Biochemical Biomarker Response of Mussel, *Unio Pictorum*, to Carbamate Pesticide Carbaryl: A Laboratory Study. Indian J Ani Res. 2019;1157:1-5. DOI: 10.18805/ijar.B1157.

[69] Faria M, Wu X, Luja-Mondragón M, Prats E, Gómez-Oliván LM, Piña B, et al. Screening anti-predator behaviour in fish larvae exposed to environmental pollutants. Science of The Total Environment. 2020;**714**:136759. DOI: 10.1016/j.scitotenv.2020.136759

[70] Crosby EB, Bailey JM, Oliveri AN, Levin ED. Neurobehavioral impairments caused by developmental imidacloprid exposure in zebrafish. Neurotoxicology and Teratology. 2015;**49**:81-90. DOI: 10.1016/j.ntt.2015.04.006

[71] Sievers M, Hale R, Swearer SE, Parris KM. Contaminant mixtures interact to impair predator-avoidance behaviours and survival in a larval amphibian. Ecotoxicology and Environmental Safety. 2018;**161**:482-488. DOI: 10.1016/j.ecoenv.2018.06.028

[72] Lee-Jenkins SS, Robinson SA. Effects of neonicotinoids on putative escape behavior of juvenile wood frogs (*Lithobates sylvaticus*) chronically exposed as tadpoles. Environmental Toxicology and Chemistry. 2018;**37**(12):3115-3123. DOI: 10.1002/etc.4284

[73] Al-Badran AA, Fujiwara M, Mora MA. Effects of insecticides, fipronil and imidacloprid, on the growth, survival, and behavior of brown shrimp *Farfantepenaeus aztecus*. PloS One. 2019;14(10):e0223641. DOI: 10.1371/journal.pone.0223641.

[74] Huang Y, Hong Y, Yin H, Yan G, Huang Q, Li Z, et al. Imidacloprid induces locomotion impairment of the freshwater crayfish. *Procambarus clarkii* via neurotoxicity and oxidative stress in digestive system. Aquatic Toxicology. 2021;**16**:238105913. DOI: 10.1016/j.aquatox.2021.105913

[75] Guerra LJ. do Amaral AMB, de Quadros VA, da Luz Fiuza T, Rosemberg DB, Prestes OD, Loro VL. Biochemical and Behavioral Responses in Zebrafish Exposed to Imidacloprid Oxidative Damage and Antioxidant Responses. Archives of Environmental Contamination and Toxicology. 2021;**81**(2):255-264. DOI: 10.1007/s00244-021-00865-9

[76] Samojeden CG, Pavan FA, Rutkoski CF, Folador A, Da Fré SP, Müller, C, Hartmann MT. Toxicity and Genotoxicity of Imidacloprid in Tadpoles of *Leptodactylus Latrans* and *Physalaemus Cuvieri* (Anura: Leptodactylidae). Ecotoxicology. DOI: 10.21203/rs.3.rs-448465/v1.

[77] Ahmad MZ, Khan A, Javed MT, Hussain I. Impact of chlorpyrifos on health biomarkers of broiler chicks. Pesticide Biochemistry and Physiology. 2015;**122**:50-58. DOI: 10.1016/j.pestbp.2014.12.024

[78] Eng ML, Stutchbury BJ, Morrissey CA. Imidacloprid and chlorpyrifos insecticides impair migratory ability in a seed-eating songbird. Scientific Reports.

2017;**7**(1):1-9. DOI: 10.1038/s41598-017-15446-x

[79] Khanam S. Behavioral Changes in Broiler Chicks Exposed to Carbaryl. Am. J. Biomed. Sci. Res. 2019;3:209-212. DOI: 10.34297/AJBSR.2019.03.000664.

[80] Addy-Orduna LM, Brodeur JC, Mateo R. Oral acute toxicity of imidacloprid, thiamethoxam and clothianidin in eared doves: a contribution for the risk assessment of neonicotinoids in birds. Science of the Total Environment. 2019;**650**:1216-1223. DOI: 10.1016/j.scitotenv.2018.09.112

[81] Eng ML, Stutchbury BJM, Morrissey CA. A neonicotinoid insecticide reduces fueling and delays migration in songbirds. Science. 2019;**365**(6458):1177-1180. DOI: 10.1126/science.aaw9419

[82] Franzen-Klein D, Jankowski M, Roy CL, Nguyen-Phuc H, Chen D, Neuman-Lee L, et al. Evaluation of neurobehavioral abnormalities and immunotoxicity in response to oral imidacloprid exposure in domestic chickens (*Gallus gallus* domesticus). Journal of Toxicology and Environmental Health, Part A. 2020;**83**(2):45-65. DOI: 10.1080/15287394.2020.1723154

[83] Silva JG, Boareto AC, Schreiber AK, Redivo DD, Gambeta E, Vergara F, et al. Chlorpyrifos induces anxiety-like behavior in offspring rats exposed during pregnancy. Neuroscience Letters. 2017;**641**:94-100. DOI: 10.1016/j.neulet.2017.01.053

[84] Lan A, Kalimian M, Amram B, Kofman O. Prenatal chlorpyrifos leads to autism-like deficits in C57Bl6/J mice. Environmental Health. 2017;**16**(1):1-10. DOI: 10.1186/s12940-017-0251-3

[85] Fereidounni S, Kumar D. Understanding the role of quercetin during neurotoxicity induced by Chlorpyrifos. The Journal of Phytopharmacology. 2018;7(1):33-39. Available online. http://www.phytopharmajournal.com/Vol7_Issue1_08.pdf

[86] Imam A, Sulaiman NA, Oyewole AL, Chengetanai S, Williams V, Ajibola MI, et al. Chlorpyrifos-and dichlorvos-induced oxidative and neurogenic damage elicits neuro-cognitive deficits and increases anxiety-like behavior in wild-type rats. Toxics. 2018;**6**(4):71. DOI: 10.3390/toxics6040071

[87] Ali SJ, Ellur G, Patel K, Sharan K. Chlorpyrifos exposure induces parkinsonian symptoms and associated bone loss in adult swiss albino mice. Neurotoxicity Research. 2019;**36**(4):700-711. DOI: 10.1007/s12640-019-00092-0

[88] Mustafa KA, Al-Baggou BK. Toxicological and neurobehavioral effects of chlorpyrifos and deltamethrin insecticides in mice. Iraqi Journal of Veterinary Sciences. 2020;34(1):189-196. DOI: 10.33899/ijvs.2019.125738.1144.

[89] Kofman O, Lan A, Raykin E, Zega K, Brodski C. Developmental and social deficits and enhanced sensitivity to prenatal chlorpyrifos in PON1−/− mouse pups and adults. Plos One. 2020;15(9):e0239738. DOI: 10.1371/journal.pone.0239738.

[90] Lee I, Eriksson P, Fredriksson A, Buratovic S, Viberg H. Developmental neurotoxic effects of two pesticides: Behavior and biomolecular studies on chlorpyrifos and carbaryl. Toxicology and Applied Pharmacology. 2015;**288**(3):429-438. DOI: 10.1016/j.taap.2015.08.014

[91] Moser VC, Phillips PM, McDaniel KL. Assessment of

biochemical and behavioral effects of carbaryl and methomyl in Brown-Norway rats from preweaning to senescence. Toxicology. 2015;**331**:1-13. DOI: 10.1016/j.tox.2015.02.006

[92] Selig M, Lewandowski A. Suspected carbaryl toxicity in a captive colony of straw-colored fruit bats (eidolon helvum). Journal of Zoo and Wildlife Medicine. 2017;**48**(4):1247-1249. DOI: 10.1638/2017-0029R.1

[93] Khalil SR, Awad A, Mohammed HH, Nassan MA. Imidacloprid insecticide exposure induces stress and disrupts glucose homeostasis in male rats. Environmental Toxicology and Pharmacology. 2017;**55**:165-174. DOI: 10.1016/j.etap.2017.08.017

[94] Abd-Elhakim YM, Mohammed HH, Mohamed WA. Imidacloprid impacts on neurobehavioral performance, oxidative stress, and apoptotic events in the brain of adolescent and adult rats. Journal of Agricultural and Food Chemistry. 2018;**66**(51):13513-13524. DOI: 10.1021/acs.jafc.8b05793

[95] Wu CH, Lin CL, Wang SE, Lu CW. Effects of imidacloprid, a neonicotinoid insecticide, on the echolocation system of insectivorous bats. Pesticide Biochemistry and Physiology. 2020;**163**:94-101. DOI: 10.1016/j.pestbp.2019.10.010

[96] Rauh VA, Garcia WE, Whyatt RM, Horton MK, Barr DB, Louis ED. Prenatal exposure to the organophosphate pesticide chlorpyrifos and childhood tremor. Neurotoxicology. 2015;51:80-86. DOI. https://doi.org/10.1016/j.neuro.2015.09.004

[97] Guo J, Zhang J, Wu C, Lv S, Lu D, Qi X, et al. Associations of prenatal and childhood chlorpyrifos exposure with Neurodevelopment of 3-year-old children. Environmental Pollution. 2019;**251**:538-546. DOI: 10.1016/j.envpol.2019.05.040

[98] Anger WK, Farahat FM, Lein PJ, Lasarev MR, Olson JR, Farahat TM, et al. Magnitude of behavioral deficits varies with job-related chlorpyrifos exposure levels among Egyptian pesticide workers. Neurotoxicology. 2020;**77**:216-230. DOI: 10.1016/j.neuro.2020.01.012

[99] El-Nahhal Y. Successful Management of Carbamate Poisoning among Children: Case Report from Gaza Strip. Occupational Diseases and Environmental Medicine. 2018;**6**(3):95-106. DOI: 10.4236/odem.2018.63008

[100] Sriapha C, Trakulsrichai S, Tongpoo A, Pradoo A, Rittilert P, Wananukul W. Acute Imidacloprid Poisoning in Thailand. Therapeutics and Clinical Risk Management. 2020;**16**:1081. DOI: 10.2147/TCRM.S269161

[101] Perananthan V, Mohamed F, Shahmy S, Gawarammana I, Dawson A, Buckley N. The clinical toxicity of imidacloprid self-poisoning following the introduction of newer formulations. Clinical Toxicology. 2021;**59**(4):347-350. DOI: 10.1080/15563650.2020.1815760

[102] Shiri-Ghaleh V, Khani S, Moradi M, Soltaninejad K. Clinical and Medicolegal Aspects of Fatal Imidacloprid Deliberate Self-Poisoning: A Case Report. International Journal of Medical Toxicology and Forensic Medicine. 2021;11:32228. DOI: 10.32598/ijmtfm.v11i.32228.

[103] Pervez M, Manzoor F. A study on lethal doses of various pesticides on honeybees (*Apis mellifera* L.) a laboratory trial. Physiological Entomology. 2021;46(1):34-44. DOI. https://doi.org/10.1111/phen.12338A

[104] Soydan E, Güler A, Bıyık S, Şentürk M, Supuran CT, Ekinci D. Carbonic anhydrase from *Apis mellifera*: purification and inhibition by

pesticides. Journal of Enzyme Inhibition and Medicinal Chemistry. 2017;**32**(1):47-50. DOI: 10.1080/14756366.2016.1232255

[105] Topal A, Alak G, Ozkaraca M, Yeltekin AC, Comaklı S, Acıl G, et al. Neurotoxic responses in brain tissues of rainbow trout exposed to imidacloprid pesticide: Assessment of 8-hydroxy-2-deoxyguanosine activity, oxidative stress and acetylcholinesterase activity. Chemosphere. 2017;**175**:186-191. DOI: 10.1016/j.chemosphere.2017.02.047

[106] Berkoz M, Ozkan-Yilmaz F, Ozluer-Hunt A, Gunduz SG, Yildirim M, Yalin S. Influence of sublethal chlorpyrifos exposure on oxidative stress and acetylcholinesterase activity in common carp (Cyprinus carpio). Feb-Fresenius Environmental Bulletin. 2019;**219**:981-988. DOI: 10.1016/j.chemosphere.2018.12.077

[107] Herbert LT, Cossi PF, Painefilú JC, Goñalons CM, Luquet CM, Kristoff G. Acute neurotoxicity evaluation of two anticholinesterasic insecticides, independently and in mixtures, and a neonicotinoid on a freshwater gastropod. Chemosphere. 2021;**265**:129107. DOI: 10.1016/j.chemosphere.2020.129107

[108] Tufi S, Leonards P, Lamoree M, de Boer J, Legler J, Legradi J. Changes in neurotransmitter profiles during early zebrafish (*Danio rerio*) development and after pesticide exposure. Environmental Science & Technology. 2016;**50**(6):3222-3230. DOI: 10.1021/acs.est.5b05665

[109] Pereira BV, Silva-Zacarin EC, Costa MJ. Dos Santos ACA, do Carmo JB, Nunes B. Cholinesterases characterization of three tropical fish species, and their sensitivity towards specific contaminants. Ecotoxicology and Environmental Safety. 2019;**173**:482-493. DOI: 10.1016/j.ecoenv.2019.01.105

[110] Tian X, Yang W, Wang D, Zhao Y, Yao R, Ma L, et al. Chronic brain toxicity response of juvenile Chinese rare minnows (*Gobiocypris rarus*) to the neonicotinoid insecticides imidacloprid and nitenpyram. Chemosphere. 2018;**210**:1006-1012. DOI: 10.1016/j.chemosphere.2018.06.083

[111] Ewere EE, Powell D, Rudd D, Reichelt-Brushett A, Mouatt P, Voelcker NH, et al. Uptake, depuration and sublethal effects of the neonicotinoid, imidacloprid, exposure in Sydney rock oysters. Chemosphere. 2019;**230**:1-13. DOI: 10.1016/j.chemosphere.2019.05.045

[112] Almeida ÉC, Passos LS, Vieira CED, Acayaba RD, Montagner CC, Pinto E, et al. Can the insecticide Imidacloprid affect the health of the Neotropical freshwater fish *Astyanax altiparanae* (Teleostei: Characidae)? Environmental Toxicology and Pharmacology. 2021;**85**:103634. DOI: 10.1016/j.etap.2021.103634

[113] Miladinović DĆ, Borozan S, Ivanović S. Involvement of cholinesterases in oxidative stress induced by chlorpyrifos in the brain of Japanese quail. Poultry Science. 2018;**97**(5):1564-1571. DOI: 10.3382/ps/pey018

[114] Oropesa AL, Sánchez S, Soler F. Characterization of plasma cholinesterase activity in the Eurasian Griffon Vulture *Gyps fulvus* and its in vitro inhibition by carbamate pesticides. Ibis. 2017;**159**(3):510-518. DOI: 10.1111/ibi.12476

[115] Rawi SM, Al-Logmani AS, Hamza RZ. Neurological alterations induced by formulated imidacloprid toxicity in Japanese quails. Metabolic Brain Disease. 2019;**34**(2):443-450. DOI: 10.1007/s11011-018-0377-1

[116] Poliserpi MB, Cristos D, Iglesias JMP, Brodeur JC. Tissue

distribution and sublethal effects of imidacloprid in the South American grayish baywing (*Agelaioides badius*). Chemosphere. 2021;**284**:131327. DOI: 10.1016/j.chemosphere.2021.131327

[117] Pallotta MM, Ronca R, Carotenuto R, Porreca I, Turano M, Ambrosino C, et al. Specific effects of chronic dietary exposure to chlorpyrifos on brain gene expression—a mouse study. International Journal of Molecular Sciences. 2017;**18**(11):2467. DOI: 10.3390/ijms18112467

[118] Ibrahim EM, Abdelrahman SM, Elhakim HK, Ragab EA. Single or combined exposure to chlorpyrifos and cypermethrin provoke oxidative stress and downregulation in monoamine oxidase and acetylcholinesterase gene expression of the rat's brain. Environmental Science and Pollution Research. 2020;**27**(11):12692-12703. DOI: 10.1007/s11356-020-07864-8

[119] Annabi A, Dhouib IB, Lamine AJ, Golli NE, Gharbi N, Fazâa SE, et al. Recovery by N-acetylcysteine from subchronic exposure to Imidacloprid-induced hypothalamic–pituitary–adrenal (HPA) axis tissues injury in male rats. Toxicology Mechanisms and Methods. 2015;**25**(7):524-531. DOI: 10.3109/15376516.2015.1045663

[120] Farag MR, Abou-EL Fotoh MF, EL-Sayed GG, EL-Sayed EW. Modulatory Effect of Ginger Aqueous Extract against Imidacloprid-Induced Neurotoxicity in Rats. Zagazig Veterinary Journal. 2019;47(4):432-446. DOI: 10.21608/zvjz.2019.14914.1061.

[121] Yamada S, Kubo Y, Yamazaki D, Sekino Y, Kanda Y. Chlorpyrifos inhibits neural induction via Mfn1-mediated mitochondrial dysfunction in human induced pluripotent stem cells. Scientific Reports. 2017;**7**(1):1-12. DOI: 10.1038/srep40925

[122] Popovska-Gorevski M, Dubocovich ML, Rajnarayanan RV. Carbamate insecticides target human melatonin receptors. Chemical Research in Toxicology. 2017;**30**(2):574-582. DOI: 10.1021/acs.chemrestox.6b00301

[123] Loser D, Hinojosa MG, Blum J, Schaefer J, Brüll M, Johansson Y, et al. Functional alterations by a subgroup of neonicotinoid pesticides in human dopaminergic neurons. Archives of Toxicology. 2021;**95**(6):2081-2107. DOI: 10.1007/s00204-021-03031-1

[124] Wu YY, Zhou T, Wang Q, Dai PL, Xu SF, Jia HR, et al. Programmed cell death in the honey bee (*Apis mellifera*) (Hymenoptera: Apidae) worker brain induced by imidacloprid. Journal of Economic Entomology. 2015;**108**(4):1486-1494. DOI: 10.1093/jee/tov146

[125] Peng YC, Yang EC. Sublethal dosage of imidacloprid reduces the microglomerular density of honey bee mushroom bodies. Scientific Reports. 2016;**6**(1):1-13. DOI: 10.1038/srep19298

[126] Özdemir S, Altun S, Özkaraca M, Ghosi A, Toraman E, Arslan H. Cypermethrin, chlorpyrifos, deltamethrin, and imidacloprid exposure up-regulates the mRNA and protein levels of bdnf and c-fos in the brain of adult zebrafish (*Danio rerio*). Chemosphere. 2018;**203**:318-326. DOI: 10.1016/j.chemosphere.2018.03.190

[127] Wani H, Rehman S, Shoukat S, Kour N, Ayoub B. Patho-Morphological Changes in Liver, Kidney and Brain of Broiler Birds Due to Chlorpyrifos Intoxication. International Journal of Livestock Research. 2018;**8**(02):266-274. DOI: 10.5455/ijlr.20170718095718

[128] Rathod AS, Ingole RS, Rathod PR, Hajare SW, Ingawale M. Individual and combined toxicopathology of chlorpyrifos and cypermethrin in broiler chickens. Indian Journal of Animal Sciences. 2020;90(5):688-692. Available online. https://www.researchgate.net/profile/Maheshkumar

[129] Singh V, Hussein M, Singh AK, Hassan MA, Gupta P. Histological and immunohistochemical changes in cerebellum of chick embryos after exposure to neonicotinoid insecticide imidacloprid. Journal of the Anatomical Society of India. 2015;**64**(2):122-127. DOI: 10.1016/j.jasi.2015.10.014

[130] Zeid EHA, Alam RT, Ali SA, Hendawi MY. Dose-related impacts of imidacloprid oral intoxication on brain and liver of rock pigeon (*Columba livia* domestica), residues analysis in different organs. Ecotoxicology and Environmental Safety. 2019;**167**:60-68. DOI: 10.1016/j.ecoenv.2018.09.121

[131] Ravikumar HA, Karapehlivan M. Chlorpyrifos-induced parkinsonian model in mice: Behavior, histopathology and biochemistry. Pesticide Biochemistry and Physiology. 2018;**144**:36-41. DOI: 10.1016/j.pestbp.2017.11.002

[132] Ravikumar Y, Madhuri D, Lakshman M, Reddy AG, Kalakumar B. Antioxidative Profile and Histopathological Alterations of Brain Induced by Cadmium (Cd) and Chlorpyrifos (CPF) in Wistar Rats. 2020. doi: http://dx.doi.org/10.5455/ijlr.20200512065339.

[133] Freeborn DL, McDaniel KL, Moser VC, Herr DW. Use of electroencephalography (EEG) to assess CNS changes produced by pesticides with different modes of action: effects of permethrin, deltamethrin, fipronil, imidacloprid, carbaryl, and triadimefon. Toxicology and Applied Pharmacology. 2015;**282**(2):184-194. DOI: 10.1016/j.taap.2014.11.011

[134] Gómez-Giménez B, Llansola M, Hernández-Rabaza V, Cabrera-Pastor A, Malaguarnera M, Agusti A, et al. Sex-dependent effects of developmental exposure to different pesticides on spatial learning. The role of induced neuroinflammation in the hippocampus. Food and Chemical Toxicology. 2017;**99**:135-148. DOI: 10.1016/j.fct.2016.11.028

[135] Zheng M, Qin Q, Zhou W, Liu Q, Zeng S, Xiao H, et al. Metabolic disturbance in hippocampus and liver of mice: A primary response to imidacloprid exposure. Scientific Reports. 2020;**10**(1):1-12. DOI: 10.1038/s41598-020-62739-9

[136] Katić A, Kašuba V, Kopjar N, Lovaković BT, Čermak AM, Mendaš G, et al. Effects of low-level imidacloprid oral exposure on cholinesterase activity, oxidative stress responses, and primary DNA damage in the blood and brain of male Wistar rats. Chemico-Biological Interactions. 2021;**338**:109287. DOI: 10.1016/j.cbi.2020.109287

[137] Meijer M, Brandsema JA, Nieuwenhuis D, Wijnolts FM, Dingemans MM, Westerink RH. Inhibition of voltage-gated calcium channels after subchronic and repeated exposure of PC12 cells to different classes of insecticides. Toxicological Sciences. 2015;**147**(2):607-617. DOI: 10.1093/toxsci/kfv154

[138] Wu X, Yang X, Majumder A, Swetenburg R, Goodfellow FT, Bartlett MG, et al. From the cover: AstrocytesAre protective against chlorpyrifos developmental neurotoxicity in human pluripotent stem cell-derived astrocyte-neuron cocultures. Toxicological Sciences. 2017;**157**(2):410-420. DOI: 10.1093/toxsci/kfx056

[139] Sandoval L, Rosca A, Oniga A, Zambrano A, Ramos JJ, González MC, et al. Effects of chlorpyrifos on cell death and cellular phenotypic specification of human neural stem cells. Science of The Total Environment. 2019;**683**:445-454. DOI: 10.1016/j.scitotenv.2019.05.270

[140] Todd SW, Lumsden EW, Aracava Y, Mamczarz J, Albuquerque EX,

Pereira EF. Gestational exposures to organophosphorus insecticides: From acute poisoning to developmental neurotoxicity. Neuropharmacology. 2020;**1**:108271. DOI: 10.1016/j.neuropharm.2020.108271

[141] Piel C, Pouchieu C, Migault L, Béziat B, Boulanger M, Bureau M, et al. Increased risk of central nervous system tumours with carbamate insecticide use in the prospective cohort agrican. International Journal of Epidemiology. 2019;**48**(2):512-526. DOI: 10.1093/ije/dyy246

[142] Paredes-Espinosa MB. Neonicotinoid neurotoxicity evaluation on human retinoic acid differentiated cholinergic neuroblastoma 5H-SY5Y cells (Bachelor's thesis, Universidad de Investigación de Tecnología Experimental Yachay). 2021. Available online: http://repositorio.yachaytech.edu.ec/handle/123456789/300.

[143] Muangphra P, Tharapoom K, Euawong N, Namchote S, Gooneratne R. Chronic toxicity of commercial chlorpyrifos to earthworm Pheretima peguana. Environ Toxicol. 2016;**31**(11):1450-1459. DOI: 10.1002/tox.22150

[144] Duarte-Restrepo E, Jaramillo-Colorado BE, Duarte-Jaramillo L. Effects of chlorpyrifos on the crustacean *Litopenaeus vannamei*. PLoS ONE. 2020;15:e0231310. DOI: 10.1371/journal.pone.0231310.

[145] Lee JW, Kim BM, Jeong CB, Won EJ, Rhee JS, Lee JS. Inhibitory effects of biocides on transcription and protein activity of acetylcholinesterase in the intertidal copepod *Tigriopus japonicus*. Comp. Biochem. Physiol. Part C Toxicol Pharmacol. 2015;**167**:147-156. DOI: 10.1016/j.cbpc.2014.10.005

[146] Morgado RG, Gomes PD, Ferreira NGC, Cardoso DN, Santos MJG, Soares AM. Toxicity interaction between chlorpyrifos, mancozeb and soil moisture to the terrestrial isopod *Porcellionides pruinosus*. Chemosphere. 2016;**144**:1845-1853. DOI: 10.1016/j.chemosphere.2015.10.034

[147] Toumi H, Burga-Perez KF, Ferard JF. Acute and chronic ecotoxicity of carbaryl with a battery of aquatic bioassays. Journal of Environmental Science and Health Part B. 2015;**51**:57-62. DOI: 10.1080/03601234.2015.1080500

[148] Tunnissen NW, Lautz LS, van Schaik TWG, Hendriks AJ. Ecological risks of imidacloprid to aquatic species in the Netherlands: Measured and estimated concentrations compared to species sensitivity distributions. Chemosphere. 2020;**126604**. DOI: 10.1016/j.chemosphere.2020.126604

[149] de Lima e Silva C, Brennan N, Brouwe, JM, Commandeur D, Verweij RA, van Gestel CAM. Comparative toxicity of imidacloprid and thiacloprid to differentspecies of soil invertebrates. Ecotoxicology. 2017;26:555-564. 10.1007/s10646-017-1790-7.

[150] Prosser RS, de Solla SR, Holman EAM, Osborne R, Robinson SA, Bartlett AJ, et al. Sensitivity of the early-life stages of freshwater mollusks to neonicotinoid and butenolide insecticides. Environ Pollut. 2016;**218**:428-435. DOI: 10.1016/j.envpol.2016.07.022

[151] Eng ML, Stutchbury BJ, Morrissey CA. A neonicotinoid insecticide reduces fueling and delays migration in songbirds. Science. 2019;**365**(6458):1177-1180. DOI: 10.1126/science.aaw9419

[152] Abd-Elhakim YM, Mohammed HH, Mohamed WAM. (2018). Imidacloprid Impacts on Neurobehavioral

Performance, Oxidative Stress, and Apoptotic Events in the Brain of Adolescent and Adult Rats. J Agric Food Chem. 2018;**66**(51):13513-13524. DOI: 10.1021/acs.jafc.8b05793

[153] Abreu-Villaca Y, Levin ED. Developmental neurotoxicity of succeeding generations of insecticides. Environment international. 2017;99, 55-77. DOI. https://doi.org/10.1016/j.envint.2016.11.019

[154] Kim KH, Kabir E, Jahan SA. Exposure to pesticides and the associated human health effects. Science of the Total Environment. 2017;575, 525-535. DOI. https://doi.org/10.1016/j.scitotenv.2016.09.009

[155] Carvalho FP. Pesticides, environment, and food safety. Food and Energy Security. 2017;6(2), 48-60. DOI. https://doi.org/10.1002/fes3.108

[156] Richardson JR, Fitsanakis V, Westerink RH, Kanthasamy AG. Neurotoxicity of pesticides. Acta Neuropathologica. 2019;138(3), 343-362. DOI. https://doi.org/10.1007/s00401-019-02033-9

[157] Jokanović M. Neurotoxic disorders and medical management of patients poisoned with organophosphorus and carbamate pesticides. The Impact of Pesticides. Academic Publishers. 2012:39-62 https://www.researchgate.net/profile/Milan-Jokanovic/publication/235974937_

[158] Jokanović M. Neurotoxic effects of organophosphorus pesticides and possible association with neurodegenerative diseases in man: a review. Toxicology. 2018;410, 125-131. DOI. https://doi.org/10.1016/j.tox.2018.09.009

[159] Keil AP, Daniels JL, Hertz-Picciotto I. Autism spectrum disorder, flea and tick medication, and adjustments for exposure misclassification: the CHARGE (CHildhood Autism Risks from Genetics and Environment) case–control study. Environmental Health. 2014;13(1), 1-10. DOI. https://doi.org/10.1186/1476-069X-13-3

[160] Am C, Boyles AL, Thayer KA, Perry MJ. Effects of neonicotinoid pesticide exposure on human health: a systematic review. Environmental Health Perspectives. 2017;125(2), 155-162. DOI. https://doi.org/10.1289/EHP515

[161] Thompson DA, Lehmler HJ, Kolpin DW, Hladik ML, Vargo JD, Schilling KE, et al. A critical review on the potential impacts of neonicotinoid insecticide use: current knowledge of environmental fate, toxicity, and implications for human health. Environmental Science: Processes & Impacts. 2020;22(6), 1315-1346. DOI. https://doi.org/10.1039/C9EM00586B

[162] Hussein RM, Mohamed WR, Omar HA. A neuroprotective role of kaempferol against chlorpyrifos-induced oxidative stress and memory deficits in rats via GSK3β-Nrf2 signaling pathway. Pesticide Biochemistry and Physiology. 2018;152, 29-37. DOI. https://doi.org/10.1016/j.pestbp.2018.08.008

[163] Abdel-Salam OM, Youness ER, Mohammed NA, Yassen NN, Khadrawy YA, El-Toukhy SE, et al. Novel neuroprotective and hepatoprotective effects of citric acid in acute malathion intoxication. Asian Pacific Journal of Tropical Medicine. 2016;9(12), 1181-1194. DOI. https://doi.org/10.1016/j.apjtm.2016.11.005

[164] Mohammadzadeh L, Hosseinzadeh H, Abnous K, Razavi BM. Neuroprotective potential of crocin against malathion-induced motor deficit and neurochemical alterations in rats. Environmental Science and Pollution Research. 2018;25(5), 4904-4914.

DOI. https://doi.org/10.1007/s11356-017-0842-0

[165] Sauer E, Moro AM, Brucker N, Nascimento S, Gauer B, Fracasso R, et al. Liver δ-aminolevulinate dehydratase activity is inhibited by neonicotinoids and restored by antioxidant agents. International Journal of Environmental Research and Public Health. 2014;11(11), 11676-11690. DOI. https://doi.org/10.3390/ijerph111111676

[166] Lonare M, Kumar M, Raut S, Badgujar P, Doltade S, Telang A. Evaluation of imidacloprid-induced neurotoxicity in male rats: a protective effect of curcumin. Neurochemistry International. 2014;78, 122-129. DOI. https://doi.org/10.1016/j.neuint.2014.09.004

[167] Waseem M, Jain S, Parvez S, Akram M. Ascorbic acid modulates non enzymatic antioxidants in swiss albino mice targeted to imidacloprid: Brain v/s Liver. (2016). https://www.thepharmajournal.com/archives/2016/vol5issue8/PartB/9-10-89-996.pdf.

[168] Farag MR, Abou-EL Fotoh MF, EL-Sayed GG, EL-Sayed EW. Modulatory Effect of Ginger Aqueous Extract against Imidacloprid-Induced Neurotoxicity in Rats. Zagazig Veterinary Journal. 2019;47(4), 432-446. DOI. http://doi.org/10.21608/zvjz.2019.14914.1061

[169] Dhouib IB, Annabi A, Doghri R, Rejeb I, Dallagi Y, Bdiri Y, et al. Neuroprotective effects of curcumin against acetamiprid-induced neurotoxicity and oxidative stress in the developing male rat cerebellum: biochemical, histological, and behavioral changes. Environmental Science and Pollution Research. 2017;24(35), 27515-27524. DOI. https://doi.org/10.1007/s11356-017-0331-5

[170] Khovarnagh N, Seyedalipour B. Antioxidant, histopathological and biochemical outcomes of short-term exposure to acetamiprid in liver and brain of rat: The protective role of N-acetylcysteine and S-methylcysteine. Saudi Pharmaceutical Journal. 2021;29(3), 280-289. DOI. https://doi.org/10.1016/j.jsps.2021.02.004

[171] Muthaiah VK, Venkitasamy L, Michael FM, Chandrasekar K, Venkatachalam S. Neuroprotective role of naringenin on carbaryl induced neurotoxicity in mouse neuroblastoma cells. Journal of Pharmacology & Pharmacotherapeutics. 2013;4(3), 192. doi: https://doi.org/10.4103/0976-500X.114599.

Chapter 5

Alzheimer-Like Cell Alterations after Vanadium Pentoxide Inhalation

Claudia Dorado-Martínez, Enrique Montiel-Flores, Oscar A. Mejía-García, José Luis Ordoñez-Librado, Ana Luisa Gutierrez-Valdez, Jesús Espinosa-Villanueva, Leonardo Reynoso-Erazo, Rocío Tron-Alvarez, Vianey Rodríguez-Lara and Maria Rosa Avila-Costa

Abstract

Vanadium (V), a widely distributed transition metal, has been considered toxic, which depends on the valence of the compound. V pentoxide (V_2O_5) is considered the most harmful. Its long-term exposure produces neurotoxicity. Mice exposed to inhaled V_2O_5 displayed less tubulin$^+$ in testicular cells and dendritic spines loss, cell death, and CA1 neuropil modifications, considered as the result of V interaction with the cytoskeleton, which made us suppose that V_2O_5 inhalation could initiate CA1 cell alterations comparable to what happen in the brains of Alzheimer disease (AD) patients. This study intends to demonstrate pyramidal CA1 cytoskeletal changes in rats which inhaled V_2O_5. Twenty rats were exposed to V_2O_5 0.02 M one hour, three times a week for several months. Our findings showed that V_2O_5-exposed rats had cell death that reached 56,57% after six months; we also observed collapsed strong argyrophilic nuclei and characteristic flame-shaped somas in all V_2O_5-exposed animals hippocampus CA1 compared to controls. We also found somatodendritic deformations. Neurite's cytoskeleton exhibited visible thickening and nodosities and prominent dendritic spine loss. Our results demonstrate that V_2O_5 induces AD-like cell death with evident cytoskeletal and synaptic alterations.

Keywords: Vanadium pentoxide, Cell death, Bielschowsky silver stain, inhalation, dendritic spines, hippocampus

1. Introduction

Vanadium (V) is a transition metal abundant in nature; its atomic number is 23. Andres Manuel Del Rio was the first who reported it in 1801. But it was actually discovered in 1830 by a Swedish chemist named Nils Sefstrom [1]. V is a bright silver-white, soft and malleable metal and the 22nd most abundant element in the earth's crust, and it has become a matter of concern among nutritionists since various marine species contain this metal as an trace element [2]. Environmental air V acts as the primary source for the general population [3].

Although V is extensively dispersed in air, its role as human nutrient is not yet confirmed. Humans are exposed to V generally through the polluted atmosphere from combustion products of vanadium-bearing fuel oils, fumes, and dust. Food contains insignificant V concentrations, frequently below 1 ng/g. V enters the organism by inhalation, skin, and gastrointestinal tract and accumulates mainly in the kidney, liver, bones, spleen, lungs and brain, accumulate fewer V concentrations [3–5].

Neurotoxic effects of V are not well recognized yet. Still, it is known that acute exposure in animals by ingestion or inhalation leads to nervous system alterations, paralysis of legs, respiratory failure, convulsions, bloody diarrhea, and death [6]. V disrupts the blood–brain barrier [7] and alters some neurotransmitters concentrations such as serotonin, norepinephrine, and dopamine, and an inhibitory effect on the uptake and release of norepinephrine were observed in the rat brain during V poisoning [8–10].

The V oxidation states of biological importance are vanadate (V^{5+}) and vanadyl (V^{4+}) and are considered harmful to mammals depending on their levels. Workers occupationally exposed to vanadium pentoxide (V_2O_5) had presented cardiovascular alterations and a variety of symptoms involving the central nervous system (CNS), gastrointestinal and respiratory systems [11]. Moreover, it has been suggested that raised tissue levels of V may be of etiological importance in manic-depressive syndrome since V reduces serotonin concentration. Blood V levels in depressed patients were greater than non-V-exposed controls [11]. Besides, reduced cognitive abilities in humans chronically exposed to this metal were found [12].

2. Vanadium sources

Metallic V is not found in nature. The most common in mining is carnotite and vanadinite. V is also found in phosphate rock, iron ores, and some crude oils in organic complexes and in small percentages of meteorites [3]. The presence of V is related to other minerals; among them is iron, aluminum, uranium, and titanium, and is frequently used as alloy steel, in combination with nickel, boron, or manganese. Extraction of V from coal or fossil fuels, such as Vanadium-rich coal tars and oil, explains the high V concentrations registered in the atmosphere [11].

V is generally employed in metallurgy in alloy with steel. And, as nonferrous metal V is considered fundamental for aircraft's manufacture, atomic and space industries. In the chemical industry, V_2O_5 and metavanadates are remarkably important for plastics and sulfuric acid production. Emissions of V may be high near producing steel alloys industries. V is also released into the air: during the re-smelting of scrap steel and the transformation of titaniferous and vanadic magnetite iron ores into steel; from the roasting of V slags; from V_2O_5 smelting furnaces; and from electric furnaces in which ferrovanadium is smelted [11, 13].

2.1 Vanadium in the environment

As a profuse element in the earth's crust, the V average varies from 159 g/t to 0.14 mg kg. The standard concentration of 135 mg/kg in soil positions V in 5th place, among all transitional metals [11, 13]. V recycling includes its release from anthropogenic and natural bases to the water, soil, and air [13–15]. Frequently, the places such as fuel plants and refineries showed the highest level of V [16, 17].

V geochemical characteristics depend on the oxidation state and pH. The moderately immobile V (III) prevails. Typically, V compounds with high oxidation states are more soluble [14]. The average concentration of V in different soils fluctuates from 10 to 220 mg kg dry mass depending on the soil types and chemical characteristics [18, 19]. The soils directly under humans' use include a much higher V concentration [17, 18]. On the other hand, what most pollutes the soil and water is the mining V-derived [20]. Vanadium is the most profuse transition metal in the aqua sphere, with an average content similar to zinc [21]. Persian Gulf sediments have very high V concentrations [22].

It seems that over the last decades, V levels in the biosphere have been significantly growing, a fact that will be of concern in the future [23]. The primary sources are mining, fossil fuel combustion, atmospheric wet and dry accumulation, etc. [24]. V remains in the water, soil, and air for long periods and may react with other elements [2, 21]. Recently, it has been shown that atmosphere V levels are increasing every day, mainly due to fossil fuel burning [11, 14, 18]. For that reason, more than 60 thousand tons of V may be released into the big cities air [14, 25].

Apparently, V concentrations in ambient air fluctuate significantly; in rural areas, V levels are under 0.001 $\mu g/m^3$, however, in areas where there is a high degree of fossil fuel burning, as in large cities, the average annual concentration goes from 0.02 $\mu g/m^3$ to 0.3 $\mu g/m^3$. It has been determined that near industrial zones, its level can reach 1 $\mu g/m^3$ [26]. Fortoul et al. [26] reported that V has increased over time in lung parenchyma from Mexico City inhabitants since it has been demonstrated that Mexican petroleum has high V concentrations.

V concentration in plants and food is very low, from less than 0.001 to 0.005 mg [14]. Some foods, including oysters, parsley, and spinach, had a relatively higher amount of V than all other foods [27].

V occupational exposure. V levels near metallurgical industries usually average about 1 mg V/m^3, whereas ambient air near industries, which produce V metal or compounds, contain a few mg V/m^3 [11]. Very high levels of V result from boiler-cleaning procedures due to the high concentration (approximately 10–25%) of V oxides in the dust. During these procedures, 50–100 mg V/m^3 are frequent, with concentrations ranging from 500 mg V/m^3 [3].

The most critical V compounds are ferrovanadium, V_2O_5, vanadium trioxide, V carbide, and salts, such as ammonium and sodium vanadate. The salts and oxides are used in powder form. It has been reported that the metallurgical industry includes the production of vapor containing V_2O_5, which condenses to form breathable aerosols. Also, residual fuels combustion with high V content have V_2O_5 aerosols [11].

2.2 Vanadium absorption, distribution and excretion

It appears that only 10% of ingested V is absorbed from the gastrointestinal tract [28]. This report suggests that most of the ingested V is transformed into the cationic vanadyl form in the stomach before being absorbed in the duodenum through an unknown mechanism [29]. In its anionic vanadate form, V is absorbed in much higher quantities (about five times more than vanadyl form) through an anionic transport system [29]. Multivalent existence of V in nature and living systems put forth the chemical complexity of this element. This multifaceted chemical character of V, in turn, echoes in its biological and biochemical properties, especially in metabolism and absorption. Again vanadate, after reaching the bloodstream, is converted into vanadyl ion, although the vanadate form also exists. Thus, vanadate (by transferrin) and vanadyl (by albumin and transferrin) are rapidly transported by blood proteins to various tissues [30]. Blood parameters showed little or no reflection of toxicity after a long-term supplementation of V compounds [31], which might be due to the transport of V from blood to the tissues. Upon supplementation, V is incorporated in various organs and tissues, including the liver, kidney, brain, heart, muscles, and bone. The kidney, spleen, bone, and liver tissues of rats have been shown to accumulate distinctly high amounts of V in chronically treated animals through oral administration [32].

The effects of V persist even after it has been withdrawn for several days [33]. Unabsorbed V is excreted in feces. When V was administrated through the parenteral route, 10% of the V was found in the feces of humans and rats [3]. V is excreted through bile and urine [34]. It is, thus, the bile route through which a significant amount of V may be eliminated through feces. Moreover, it may be suggested that V content in feces does not reflect V absorbed or unabsorbed (1).

The toxicity of V depends on various factors, including the administration route and the V compound toxicity. In general, the toxicity of V is low, and its toxicity is least following ingestion and greatest following parenteral administration. Inhalation is a route of exposure that produces intermediate toxicity [3, 11]. The toxicity of V increases with higher valences, and the pentavalent compounds (as V pentoxide) are usually the most toxic [3].

2.3 Vanadium effects in the nervous system

V crosses the blood–brain barrier [7], and its compounds can induce neurologic alterations through different routes of administration [3, 11]. It has been reported that V-exposed lactating rat pups developed neurological deficits [35]; other authors described neurological alterations and increased brain V concentration after sodium metavanadate intraperitoneal administration [36–38]. Also, our group [7, 8] reported neuroinflammation in the brain of mice that inhale V_2O_5. We found a seven-fold peak increase in V brain concentration after one week of inhalation and remained constant (0.10–0.12 mg/g dry weight tissue) during eight weeks of V_2O_5 inhalation. The inhalation route seems to induce neurotoxicity [6], which is epidemiologically relevant since this is the main route to the brain during occupational and environmental exposure.

One of the first studies on the V neurological effects was made by Done [39], who found that humans exposed to V displayed tremor and depression. Other researchers demonstrated that occupationally exposed people present alterations in cognitive ability tasks [40]. Despite the route, duration, and compound, V exposure has affected nerve cells and glia. In a study of chronic intraperitoneal exposure at 3 mg/kg in mice, Folarin et al. [36] reported that the brain accumulates large amounts of V, mainly in the brain stem, cerebellum, and olfactory bulb. This study described disruption of the layering pattern in the prefrontal cortex with nuclear pyknosis, loss of pyramidal neurons and reduced apical dendrites in the hippocampal CA1, and loss of cerebellar Purkinje cells. These morphological alterations were accompanied by astrogliosis and microgliosis.

Demyelination has also been reported after drinking milk from mothers exposed to sodium metavanadate [41]. Our group also described that in male CD-1 mice exposed by inhalation to 0.02 M V_2O_5 2 h twice a week for four weeks, Golgi staining revealed a severe loss in dendritic spines in the striatum compared to the controls, showing that the inhalation of V_2O_5 causes severe neuronal damage in this nucleus [8]. We observed fewer dendritic spines in the olfactory bulb granule cells after three months of exposure using the same inhalation protocol, and electron microcopy alterations consisted in swelled mitochondria and endoplasmic reticulum, and neuronal death that can be correlated with the olfactory dysfunction [42]. In the hippocampus, we found a decrease in dendritic spines and necrosis of the pyramidal CA1 neurons, modifications that could be associated with spatial memory impairment [43].

2.4 Mechanisms of vanadium neurotoxicity

It has been reported that V induces reactive oxygen species (ROS) production, which several authors have proposed as a reasonable basis for its neurotoxicity [6, 44, 45]. V, as other catalytic transition metals, participate in the Fenton reaction [46]. V in body fluids exists mainly in the 5^+ oxidation state as V pentoxide (V_2O_5) [47]. V enters the cell as vanadate via anion channels while as vanadyl ions by passive diffusion and endocytosis bound to transferrin [48]. When entering the cell, vanadate is reduced by intracellular antioxidants to vanadyl, with subsequent production of ROS [49]. H_2O_2 then oxidizes vanadyl into vanadate in a Fenton-like reaction with the consequent hydroxyl radical production [50]. With higher V levels, these reactions result in oxidative stress and toxic effects on lipids, proteins, and nucleic acids. With its high lipid content, the brain is vulnerable to oxidant-induced lipid peroxidation [51], and as such, V neurotoxicity is related to myelin deficits [45]. Moreover, as we mentioned above, earlier results from our group revealed substantia nigra tyrosine hydroxylase cell loss, and therefore, dendritic spine loss in the striatum medium-size spiny neurons [8], blood–brain barrier disruption [7], and hippocampal cells alterations [43].

Besides oxidative stress, it has been demonstrated that the cytoskeleton is an important target of V toxicity because of its ability to compete with phosphatases; due to this, V inhibits actin polymerization through the tyrosine phosphatases inhibition [52, 53], which, in consequence, by decreasing gamma-tubulin disturbs microtubules function and formation [54]. It is also well known that actin polymerization establishes the morphology of dendrites and dendritic spines [55]. These facts make us consider the possibility that V_2O_5 inhalation might induce hippocampus cell death similar to that seen in Alzheimer disease (AD).

2.5 Alzheimer disease

Today, aging human populations worldwide face an epidemic of AD, with an increasing number of cases to nearly 106 million by 2050 [56]. Several factors have been described to participate in the AD etiology including, aging, genetics [57], head injury [58], and exposure to certain chemicals and compounds [59].

AD is a neurodegenerative disease that represents the most common cause of dementia. Symptoms associated with dementia vary from difficulties with orientation, language, and problem-solving to memory alterations and other cognitive skill deficits that affect a person's ability to perform daily life activities [60]. The most noticeable symptoms at the beginning of the disease are disorientation and episodic and spatial memory loss [61]. The medial temporal lobe region, consisting of the hippocampal formation and related cortices, are essential for the adequate functioning of spatial and declarative memory systems [62, 63] and are the first areas affected in the progression of the disease [64].

Synaptic failure has been suggested as the leading cause of AD pathology [65]. The principal neuropathological hallmarks of the disease are the neurofibrillary tangles (NFTs) associated with abnormal phosphorylated tau protein and the accumulation of aberrant amyloid-β, features also found in the brains of old patients without cognitive impairments or AD [66]. Nonetheless, directly or indirectly, these proteins induce synapsis alterations by changing dendritic spines morphology or causing their loss and neuronal degeneration [67, 68].

The development of intraneuronal lesions at selectively vulnerable brain structures is central to the pathological process in AD [69–71]. The lesions consist mainly of hyperphosphorylated tau protein. They include tangle material, NFTs in cell bodies, neuropil threads (NTs) in neuronal processes, and material in dystrophic nerve cell processes of neuritic plaques (NPs) [72–74].

2.6 Alzheimer's disease experimental models

Experimental models are crucial in understanding AD pathogenesis for implementing novel therapeutics. So far, AD experimental models consist almost exclusively of transgenic mammals that express the human genes that result in the formation of amyloid plaques (by expression of human APP alone or in combination with human PSEN1) and NFTs (by the expression of human MAPT) [75–78]. Other experimental models have used invertebrates such as C. *elegans and Drosophila melanogaster* and vertebrates such as zebrafish; nevertheless, these models are very different from human physiology and less extensively used [79]. Nevertheless, some issues have been raised about this model's validity, mainly because the efficacy in clinical trials has been very low [80, 81]. Facts that make us wonder if the animals in the experimental models actually have AD, considering only the specific pathological features. Most animal models develop only the amyloid accumulation that defines AD. This often gives rise to specific memory-associated cognitive alterations. However, these models normally preset the absence of the main AD pathological features, including cell death and, most importantly, NFTs development [79]. The lack of NFTs could partly explain the failure between pre-clinical and clinical trials [80].

Therefore, in this chapter, we intend to demonstrate that the inhalation of V_2O_5 produces cellular alterations like those observed in AD, with synaptic alterations (shown by the loss of dendritic spines) and by the presence of NFTs, due to V directly interacts with the cytoskeletal components, and is a potent inhibitor of tyrosine phosphatases.

3. Experimental procedures

The experiments were accomplished in 24 male Wistar rats weighing 180–200 g at the beginning of the study. The rats were individually placed in plastic cages with controlled light conditions (12 h light/12 h dark) and fed with Purina Rat Chow and water *ad libitum*. Body weight was recorded daily. The experimental protocol was carried out following the Animal Act of 1986 for Scientific Procedures and the Rules for Research in Health Matters (Mexico). We made efforts to minimize the number of animals used and their suffering.

3.1 Vanadium pentoxide inhalation

V_2O_5 inhalations were performed as described by our group [8]. As part of our experiment with V, a pilot study was implemented with 0.005 and 0.01 M V_2O_5, and we found no changes using light microscopy in lung tissue; therefore, a higher dose was utilized, 0.02 M, realizing that V half-life about 48 h [11] we designed a three times a week exposure protocol.

Twelve rats were placed in an acrylic chamber inhaling 0.02 M V_2O_5 (Sigma, St. Louis, MO, USA) (Sigma Aldrich, Co. Mexico) 1 h three times a week for two and six months. Twelve control rats inhaled only the vehicle—deionized water—for the same time. Inhalations were performed in closed acrylic boxes (40 cm wide x 70 cm long and 25 cm high) attached to an ultra-nebulizer (Shinmed, Taiwan), with 10 l/min continuous flux. The ultra-nebulizer is designed to produce droplets in a 0.5–5 μm range. A trap for the vapor was located on the opposite side with a solution of sodium bicarbonate to precipitate the remaining metal. During the inhalation, animals were constantly monitored for respiration rate, depth, and regularity. The exposure system was monitored for temperature, oxygen level, and V concentration.

After two or six months, rats were sacrificed under sodium pentobarbital anesthesia (lethal dose) and perfused via the aorta with a saline solution followed by the fixative containing 10% formaldehyde in 0.2 M-phosphate buffer. The brains were removed and placed in the fixative solution for one hour.

3.2 Bielschowsky silver impregnation

After the routine paraffin processing, serial coronal brain sections were cut at 8 μm thickness in a sliding microtome (Leica SM2010 R, Germany). Brain sections were deparaffinized in xylene and alcohol before being disposed into 20% silver nitrate solution for 20 min at 37°C. After washing with distilled water, slides were submerged in 20% silver nitrate solution titrated with fresh sodium hydroxide and evaporated ammonia. After 15 min, slides were washed with ammonia before being individually revealed with 100 ml of a developer (20 ml of formaldehyde, 100 ml distilled water, 20 μl concentrated nitric acid, and 0.5 g citric acid) and then added to 50 ml of titrated silver nitrate solution. Slides were then rinsed in tap water, fixed in 5% sodium thiosulfate, and dehydrated through alcohols and xylene [82]. The hippocampus CA1 pyramidal cells were evaluated under a light Optiphot 2 microscope (Nikon, Japan).

3.3 Golgi stain

Brain tissue from the hippocampus CA1 was cut into 90 mm- thick sections and processed for the rapid Golgi method [83]. The histological analysis consisted in counting the number of dendritic spines in a 10 mm-long area from five secondary dendrites from 20 CA1 pyramidal neurons from each rat [8, 84].

Means from each group were compared for statistical differences by one-way ANOVA test ($p < 0.05$) followed by *posthoc* comparisons with Tukey test. The statistical analyses were conducted with GraphPad Prism 9 for Mac Software.

4. Results

The animals that inhaled V_2O_5 did not show changes in their weight or clinical alterations compared to the control group.

4.1 Dendritic spines

Brain sections were treated with the Golgi stain to determine if V_2O_5 inhalation induces synaptic alterations in the hippocampus CA1. The synaptic damage resulted in significant CA1 pyramidal neurons dendritic spine loss of exposed rats compared to controls (**Figures 1** and **2B, C**). As it is shown in **Figure 1**, spine loss was more evident with longer inhalation time.

4.2 Hippocampus CA1 neuronal alterations

With the Bielschowsky method, we found that rats exposed to V_2O_5 after two months have substantial CA1 pyramidal cell death (25%) (**Figures 3** and **5**), and after six months, the cell death reached 56.57%, being statistically different vs.

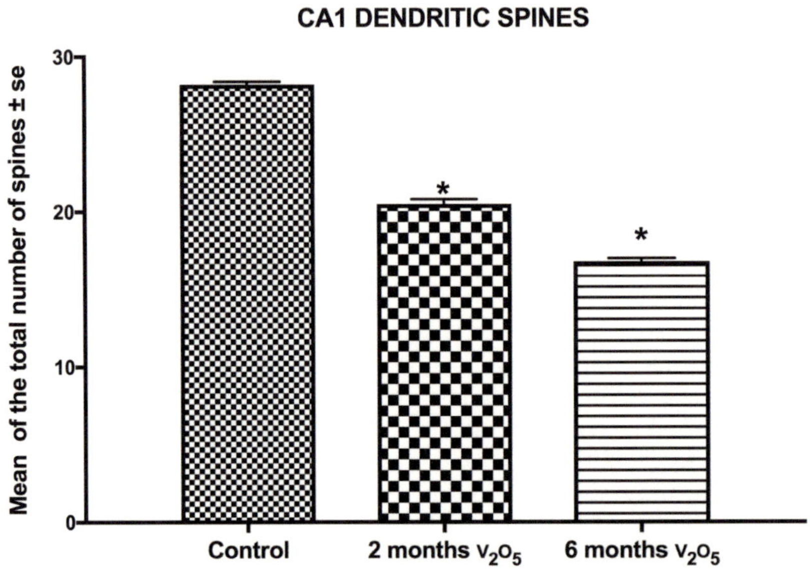

Figure 1.
*The number of pyramidal CA1 neurons dendritic spines, contrasting control and exposed rats after two and six months of V_2O_5 inhalation. One way ANOVA, *p < 0.05 vs. control group.*

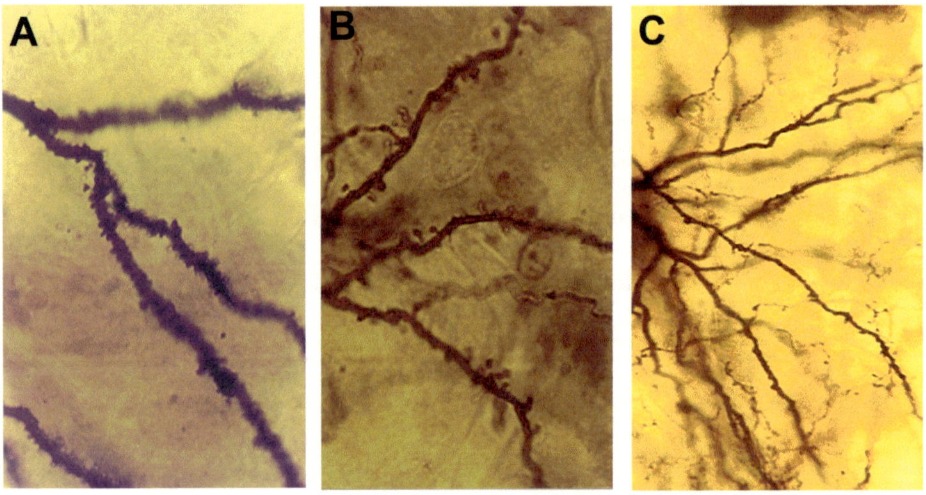

Figure 2.
Dendritic spine density. Representative Golgi-stained pyramidal CA1 neurons of the control group (A), two months (B), and six months of V_2O_5 inhalation (C). Both exposure times provoked a significant decrease in the total number of spines, mainly after six months. (magnification 40X).

two months and control groups (**Figures 3** and **4**); we observed that in all V_2O_5-exposed rats the pyramidal hippocampus CA1 cells displayed strong argyrophilic and collapsed somas compared to control rats, the somas also revealed the typical flame-shaped (**Figures 4–6**). Also, somatodendritic deformations were identified. Axons and dendrites exhibited thick dark bands resembling thickening nodosities and fibrillary cytoskeleton proteins linear traces. The neurofibrils were fused, disordered, thickened, and crowded together into broadband, and the neurites were deeply stained; we also noticed curly fibers. Some neurites displayed neurofibrillary-type tangles (**Figure 6**).

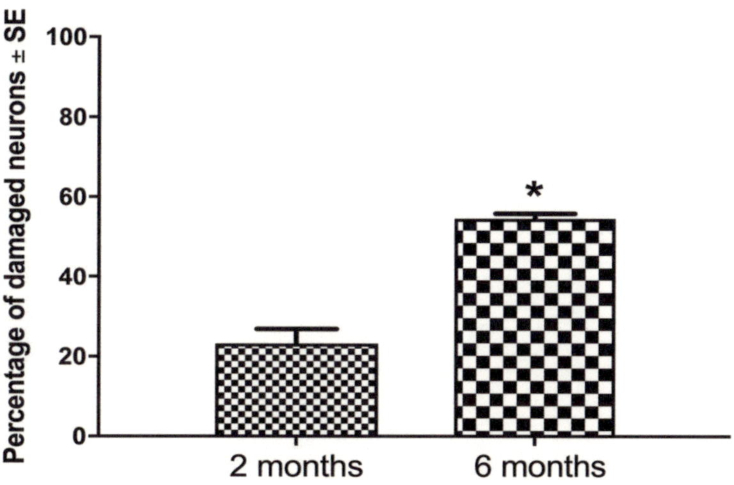

Figure 3.
*Damaged pyramidal hippocampus CA1 neurons percentage after two or six months of V_2O_5 inhalation. *P < 0.05 vs. two months group.*

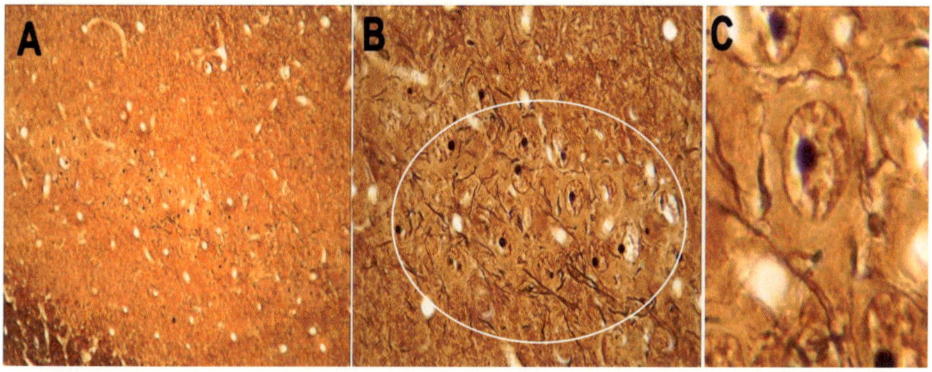

Figure 4.
Representative photomicrographs of Hippocampus CA1 control group stained with the Bielschowsky method. As can be seen in B (white oval), the pyramidal neurons of the hippocampus CA1 are healthy, in terms of size and shape. Figure C depicts the detail of B white oval. A 10X, B 40X and C 100X.

5. Discussion

Our results show significant alterations in the cytoskeleton and synaptic activity, demonstrated by the loss of dendritic spines and Alzheimer-like fibrillary tangles.

It is essential to stand out that V concentrations in the environment vary substantially; in rural areas, V concentrations are below 0.001 μg/m^3, in big cities, where there are high levels of fossil fuel burning, the average V concentration range from 0.02 μg/m^3 to 0.3 μg/m^3. It has been shown that near industrial zones, its concentrations can reach 1 μg/m^3. In this experiment, V concentrations in the inhalation chamber was 1436 μg/m^3 [54], exceeding the highest concentration reported in ambient air (1 μg/m^3). In this regard, we know that the concentrations used here are higher than those subjects with occupational exposure, but animal models permit amplifying the impact that V has on the nervous system.

Our results demonstrated that V_2O_5 inhalation generates a significant loss of pyramidal CA1 neurons dendritic spines and notorious cytoskeleton distortions resulting in the alteration of the synaptic transmission and, therefore, possibly in

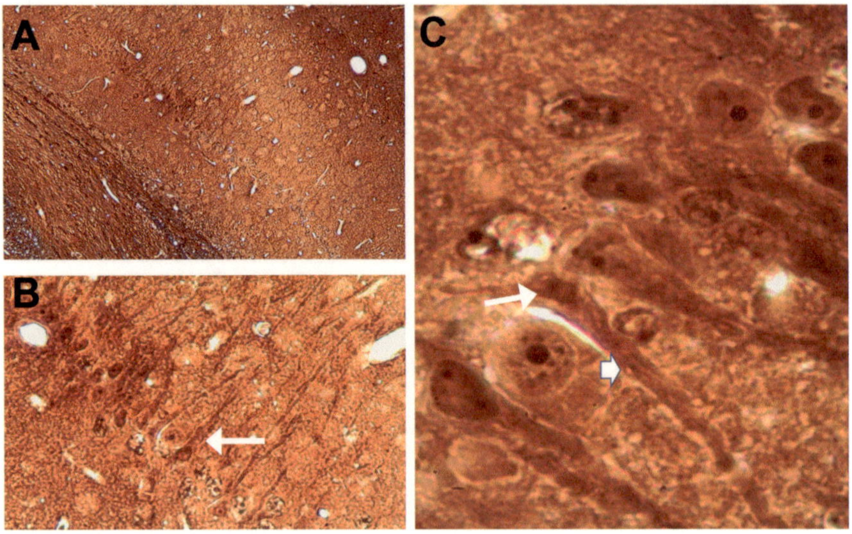

Figure 5.
Representative photomicrographs of Hippocampus CA1 Bielschowsky staining from the experimental group after two months of V_2O_5 inhalation. Neuronal soma deformation is observed (arrows). The axons displayed thicker and darker bands (arrowhead); A (10x), B (40x), and C (100x)

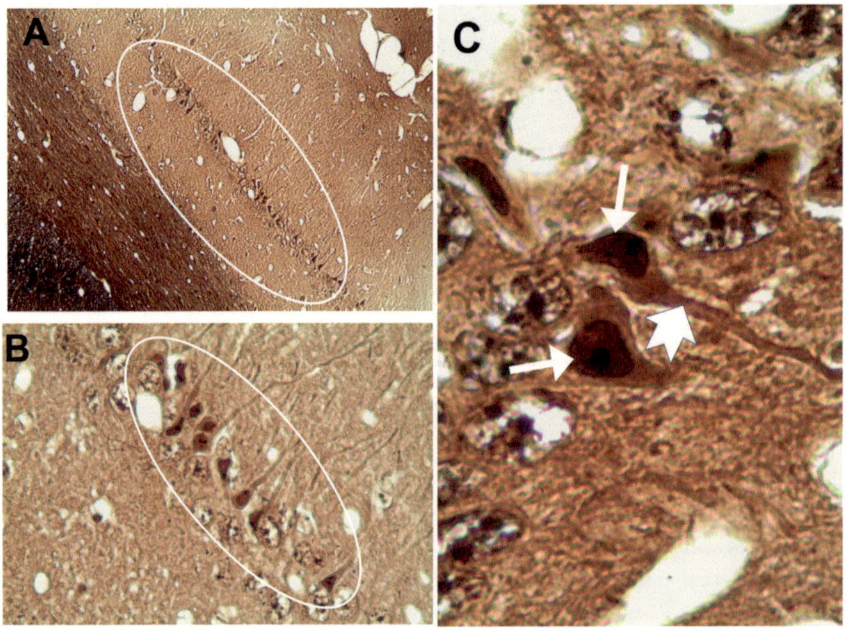

Figure 6.
Hippocampus CA1 representative photomicrographs of Bielschowsky staining from the experimental group after six months of V_2O_5 inhalation. It can be observed strong argyrophilic nuclei (white oval in a and B; arrows in C) typical flame-shaped and intensely stained neurites (white oval in a, B and C), forming similar structures to neurofibrillary tangles (arrowhead); A (10x), B (40x), and C (100x).

memory disturbances. It is well known that many neurological conditions lead to a decreased number of dendritic spines [85], for instance, epilepsy, alcoholism, and others disorders, imply that the decline in the number and availability of axo-spinous synapses are the consequence of the dendritic spines loss (85). Previously, our group informed significant dendritic spine loss after ozone inhalation in the hippocampus, correlated with memory alterations [84], also, dendritic spines loss in the corpus striatum and cerebral cortex with motor impairments [86] as well as olfactory bulb modifications [87]. Furthermore, we found dendritic spine loss in the corpus striatum after V_2O_5 inhalation [8]. Since V interacts with the cytoskeleton, this interaction may be the cause of dendritic spine loss since it seems that actin is a critical element for dendritic spine architecture preservation. It orchestrates the spine's morphology and number [88]. In this context, Pelucchi and cols. [88] mention that Rho activation is essential for the dendritic spine functionality, cofilin phosphorylation, and, consequently, spine actin stabilization. According to Wang et al. [89], cofilin phosphorylation prevents binding to the F- and G-actin binding, and only a dephosphorylated cofilin can initiate the actin-binding. Consequently, their activity is synchronized by phosphorylation/dephosphorylation. It is important to mention again that V is practically a structural and electronic phosphate analog and a phosphatase inhibitor [90]. In humans, the resemblance between phosphate and V explains V and phosphate-dependent enzymes interplay. Therefore, V may achieve a regulatory function in phosphate-depending metabolic processes [90].

It is well known that V neurotoxic properties have been predominantly attributed to its capacity to induce oxidative stress by the generation of ROS, which in turn initiates the peroxidative decomposition of the cellular membranes

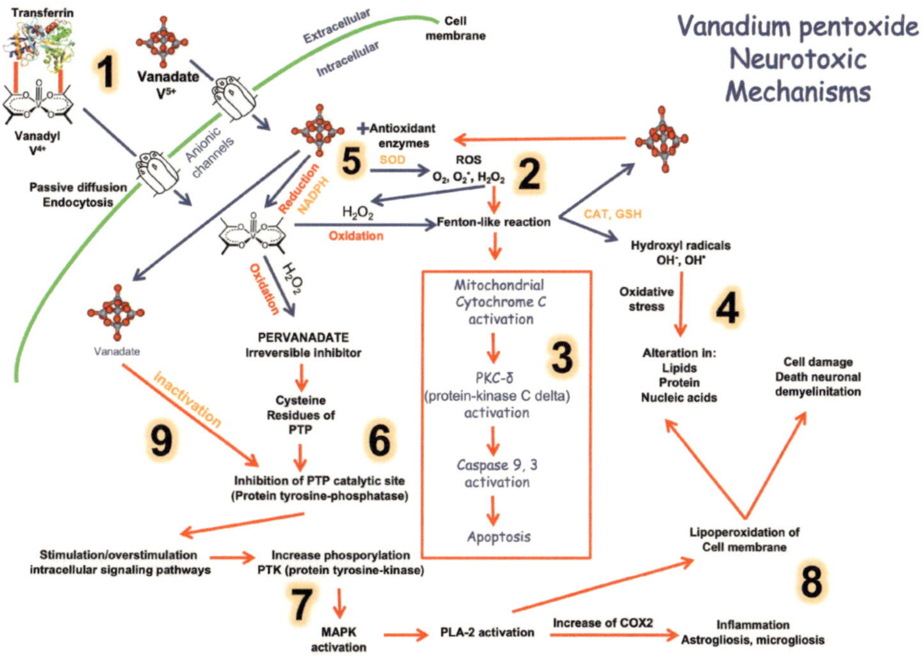

Figure 7.
*When vanadium enters the body, it enters as a tetravalent ((vanadyl) or as a pentavalent (V^{5+}) [3]; then, it is transported via the blood by albumin and transferrin (**1**). V with these two valences enters cells through anionic channels. These two forms arrive the cells through anionic channels; once in the cell, V^{5+} reacts with some antioxidant enzymes such as superoxide dismutase (SOD) (**2**) [12], producing H_2O_2 through Fenton-like reaction, where the mitochondrion initiates the cytochrome C pathway inducing the apoptosis route through the activation of caspases 3 and 9 (**3**) [95], then, vanadate generates free radicals (OH+ OH-) by reacting with GSH and CAT enzymes (**4**) [94], stimulating oxidative stress triggering lipids, proteins, and DNA alterations. V^{5+} reduces to vanadyl through NADPH-oxidase (**5**), which in turn, forms pervanadate, oxidized by H_2O_2, that will permanently inhibit protein tyrosine phosphatases (PTP) [96] (**6**), which will aggregate the phosphorylated protein tyrosine kinase (PTK) activating intracellular signaling pathways (**7**) [1], triggering the inflammation mechanisms through phospholipase-A2 (PLA-A2) and COX-2 formation, activating the gliosis process (**8**) [97], similarly DNA, cell death, demyelination and damage to proteins through lipid peroxidation. Finally, the PTP is inactivated by vanadate (**9**) [98], which results in the activation of intracellular death signaling pathways.*

phospholipids [6, 44, 45] and neuron inflammation [91]. It is also associated with hypomyelination correlated with oxidative stress [92] and a decrease in myelin essential protein [93]. It has also been reported that V produces DNA cleavage, apoptosis and induces iron-mediated oxidative stress in brain cell cultures [94] and hippocampus neuronal death [36]. Likewise, it has been reported that V inactivates protein-tyrosine-phosphatases (PTP) because it binds to the cysteine catalytic residue, which leads to an increase in phosphorylation of PTP, increasing the phosphorylation of the MAPK pathways, which probably causes tau protein hyperphosphorylation, to generate or induce neurofibrillary tangles (NFTs) [94]. Thus, according to our findings and the revised literature, V neurotoxic effects are summarized in **Figure** 7.

Likewise, an increased body of evidence implicates oxidative stress as involved in at least the propagation of cellular injury, which leads to neuropathology in various conditions, such as AD. Moreover, oxidative stress is intimately linked with an integrated series of cellular phenomena, which all seem to contribute to neuronal death [51, 99].

The facts mentioned above provide evidence that V_2O_5 disrupts critical neuronal processes and leads to alterations that include ROS generation, producing cell death. Further work should be done to answer questions, such as identifying the signaling pathways that induced the changes reported here.

Furthermore, as formerly reported, V_2O_5 modifies cytoskeletal proteins such as γ-tubulin [54], inducing actin alterations [52]. Some studies have demonstrated the interaction between V with actin. V has a high affinity for cytoskeletal actin-binding sites. G- and F- actin interact with oxovanadium (IV), with 4:1 and 1:1 stoichiometries, respectively, and it has been demonstrated that G-actin-V interaction might occur close to the actin adenosine triphosphate binding position [100–102]. Likewise, decavanadate can modify actin's structure by oxidizing its cysteines in its polymerized form [103].

Remarkably, earlier results demonstrate that V induces Tau hyperphosphorylation [104, 105], ROS, and neuronal inflammation [106], occasioning AD-like damage. Moreover, the substantial hippocampal CA1 cell damage might result from the affinity of G-actin for V, and its association with the metal, since neurons have a particularly dynamic cytoskeleton, which requires continuous polymerization of actin filaments [107].

6. Conclusion

Our results show that vanadium pentoxide, when inhaled, produces important synaptic alterations, manifested in this case, by the significant loss of dendritic spines of CA1 pyramidal neurons and by the presence of Alzheimer-type fibrillar tangles, an aspect considered to be the main neuropathological feature in AD [107], related to the evident alterations of the cytoskeleton. Therefore, more research is needed to establish the relationship between V_2O_5 and Tau hyperphosphorylation, not only in the hippocampus but also in the amygdala, neocortex, and entorhinal, structures involved in AD [108, 109], and whether spatial memory is altered.

Moreover, these data must encourage research efforts towards environmental health effects, with the final purpose of intervening in decrease metals atmospheric pollution such as V. We have to promote viable schemes to safeguard the CNS from toxicants, which have redoubled in the atmosphere during the last decades and represent an important health challenge since metal pollution has been related to neurodegenerative diseases.

Acknowledgements

This work was supported by the research grants from PAPCA–Iztacala UNAM 2016-2113 and PAPIIT-DGAPA IN216821.

We are very grateful to Veronica Rodríguez Mata and Patricia Aley Medina for their excellent photographic and technical assistance.

Conflict of interest

The authors declare no conflict of interest.

Author details

Claudia Dorado-Martínez[1], Enrique Montiel-Flores[1], Oscar A. Mejía-García[1], José Luis Ordoñez-Librado[1], Ana Luisa Gutierrez-Valdez[1], Jesús Espinosa-Villanueva[1], Leonardo Reynoso-Erazo[2], Rocío Tron-Alvarez[2], Vianey Rodríguez-Lara[3] and Maria Rosa Avila-Costa[1*]

1 Neuromorphology Lab, Facultad de Estudios Superiores Iztacala, UNAM, Tlalnepantla, Edo. Mex., Mexico

2 Health Education Project, Facultad de Estudios Superiores Iztacala, UNAM, Tlalnepantla, Edo. Mex., Mexico

3 Faculty of Medicine, Department of Cell and Tissue Biology, UNAM, Mexico City, Mexico

*Address all correspondence to: nigraizo@unam.mx

References

[1] Mukherjee B, Patra B, Mahapatra S, Banerjee P, Tiwari A, Chatterjee M. Vanadium--an element of atypical biological significance. Toxicol Lett. 2004;150(2):135-143 DOI: 10.1016/j.toxlet.2004.01.009.

[2] Almeida M, Filipe S, Humanes M, Maia MF, Melo R, Severino N, et al. Vanadium haloperoxidases from brown algae of the Laminariaceae family. Phytochemistry. 2001;57(5):633-642. DOI: 10.1016/S0031-9422(01)00094-2

[3] Barceloux DG. Vanadium. J Toxicol. Clin Toxicol. 1999;37(2):265-278. DOI: 10.1081/CLT-100102425

[4] Hansen TV, Aaseth J, Alexander J. The effect of chelating agents on vanadium distribution in the rat body and on uptake by human erythrocytes. Arch Toxicol. 1982;50(3-4):195-202. DOI: 10.1007/bf00310851

[5] Bracken WM, Sharma RP, Elsner YY. Vanadium accumulation and subcellular distribution in relation to vanadate induced cytotoxicity in vitro. Cell Biol Toxicol. 1985;1(4):259-268. DOI: 10.1007/BF00118191

[6] Olopade JO, Connor JR. Vanadium and neurotoxicity: a review. Curr Topics Toxicol. 2011; 1;7:33-39.

[7] Avila-Costa MR, Colín-Barenque L, Zepeda-Rodríguez A, Antuna SB, Saldivar L, Espejel-Maya et al. Ependymal epithelium disruption after vanadium pentoxide inhalation: a mice experimental model. Neurosci Lett. 2005. 10;381(1-2):21-5. DOI: 10.1016/j.neulet.2005.01.072

[8] Avila-Costa MR, Montiel Flores E, Colin-Barenque L, Ordoñez JL, Gutiérrez AL, Niño-Cabrera HG, et al. Nigrostriatal modifications after vanadium inhalation: an immunocytochemical and cytological approach. Neurochem Res. 2004;29(7):1365-1369. DOI: 10.1023/B:NERE.0000026398.86113.7d

[9] Witkowska D, Brzezinski J. Alteration of brain noradrenaline, dopamine and 5-hydroxytryptamine levels during vanadium poisoning. Pol J Pharmacol Pharm. 1979;31(4):393-398. PMID: 523342

[10] Witkowska D, Brzezinski J. Effect of metavanadate on the uptake and release of noradrenaline in rat brain cerebral cortex slices. Toxicol Lett. 1983;17 (3-4):223-231. DOI: 10.1016/0378-4274(83)90230-8

[11] World Health Organization. Vanadium-Environmental Health Criteria 81. 1988.

[12] Barth A, Schaffer AW, Konnaris C, Blauensteiner R, Winker R, Osterode W, et al. Neurobehavioral effects of vanadium. J Toxicol Environ Health A. 2002;65(9):677-683. DOI: 10.1080/15287390252900377

[13] Fortoul TI, Rojas-Lemus M, Rodriguez-Lara V, Gonzalez-Villalva A, Ustarroz-Cano M, Cano-Gutierrez G, et al. Overview of environmental and occupational vanadium exposure and associated health outcomes: an article based on a presentation at the 8th International Symposium on Vanadium Chemistry, Biological Chemistry, and Toxicology, Washington DC, August 15-18, 2012. J Immunotoxicol. 2014;11(1):13-18. DOI: 10.3109/1547691x.2013.789940

[14] Imtiaz M, Rizwan MS, Xiong S, Li H, Ashraf M, Shahzad SM, et al. Vanadium, recent advancements and research prospects: A review. Environ Int. 2015;80:79-88. DOI: 10.1016/j.envint.2015.03.018

[15] Amorim FA, Welz B, Costa AC, Lepri FG, Vale MG, Ferreira SL.

Determination of vanadium in petroleum and petroleum products using atomic spectrometric techniques. Talanta. 2007;72(2):349-359. DOI: 10.1016/j.talanta.2006.12.015

[16] Khan S, Kazi TG, Kolachi NF, Baig JA, Afridi HI, Shah AQ, et al. Hazardous impact and translocation of vanadium (V) species from soil to different vegetables and grasses grown in the vicinity of thermal power plant. J Hazard Mater. 2011;190(1-3):738-743. DOI: 10.1016/j.jhazmat.2011.03.105

[17] Teng Y, Yang J, Sun Z, Wang J, Zuo R, Zheng J. Environmental vanadium distribution, mobility and bioaccumulation in different land-use districts in Panzhihua Region, SW China. Environ Monit Assess. 2011;176(1-4):605-620. DOI: 10.1007/s10661-010-1607-0

[18] Panichev N, Mandiwana K, Moema D, Molatlhegi R, Ngobeni P. Distribution of vanadium(V) species between soil and plants in the vicinity of vanadium mine. J Hazard Mater. 2006;137(2):649-653. DOI: 10.1016/j.jhazmat.2006.03.006

[19] McLauchlan CC, Murakami HA, Wallace CA, Crans DC. Coordination environment changes of the vanadium in vanadium-dependent haloperoxidase enzymes. J Inorg Biochem. 2018;186:267-279. DOI: 10.1016/j.jinorgbio.2018.06.011

[20] Ortiz-Bernad I, Anderson RT, Vrionis HA, Lovley DR. Vanadium respiration by Geobacter metallireducens: novel strategy for in situ removal of vanadium from groundwater. Appl Environ Microbiol. 2004;70(5):3091-3095. DOI: 10.1128/aem.70.5.3091-3095.2004

[21] Kustin K. Aqueous vanadium ion dynamics relevant to bioinorganic chemistry: A review. J Inorg Biochem. 2015;147:32-38. DOI: 10.1016/j.jinorgbio.2014.12.009

[22] Pourang N, Nikouyan A, Dennis JH. Trace element concentrations in fish, surficial sediments and water from northern part of the Persian Gulf. Environ Monit Assess. 2005;109(1-3):293-316. DOI: 10.1007/s10661-005-6287-9

[23] Ringelband U, Hehl O. Kinetics of Vanadium Bioaccumulation by the brackish water hydroid Cordylophora caspia (Pallas). Bull Environ Contam Toxicol. 2000;65(4):486-493. DOI: 10.1007/s001280000150

[24] Morrell BG, Lepp NW, Phipps DA. Vanadium uptake by higher plants: Some recent developments. Environ Geochem Health. 1986;8(1):14-18. DOI: 10.1007/bf02280116

[25] Aragon AM, Altamirano-Lozano M. Sperm and testicular modifications induced by subchronic treatments with vanadium (IV) in CD-1 mice. Reprod Toxicol. 2001;15(2):145-151. DOI: 10.1016/s0890-6238(01)00117-4

[26] Fortoul TI, Quan-Torres A, Sanchez I, Lopez IE, Bizarro P, Mendoza ML, et al. Vanadium in ambient air: concentrations in lung tissue from autopsies of Mexico City residents in the 1960s and 1990s. Arch Environ Health. 2002;57(5):446-449. DOI: 10.1080/00039890209601436

[27] Myron DR, Givand SH, Nielsen FH. Vanadium content of selected foods as determined by flameless atomic absorption spectroscopy. J Agric Food Chem. 1977;25(2):297-300. DOI: 10.1021/jf60210a036

[28] Poucheret P., Verma S., Grynpas M.D., McNeill J.H. (1998) Vanadium and diabetes. In: Pierce G.N., Izumi T., Rupp H., Grynberg A. (eds) Molecular and Cellular Effects of Nutrition on Disease Processes.

Developments in Molecular and Cellular Biochemistry, vol 26. Springer, Boston, MA. DOI: 10.1007/978-1-4615-5763-0_9

[29] Hirano S, Suzuki KT. Exposure, metabolism, and toxicity of rare earths and related compounds. Environ Health Perspect. 1996;104 Suppl 1:85-95. DOI: 10.1289/ehp.96104s185

[30] Fantus I.G., Deragon G., Lai R., Tang S. (1995) Modulation of insulin action by vanadate: evidence of a role for phosphotyrosine phosphatase activity to alter cellular signaling. In: Srivastava A.K., Chiasson JL. (eds) Vanadium Compounds: Biochemical and Therapeutic Applications. Developments in Molecular and Cellular Biochemistry, vol 16. Springer, Boston, MA. DOI: 10.1007/978-1-4613-1251-2_12

[31] Fawcett JP, Farquhar SJ, Thou T, Shand BI. Oral vanadyl sulphate does not affect blood cells, viscosity or biochemistry in humans. Pharmacol Toxicol. 1997;80(4):202-206. DOI: 10.1111/j.1600-0773.1997.tb00397.x

[32] Hamel F.G., Duckworth W.C. (1995) The relationship between insulin and vanadium metabolism in insulin target tissues. In: Srivastava A.K., Chiasson JL. (eds) Vanadium Compounds: Biochemical and Therapeutic Applications. Developments in Molecular and Cellular Biochemistry, vol 16. Springer, Boston, MA. DOI: 10.1007/978-1-4613-1251-2_11

[33] Cam MC, Brownsey RW, McNeill JH. Mechanisms of vanadium action: insulin-mimetic or insulin-enhancing agent? Can J Physiol Pharmacol. 2000;78(10):829-847. DOI: 10.1139/y00-053

[34] Alimonti A, Petrucci F, Krachler M, Bocca B, Caroli S. Reference values for chromium, nickel and vanadium in urine of youngsters from the urban area of Rome. J Environ Monit. 2000;2(4):351-354. DOI: 10.1039/b001616k

[35] Edel J, Sabbioni E. Vanadium transport across placenta and milk of rats to the fetus and newborn. Biol Trace Elem Res. 1989;22(3):265-275. DOI: 10.1007/BF02916615

[36] Folarin OR, Snyder AM, Peters DG, Olopade F, Connor JR, Olopade JO. Brain Metal Distribution and Neuro-Inflammatory Profiles after Chronic Vanadium Administration and Withdrawal in Mice. Front Neuroanat. 2017;11:58. DOI: 10.3389/fnana.2017.00058

[37] Mustapha O, Oke B, Offen N, Siren AL, Olopade J. Neurobehavioral and cytotoxic effects of vanadium during oligodendrocyte maturation: a protective role for erythropoietin. Environ Toxicol Pharmacol. 2014;38(1):98-111. DOI: 10.1016/j.etap.2014.05.001

[38] Ladagu AD, Olopade FE, Folarin OR, Elufioye TO, Wallach JV, Dybek MB, et al. Novel NMDA-receptor antagonists ameliorate vanadium neurotoxicity. Naunyn Schmiedebergs Arch Pharmacol. 2020;393(9):1729-1738. DOI: 10.1007/s00210-020-01882-6

[39] Done A. Of metals and chelation. Emer Med. 1979;11:186-218.

[40] Li H, Zhou D, Zhang Q, Feng C, Zheng W, He K, et al. Vanadium exposure-induced neurobehavioral alterations among Chinese workers. Neurotoxicology. 2013;36:49-54. DOI: 10.1016/j.neuro.2013.02.008

[41] Mustapha O, Oke B, Offen N, Sirén A-l, Olopade J. Neurobehavioral and cytotoxic effects of vanadium during oligodendrocyte maturation: a protective role for erythropoietin. Environ Toxicol Pharmacol. 2014;38(1):98-111. DOI: 10.1016/j.etap.2014.05.001

[42] Fortoul TI, Rodriguez-Lara V, Gonzalez-Villalva A, Rojas-Lemus M, Cano-Gutierrez G, Ustarroz-Cano M, et al. Vanadium inhalation in a mouse model for the understanding of air-suspended particle systemic repercussion. J Biomed Biotechnol. 2011;2011:951043. DOI: 10.1155/2011/951043

[43] Avila-Costa MR, Fortoul TI, Niño-Cabrera G, Colín-Barenque L, Bizarro-Nevares P, Gutiérrez-Valdez AL, et al. Hippocampal cell alterations induced by the inhalation of vanadium pentoxide (V2O5) promote memory deterioration. Neurotoxicology. 2006;27(6):1007-1012. DOI: 10.1016/j.neuro.2006.04.001

[44] Cuesta S, Proietto R, Garcia GB. Astrogliosis and HSP 70 activation in neonate rats' brain exposed to sodium metavanadate through lactation. Neurotoxicol Teratol. 2013;37:57-62. DOI: 10.1016/j.ntt.2013.03.002

[45] Todorich B, Olopade JO, Surguladze N, Zhang X, Neely E, Connor JR. The mechanism of vanadium-mediated developmental hypomyelination is related to destruction of oligodendrocyte progenitors through a relationship with ferritin and iron. Neurotox Res. 2011;19(3):361-373. DOI: 10.1007/s12640-010-9167-1

[46] Valko M, Morris H, Cronin MT. Metals, toxicity and oxidative stress. Curr Med Chem. 2005;12(10):1161-1208. DOI: 10.2174/0929867053764635

[47] Nechay BR. Mechanisms of action of vanadium. Annu Rev Pharmacol Toxicol 1984;24:501-24. DOI: 10.1146/annurev.pa.24.040184.002441

[48] Yang X, Wang K, Lu J, Crans DC. Membrane transport of vanadium compounds and the interaction with the erythrocyte membrane. Coord Chem Rev. 2003;237(1-2):103-111. DOI: 10.1016/S0010-8545(02)00247-3

[49] Ding M, Gannett PM, Rojanasakul Y, Liu K, Shi X. One-electron reduction of vanadate by ascorbate and related free radical generation at physiological pH. J Inorg Biochem. 1994;55(2):101-112. DOI: 10.1016/0162-0134(94)85032-1

[50] Capella LS, Gefé MR, Silva EF, Affonso-Mitidieri O, Lopes AG, Rumjanek VM, et al. Mechanisms of vanadate-induced cellular toxicity: role of cellular glutathione and NADPH. Arch Biochem Biophys. 2002;406(1):65-72. DOI: 10.1016/s0003-9861(02)00408-3

[51] Wang X, Michaelis EK. Selective neuronal vulnerability to oxidative stress in the brain. Front Aging Neurosci. 2010;2:12. DOI: 10.3389/fnagi.2010.00012

[52] Rodríguez-Lara V, Morales-Rivero A, Rivera-Cambas AM, Fortoul TI. Vanadium inhalation induces actin changes in mice testicular cells. Toxicol Ind Health. 2016;32(2):367-374. DOI: 10.1177/0748233713501364

[53] Mailhes JB, Hilliard C, Fuseler JW, London SN. Vanadate, an Inhibitor of Tyrosine Phosphatases, Induced Premature Anaphase in Oocytes and Aneuploidy and Polyploidy in Mouse Bone Marrow Cells. Mutat Res. 2003;538(1-2):101-107. DOI: 10.1016/s1383-5718(03)00108-6

[54] Mussali-Galante, P., Rodríguez-Lara, V., Hernández-Tellez, B., Ávila-Costa, M.R., Colín-Barenque, L., Bizarro-Nevarez, P., et al. Inhaled vanadium pentoxide decrease gamma-tubulin of mouse testes at different exposure times. Toxicol Ind Health. 2005; 21(7-8), pp.215-222. DOI: 10.1191/0748233705th232oa

[55] Lee JR. Protein tyrosine phosphatase PTPRT as a regulator of synaptic formation and neuronal development.

BMB Reports. 2015;48(5):249. DOI: 10.5483/BMBRep.2015.48.5.037

[56] Brookmeyer R, Johnson E, Ziegler-Graham K, Arrighi HM. Forecasting the global burden of Alzheimer's disease. Alzheimers Dement. 2007;3(3):186-191. DOI: 10.1016/j.jalz.2007.04.381

[57] Coon KD, Myers AJ, Craig DW, Webster JA, Pearson JV, Lince DH, et al. A high-density whole-genome association study reveals that APOE is the major susceptibility gene for sporadic late-onset Alzheimer's disease. J Clin Psychiatry. 2007;68(4): 613-618. DOI: 10.4088/jcp.v68n0419.

[58] Guo Z, Cupples L, Kurz A, Auerbach S, Volicer L, Chui H, et al. Head injury and the risk of AD in the MIRAGE study. Neurology. 2000;54(6):1316-1323. DOI: 10.1212/wnl.54.6.1316

[59] Calderón-Garcidueñas L, Reed W, Maronpot RR, Henriquez-Roldán C, Delgado-Chavez R, Calderón-Garcidueñas A, et al. Brain inflammation and Alzheimer's-like pathology in individuals exposed to severe air pollution. Toxicol Pathol. 2004;32(6):650-658. DOI: 10.1080/01926230490520232

[60] Alzheimer's Association. 2018 Alzheimer's disease facts and figures. Alzheimer's & Dementia. 2018;14(3):367-429. DOI: 10.1016/j.jalz.2018.02.001

[61] Wilson RS, Arnold SE, Schneider JA, Kelly JF, Tang Y, Bennett DA. Chronic psychological distress and risk of Alzheimer's disease in old age. Neuroepidemiology. 2006;27(3):143-153. DOI: 10.1159/000095761

[62] Dickerson BC, Eichenbaum H. The episodic memory system: neurocircuitry and disorders. Neuropsychopharmacology. 2010;35(1):86-104. DOI: 10.1038/npp.2009.126

[63] Serrano-Pozo A, Frosch MP, Masliah E, Hyman BT. Neuropathological alterations in Alzheimer disease. Serrano-Pozo A, Frosch MP, Masliah E, Hyman BT. Neuropathological alterations in Alzheimer disease. Cold Spring Harb Perspect Med. 2011;1(1):a006189. DOI: 10.1101/cshperspect.a006189. 2011;1(1):a006189. DOI: 10.1101/cshperspect.a006189

[64] Braak H, Braak E. Neuropathological stageing of Alzheimer-related changes. Acta Neuropathol. 1991;82(4):239-259. DOI: 10.1007/BF00308809

[65] Selkoe DJ. Alzheimer's disease is a synaptic failure. Science. 2002;298(5594):789-791. DOI: 10.1126/science.1074069

[66] Ferrer I. Defining Alzheimer as a common age-related neurodegenerative process not inevitably leading to dementia. Prog Neurobiol. 2012;97(1):38-51. DOI: 10.1016/j.pneurobio.2012.03.005

[67] Forner S, Baglietto-Vargas D, Martini AC, Trujillo-Estrada L, LaFerla FM. Synaptic impairment in Alzheimer's disease: a dysregulated symphony. Trends Neurosci. 2017;40(6):347-357. DOI: 10.1016/j.tins.2017.04.002

[68] Chen Y, Fu AK, Ip NY. Synaptic dysfunction in Alzheimer's disease: mechanisms and therapeutic strategies. Pharmacol Ther. 2019;195:186-198. DOI: 10.1016/j.pharmthera.2018.11.006

[69] Duyckaerts C, Delaère P, He Y, Camilleri S, Braak H, Piette F, Hauw JJ (1995) The relative merits of tau- and amyloid markers in the neuropathology of Alzheimer's disease. In: Bergener M,

Finkel SI (eds) Treating Alzheimer's and other dementias. Springer, Heidelberg Berlin New York, pp 81-89.

[70] Feany MB, Dickson DW. Neurodegenerative disorders with extensive tau pathology: a comparative study and review. Ann Neurol. 1996;40(2):139-148. DOI: 10.1002/ana.410400204

[71] Goedert M. Tau protein and the neurofibrillary pathology of Alzheimer's disease. Trends Neurosci. 1993;16(11):460-465. DOI: 10.1016/0166-2236(93)90078-z

[72] Bancher C, Brunner C, Lassmann H, Budka H, Jellinger K, Wiche G, et al. Accumulation of abnormally phosphorylated tau precedes the formation of neurofibrillary tangles in Alzheimer's disease. Brain Res. 1989;477(1-2):90-99. DOI: 10.1016/0006-8993(89)91396-6

[73] Braak F, Braak H, Mandelkow E-M. A sequence of cytoskeleton changes related to the formation of neurofibrillary tangles and neuropil threads. Acta Neuropathol. 1994;87(6):554-567. DOI: 10.1007/BF00293315

[74] Braak H, Braak E, Grundke-Iqbal I, Iqbal K. Occurrence of neuropil threads in the senile human brain and in Alzheimer's disease: a third location of paired helical filaments outside of neurofibrillary tangles and neuritic plaques. Neurosci Lett. 1986;65(3):351-355. DOI: 10.1016/0304-3940(86)90288-0

[75] Boutajangout A, Wisniewski T. Tau-based therapeutic approaches for Alzheimer's disease-a mini-review. Gerontology. 2014;60(5):381-385. DOI: 10.1159/000358875

[76] Dujardin S, Colin M, Buee L. Animal models of tauopathies and their implications for research/translation into the clinic. Neuropathol Appl Neurobiol. 2014. DOI: 10.1111/nan.12200

[77] Barrett J, McGonigle P. Rodent models for Alzheimer's disease in drug discovery. In: Adeboye Adejare (Ed.) Drug Discovery Approaches for the Treatment of Neurodegenerative Disorders: Academic Press, 2017. p. 235-247. DOI: 10.1016/B978-0-12-802810-0.00012-X

[78] Wisniewski T, Goñi F. Immunotherapeutic approaches for Alzheimer's disease. Neuron. 2015;85(6):1162-1176. DOI: 10.1016/j.neuron.2014.12.064

[79] Drummond E, Wisniewski T. Alzheimer's disease: experimental models and reality. Acta Neuropathol. 2017;133(2):155-175. DOI: 10.1007/s00401-016-1662-x

[80] Banik A, Brown RE, Bamburg J, Lahiri DK, Khurana D, Friedland RP, et al. Translation of Pre-Clinical Studies into Successful Clinical Trials for Alzheimer's Disease: What are the Roadblocks and How Can They Be Overcome? 1. J Alzheimers Dis. 2015;47(4):815-843. DOI: 10.3233/JAD-150136

[81] Schneider LS, Mangialasche F, Andreasen N, Feldman H, Giacobini E, Jones R, et al. Clinical trials and late-stage drug development for A lzheimer's disease: an appraisal from 1984 to 2014. J Intern Med. 2014;275(3):251-283. DOI: 10.1111/joim.12191

[82] Nobakht M, Hoseini SM, Mortazavi P, Sohrabi I, Esmailzade B, Roosh NR, Omidzahir S. Neuropathological changes in brain cortex and hippocampus in a rat model of Alzheimer's disease. Iranian Biomed J. 2011;15(1-2):51. PMCID: PMC3639737

[83] Valverde F. The Golgi Method. A Tool for Comparative Structural

Analyses. In: Nauta WJH, Ebbesson SOE, editors. Contemporary Research Methods in Neuroanatomy. Berlin, Heidelberg: Springer Berlin Heidelberg; 1970. p. 12-31.

[84] Avila-Costa MR, Colin-Barenque L, Fortoul TI, Machado-Salas P, Espinosa-Villanueva J, Rugerio-Vargas C, et al. Memory deterioration in an oxidative stress model and its correlation with cytological changes on rat hippocampus CA1. Neurosci Lett. 1999;270(2):107-109. DOI: 10.1016/s0304-3940(99)00458-9

[85] Fiala JC, Spacek J, Harris KM. Dendritic spine pathology: cause or consequence of neurological disorders? Brain Res Rev. 2002;39(1):29-54. DOI: 10.1016/s0165-0173(02)00158-3

[86] Avila-Costa MR, Colín-Barenque L, Fortoul TI, Machado-Salas JP, Espinosa-Villanueva J, Rugerio-Vargas C, et al. Motor impairments in an oxidative stress model and its correlation with cytological changes on rat striatum and prefrontal cortex. Int J Neurosci. 2001;108(3-4):193-200. DOI: 10.3109/00207450108986514

[87] Colín-Barenque L, Avila-Costa M, Fortoul T, Rugerio-Vargas C, Machado-Salas J, Espinosa-Villanueva J, et al. Morphologic alteration of the olfactory bulb after acute ozone exposure in rats. Neurosci Lett. 1999;274(1):1-4. DOI: 10.1016/s0304-3940(99)00639-4

[88] Pelucchi S, Stringhi R, Marcello E. Dendritic spines in Alzheimer's disease: how the actin cytoskeleton contributes to synaptic failure. International Journal of Molecular Sciences. 2020;21(3):908. DOI: 10.3390/ijms21030908

[89] Wang Q, Yuan W, Yang X, Wang Y, Li Y and Qiao H. Role of Cofilin in Alzheimer's Disease. Front. Cell Dev. Biol. 2020; 8:584898. DOI: 10.3389/fcell.2020.584898

[90] Hanus-Fajerska E, Wiszniewska A, Kamińska I. A Dual Role of Vanadium in Environmental Systems-Beneficial and Detrimental Effects on Terrestrial Plants and Humans. Plants (Basel). 2021;10(6):1110. DOI:10.3390/plants10061110

[91] Jaiswal MR, Kale PP. Mini review–vanadium-induced neurotoxicity and possible targets. Neurol Sci. 2020;41(4):763-768. DOI: 10.1007/s10072-019-04188-5

[92] Sasi MM, Haider SS, El-Fakhri M, Ghwarsha KM. Microchromatographic analysis of lipids, protein, and occurrence of lipid peroxidation in various brain areas of vanadium exposed rats: a possible mechanism of vanadium neurotoxicity. Neurotoxicology. 1994;15(2):413-420. PMID: 7991230.

[93] Adebiyi OE, Olayemi FO, Olopade JO, Tan NH. Beta-sitosterol enhances motor coordination, attenuates memory loss and demyelination in a vanadium-induced model of experimental neurotoxicity. Pathophysiology. 2019; 26(1):21-29. DOI: 10.1016/j.pathophys.2018.12.002

[94] Fatola OI, Olaolorun FA, Olopade FE, Olopade JO. Trends in vanadium neurotoxicity. Brain Res Bull. 2019;145:75-80. DOI: 10.1016/j.brainresbull.2018.03.010

[95] Goc A. Biological activity of vanadium compounds. Cent Eur J Biol. 2006;1(3):314-332. DOI: 10.2478/s11535-006-0029-z

[96] Glenner GG, Wong CW. Alzheimer's disease: initial report of the purification and characterization of a novel cerebrovascular amyloid protein. Biochem Biophys Res Commun. 1984;120(3):885-890. DOI: 10.1016/s0006-291x(84)80190-4

[97] Tsave O, Petanidis S, Kioseoglou E, Yavropoulou MP, Yovos JG, Anestakis D,

et al. Role of vanadium in cellular and molecular immunology: association with immune-related inflammation and pharmacotoxicology mechanisms. Oxid Med Cell Longev. 2016;2016:4013639. DOI: 10.1155/2016/4013639

[98] Irving E, Stoker AW. Vanadium compounds as PTP inhibitors. Molecules. 2017;22(12):2269. DOI: 10.3390/molecules22122269

[99] Andersen JK. Oxidative stress in neurodegeneration: cause or consequence? Nat Med. 2004;10 Suppl: S18-S25. DOI: 10.1038/nrn1434.

[100] Combeau C, Carlier MF. Probing the mechanism of ATP hydrolysis on F-actin using vanadate and the structural analogs of phosphate BeF-3 and A1F-4. The J Biol Chem. 1988;263(33):17429-17436. DOI: 10.1016/S0021-9258(19)77854-5.

[101] Ramos S, Almeida RM, Moura JJ, Aureliano M. Implications of oxidovanadium(IV) binding to actin. J Inorg Biochem. 2011;105(6):777-783. DOI: 10.1016/j.jinorgbio.2011.02.010

[102] Ramos S, Manuel M, Tiago T, Duarte R, Martins J, Gutierrez-Merino C, et al. Decavanadate interactions with actin: inhibition of G-actin polymerization and stabilization of decameric vanadate. J Inorg Biochem. 2006;100(11):1734-1743. DOI: 10.1016/j.jinorgbio.2006.06.007

[103] Ramos S, Duarte RO, Moura JJ, Aureliano M. Decavanadate interactions with actin: cysteine oxidation and vanadyl formation. Dalton Trans. 2009(38):7985-7994. DOI: 10.1039/b906255f

[104] Derkinderen P, Scales TM, Hanger DP, Leung KY, Byers HL, Ward MA, et al. Tyrosine 394 is phosphorylated in Alzheimer's paired helical filament tau and in fetal tau with c-Abl as the candidate tyrosine kinase. J Neurosci. 2005;25(28):6584-6593. DOI: 10.1523/JNEUROSCI.1487-05.2005

[105] Jhang KA, Park J-S, Kim H-S, Chong YH. Resveratrol Ameliorates Tau Hyperphosphorylation at Ser396 Site and Oxidative Damage in Rat Hippocampal Slices Exposed to Vanadate: Implication of ERK1/2 and GSK-3β Signaling Cascades. J Agric Food Chem. 2017;65(44):9626-9634. DOI: 10.1021/acs.jafc.7b03252

[106] Korbecki J, Baranowska-Bosiacka I, Gutowska I, Chlubek D. Vanadium compounds as pro-inflammatory agents: effects on cyclooxygenases. Int J Mol Sci. 2015;16(6):12648-12668. DOI: 10.3390/ijms160612648

[107] Coles CH, Bradke F. Coordinating neuronal actin-microtubule dynamics. Curr Biol. 2015;25(15):R677-R691. DOI: 10.1016/j.cub.2015.06.020

[108] Kiuchi A, Otsuka N, Namba Y, Nakano I, Tomonaga M. Presenile appearance of abundant Alzheimer's neurofibrillary tangles without senile plaques in the brain in myotonic dystrophy. Acta Neuropathol. 1991;82(1):1-5. DOI: 10.1007/BF00310916

[109] Serrano-Pozo A, Frosch MP, Masliah E, Hyman BT. Neuro pathological alterations in Alzheimer disease. Cold Spring Harb Perspect Med. 2011;1(1):a006189-a. DOI: 10.1101/cshperspect.a006189

Chapter 6

Chemotherapy-Induced Peripheral Neuropathy: Mechanisms and Clinical Assessment

Jordi Casanova-Mollà

Abstract

Antineoplastic drugs may be neurotoxic and the clinical features frequently include distal sensory loss and neuropathic pain. This is related to a direct damage in sensory neurons and non-selective degeneration of sensory nerve fibers. Due to different mechanisms, there are agents that affects also motor or autonomic nerves. In the case of immune checkpoint inhibitors, an inflammatory response attacks the muscle, motor neurons or neuromuscular transmission. We present an easy-to-read article to understand first symptoms of chemotherapy-induced neuropathy (CIN) with describing each agent and the course of neuropathy as well as the clinical assessment with neurophysiological techniques. In addition, skin biopsy allows us to examine histological changes such as reinnervation. Neuroprotection with antioxidant therapy is possible but more effort in this field is needed.

Keywords: chemotherapy-induced neuropathy, oxaliplatin-induced neuropathy, neurotoxicity, polyneuropathy, toxic neuropathy

1. Introduction

Currently the chemotherapeutic drugs are part of cancer treatment. Among their side effects, neurotoxicity at peripheral nervous system is a well recognize dose-limiting side effect. It is relevant because it causes persistent pain and sensory loss in cancer survivors. The prevalence of chemotherapy-induced peripheral neuropathy (CIPN) has been reported around 30% of patients at 6 months after treatment. It reaches up to 40% when patients are also examined with nerve conduction studies [1]. It is important to note that neurotoxicity could be subclinical, it means that it may start before patient starts to be symptomatic.

The clinical picture at presentation of CIPN is a length-dependent sensory polyneuropathy despite other combination of sensory, motor and autonomic nerve dysfunction are possible. It is important to recognize different types of sensory nerve fibers which are specific to different sensory modalities (touch, vibration, temperature and pain). All of these neurons have their cell bodies in the dorsal root ganglion (DRG). The thin-myelinated Aδ fibers and unmyelinated C fibers are known as small nerve fibers carrying thermal and painful stimulus to the brain. We need selective neurophysiological and histological techniques to evaluate them as well as to examine the function of the autonomic nervous system [2].

IntechOpen

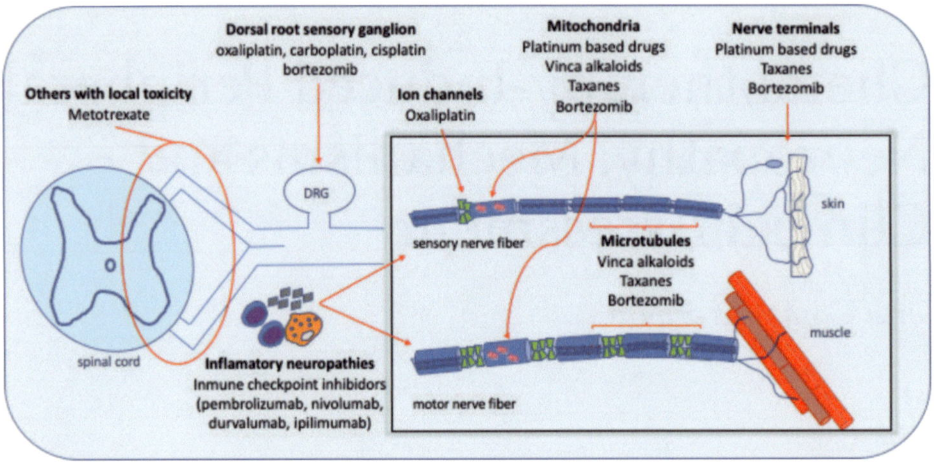

Figure 1.
Different targets to produce neurotoxicity by chemotherapy.

Drug	Main mechanism of action	Mechanism of neurotoxicity	Tumor
Platinum salts (oxaliplatin, carboplatin, cisplatin)	Alkylation of DNA	Ion channels hyperexcitability, neuronal DNA damage, loss of axonal transport, mitochondrial dysfunction, neuroinflammation	digestive tract tumors, pulmonary, ovarian, testicular, uterine, SCLC
Taxanes (paclitaxel, docetaxel)	Microtubule stabilizer	Loss of axonal transport, neuroinflammation, damage of mitochondrial DNA, ion channel hyperexcitability	breast, gynecologic, gastric, NSCLC prostate, sarcomas
Vincristine, Vinblastine	Microtubule stabilizer	Loss of axonal transport, neuroinflammation	lymphoma, testicular, NSCLC
Bortezomib	Proteasome inhibitor; microtubule stabilizer	Mitochondrial damage, accumulation of aggregates, DNA damage, increase sphingolipid metabolism	multiple myeloma, lymphomas
Thalidomide, Lenalidomide,	Immunomodulator and antiangiogenic effect	Oxidative stress, downregulation of TNF-α, inhibits NF-κB	multiple myeloma
Brentuximab	Immunomodulator (anti-CD30)	Loss of axonal transport	lymphomas
Check-point inhibitors (ipilimumab, pembrolizumab, avelumab)	Immunomodulator effect against cytotoxic T-lymphocyte	Immune-related neuropathies; vasculitic neuropathy (pembrolizumab)	melanoma
Methotrexate or Cytarabine intrathecal	Dihydrofolate reductase inhibitor	Spinal cord and proximal roots demyelination	leukemia and lymphomas

SCLC = small-cell lung cancer; NSCLC: non-small cell lung cancer.

Table 1.
Classification of commonly used chemotherapy drugs related to elevated risk of CIPN.

The most neurotoxic families of chemotherapeutic drugs are the platinum derivates (e.g. oxaliplatin, carboplatin or cisplatin), taxanes (e.g. paclitaxel and docetaxel), vinca alkaloids (e.g. vincristine), proteasome inhibitors (e.g. bortezomib) and immunomodulators (e.g. thalidomide and checkpoint inhibitors). Others, as methotrexate or arsenic salts are less frequently used. See **Figure 1** a general schema with different targets on the peripheral nervous system and in **Table 1** a list of them with their mechanism of neurotoxicity.

2. Acute neurotoxicity

There are drugs that can produce acute neurotoxicity, a side effect commonly seen with oxaliplatin. It is characterized by transient paresthesia, dysesthesia and muscle cramps induced by cold exposure, a phenomenon often called cold allodynia that typically appears during or immediately after infusion of the treatment. It usually resolves within a few hours or days before the next oxaliplatin cycle [3]. Symptoms reported by patients include tingling paresthesia in the hands (100%), feet (42%) and orofacial area (50%) and also, pharyngeal or laryngeal regions, all of them triggered by cold (especially when drinking). More infrequently, patients report fasciculations (29%), jaw spasms (26%), cramps (20%), difficulty of swallowing (18%) and neuromyotonia-like syndrome. All these phenomena reveal an increase in sensory and motor nerve excitability related to the impairment of voltage-gated sodium channels induced by oxaliplatin [4]. A functional study demonstrated that oxaliplatin induces reversible slowing of sodium channel inactivation [5]. We know that it does not require discontinuation of treatment or dose reduction, but prolonging the time of infusion from 2 h to 4 or 6 h is recommended [6]. Some authors have found a relationship to later develop of chronic neuropathy [7, 8]. In particular when cold allodynia persists for days or weeks after infusion. Even some patients, continued to report residual symptoms in subsequent doses of oxaliplatin [9]. Another symptom that patients frequently ask is the Lhermitte's sign, a sudden lightening sensation radiate out into both arms or feet when neck flexion is forced. The mechanism to produce it at cervical spinal cord is unknown but usually self-limited despite in some exceptional cases it could appear lately and be persistent during months [10, 11].

It has been described in addition acute sensitization of nociceptors with paclitaxel, the paclitaxel-associate acute pain syndrome. It consists of aching or other pain sensations mainly at lower legs peaked on day 4 after paclitaxel initiation. This is related to fast infusion of treatment (3 hours) but also, indicates more risk to sensory neuropathy after 12 weeks of therapy [12].

3. Targets of neurotoxicity at peripheral nerves

Even when all body is exposed to chemotherapy, there are tissues more vulnerable to chemotherapy than others. This is the case of sensory neurons located at dorsal root ganglion (DRG) which are outside the protection of the blood–brain barrier. They are the principal targets of platinum derivates such us oxaliplatin, cisplatin or other platinum agents. Thus, neurons are damaged directly at DRG producing a progressive sensory neuronopathy. However, neurotoxicity also causes multiple lesions within the axons both for platinum agents and for other drugs as taxanes generating distal axonopathy. This will have different consequences for patients.

On one hand, the myelinated sensory nerve fibers lose their function. This is noted by many patients in a "glove and stocking" pattern of sensory loss involving hands and feet. They frequently refer reduced precision to make fine movements with tip of the fingers which is noted by having less ability to cross buttons when dressing or when typing the computer. Also, gait disturbances affect their daily activities because of instability when walking in irregular ground or for descending stairs. On the other hand, thin myelinated (Aδ fibers) and unmyelinated (C fibers) carrying the information of temperature and pain are also damaged. A combination of negative and positive symptoms (see **Figure 2**) contributes to sensory disturbances. The unpleasant dysesthesias and neuropathic pain are consequence of the gain of function in damaged sensory nerve fibers that increases their excitability by producing spontaneous burning sensation or electric shock-like pain.

This clinical picture is common for all chemotherapy agents despite the mechanisms may differ among them. Also, it may determine the severity of axonal loss and its recovery since regeneration is expected to occur if the axon is affected distally whereas poor should be assumed in a neuronopathy. In general, we use the term sensory polyneuropathy for CINP when symptoms have a characteristic distance-dependent pattern even when we know that it is combined with sensory neuronopathy which has been demonstrated for oxaliplatin and cisplatin [13, 14].

There are other drugs such as vincristine, bortezomib or arsenic salts with ability to produce a more generalized axonal damage in all nerves. In this case, sensory deficits are accompanied by frequent muscular cramps, predominantly at night in both legs as well as distal weakness in upper and lower extremities because of motor neuropathy. Moreover, the failure in autonomic nerves leads to chronic constipation, reduced distal sweating and dizziness when standing (orthostatic hypotension) due to autonomic neuropathy or dysautonomia.

More recently, the introduction of the checkpoint inhibitors as a treatment for advance melanoma have opened the possibility of different immune-mediated neuromuscular manifestations reported as complication of the treatment in 75% of

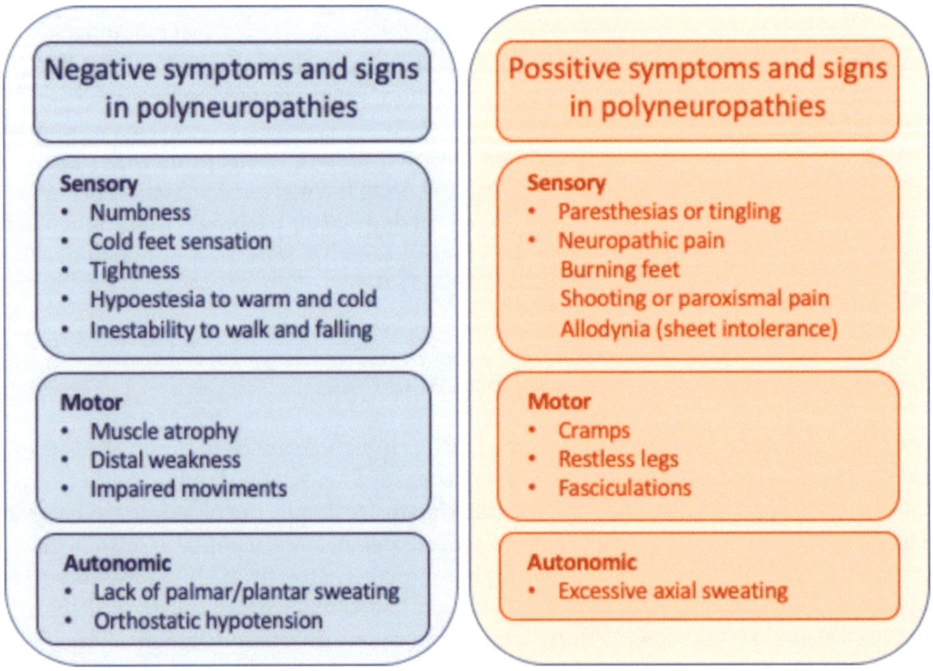

Figure 2.
Comparison of positive and negative symptoms in CIPN.

patients [15]. In this case acute demyelinating polyneuropathy (Guillain-Barré syndrome), demyelinating sensorimotor neuropathy, myositis or myasthenic syndrome have to be considered.

The combination of peripheral and central neurotoxicity at spinal cord should be considered in intrathecal infusion of chemotherapy. This is necessary for patients with acute leukemia treated with methotrexate. It has been described also after vincristine treatment. In this case, proximal motor roots can be unexpectedly block with a variable extension of myelitis at the level of lumbar infusion producing a complete paresis in lower limbs (paraparesis) with a lower abdomen level of sensory loss together with urinary dysfunction. This is a devastating situation that has been reported in few cases with poor prognosis for recovery [16, 17].

4. Risks and other conditionings for CIPN

It is difficult to establish in humans exactly the timing of changes on peripheral nerves after a pharmacological insult. Even though we know the day chemotherapy starts, there are different risk factors than makes neuropathy more probable in one patient than another. In **Table 2** are listed the most known of them. In particular, one of such factors is the cumulative dose, especially for platinum agents. It was demonstrated that high-dose cisplatin was intrinsically more neurotoxic [23]. There is a range between 300 and 400 mg/m^2 from which sensory symptoms starts to be persistent and from 540 to 850 mg/m^2 from which the CIPN is generally stablished with high risk to be a long-term condition. However, we know now that there is no specific dose to be secure and probable neurotoxicity starts from first dose with a cumulative effect within sensory neurons.

Factors associated to higher risk of CIPN	Evidence	Type of study	Reference
Age	Low	Retrospective	[18]
Type of cancer	No evidence	Observational	[10]
Smoker	No evidence	Observational	[10]
Alcoholic	No evidence	Observational	[10]
Pre-chemotherapy neuropathy			
Diabetes	High if diabetic neuropathy	Retrospective	[6, 18]
Hereditary neuropathy	High	Retrospective	vincristine [19]
Cancer-induced neuropathy	High	Observational	[10, 20–22]
Dose of chemotherapy	Very High	Observational Experimental	[13, 14, 23]
Acute cold allodynia	High	Retrospective Observational	[7, 8, 9]
Repeated chemotherapy	Moderate	Observational	oxaliplatin [24]
Association with other chemotherapy	Very High		cisplatin+vincristine [18] cisplatin+paclitaxel [25] bortezomib-thalidomide [26]

Table 2.
General risk factors for CIPN.

One phenomenon that usually appears with platinum agents (cisplatin and oxaliplatin) is the coasting effect. It refers to the further progression of neurotoxicity during 3 to 6 months after stopping the treatment that results from its capacity to accumulate in DRG for a long time. It was described first for cisplatin [18, 27, 28] and later for oxaliplatin [9, 29, 30]. This surprises the patient who frequently ask worried because of deterioration of their sensory deficits after treatment was stopped.

5. Clinical assessment for early detection of CIPN

A good complement for clinical examination is the use of validated scales. It allows systematic data acquisition which is comparable in the follow-up of patients and also, their inclusion in research studies. There are different types of scales, ones are self-administered, others are based on clinical examination or they include a combination of clinical and results of complementary tests. We will comment two of the most used scales for CIPN and one self-administered scale.

The National Cancer Institute-Common Terminology Criteria for Adverse Events (NCI-CTCAE) includes a scale based on the degree of impact of peripheral sensory neuropathy which is the most widely used scale used by oncologists [31]. It grades from 1 to 5 patient's functionality disturbance due to sensory symptoms of neuropathy. There are different versions which are updated by the Division of Cancer Treatments and Diagnosis. The version 4.03 published in 2009 is currently the most referenced in last publications. The 5 grades are: 1) asymptomatic (weakness or loss of tendon reflex on examination) or paresthesia not interfering with function; 2) symptomatic or sensory alterations interfering with function but not with daily activities; 3) weakness or sensory alterations interfering with daily activities; 4) life threatening disabling; 5) death.

	0	1	2	3	5
Sensory symptoms	None	Symptoms limited to fingers or toes	Symptoms extends to ankle or wrist	Symptoms extends to knee or elbow	Symptoms above knees or elbows, or functionally disabling
Motor symptoms	None	Slight difficulty	Moderate difficulty	Require help/ assistance	Paralysis
Autonomic symptoms	0	1	2	3	4 or 5
Pin sensibility	Normal	Reduced in fingers or toes	Reduced up to wrist/ ankle	Reduced up to elbow/knee	Reduced above elbow/knee
Vibration sensibility	Normal	Reduced fingers or toes	Reduced up to writs/ ankle	Reduced up to elbow/knee	Reduced above elbow/knee
Strenght	Normal	Mild weakness	Moderate weakness	Severe	Paralysis
Tendon reflex	Normal	Ankle reflex reduced	Ankle reflex abset	Only	All reflexes absent

Note: Ranged from 0 to 28. CINP is significant if score > 5 points [32].

Table 3.
TNS clinical (TNSc) scale useful for the follow-up of patients.

The second most used scale for CIPN is the total neuropathy score (TNS). Its complete version was originally developed and validated for diabetic neuropathy. It combines clinical information obtained from grading symptoms and signs with neurophysiological parameters as nerve conduction studies and quantitative evaluation of sensory modalities. The clinical version (TNSc) includes the first 7 items (range 0 to 28) which are based only on clinical examination. It is showed in **Table 3**. A good correlation was reported between both, TNSc vs. NCI-CTCAE [32] even when TNSc is more sensitive in detecting mild sensory damage [33].

However, assessment of CIPN needs to involve subjective and objective information as well as the impact of the symptoms on functional activity. With this purpose, the European Organization for Research and Treatment of Cancer (EORTC) developed the self-administered scale QLQ-CIPN20. It includes 20 items in the form of auto-administered questions consisting of 3 scales (sensory, motor and autonomic). Each item range 1 (not at all) to 4 (very much) and a higher score is equivalent to worse or more symptoms during the past week. It should provide valuable information on CIPN-related symptoms and functional limitations of patients at risk [34].

6. Neurophysiological assessment for early detection of CIPN

There are different non-invasive techniques that provide information regarding the type of nerves (motor, sensory or autonomic) involved in CIPN. This is important to confirm the diagnosis but also to identify early markers of axonal damage and additionally, it may help to establish the prognosis for recovery.

6.1 Nerve conduction studies (NCS)

Peripheral nerves usually can be easily stimulated by electrical stimulus and brought to action potential. It can be applied to sensory or motor nerves. We measure the amplitude which reflects the amount of excitable axons, and the latency of the response to calculate the velocity conduction. It is essential to note that both, latency and velocity conduction reflect only the fastest conducting fibers. On the other hand, low amplitude of the sensory nerve potential indicates severe axonal loss [35]. In **Figure 3** there are examples of sensory nerve action potentials from a patient with sensory polyneuropathy after treatment with oxaliplatin.

The reduced amplitudes at sensory nerves with no significative changes in velocity conduction and motor responses are the common finding after treatment with platinum agents and taxanes. It affects distally sensory nerves at both sides in feet and hands. The sural nerve measured at ankle shows higher changes that other nerves such us radial or cubital nerves [36]. However, it is possible that the amplitude for sural nerve will fall within normal reference values, especially after treatment with oxaliplatin and taxanes in which sensory damage is limited to fingers or sole of the foot. The recording of the dorsal sural nerve is also recommendable to demonstrate low amplitudes in sensory distal polyneuropathy [37] (see **Figure 3a**). Nevertheless, not having normative values for such a distal nerve and the absence of response expected in the majority of the patients with CIPN makes results in amplitude necessary to be interpreted in relation to those obtained proximally at sural nerve in the same patient. If sensory symptoms are limited to hands, median entrapment neuropathy should be also rule out. Long-term follow up of patients after oxaliplatin showed persistent low amplitudes at sensory nerves 3 year after treatment [38].

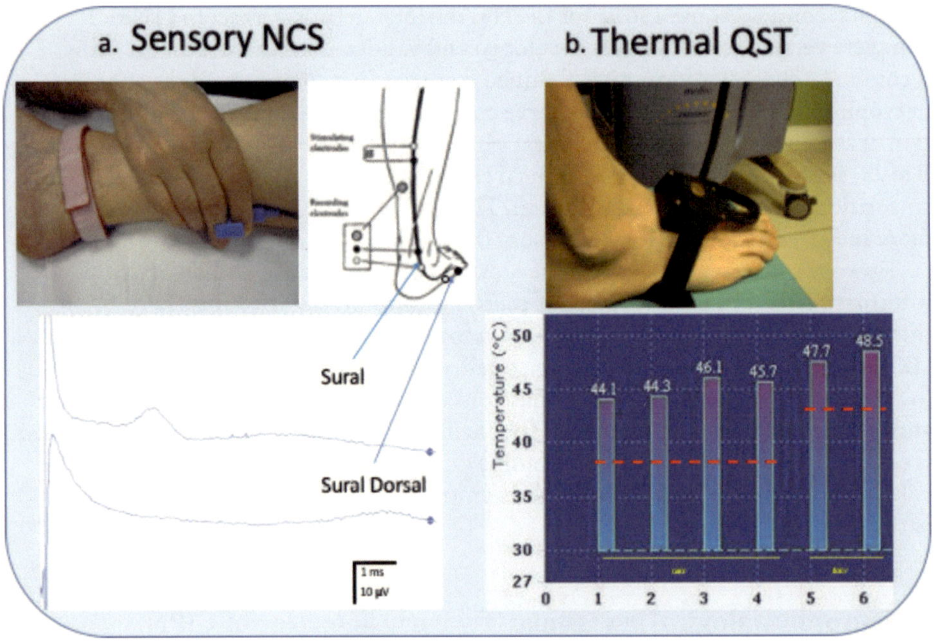

Figure 3.
Different techniques for diagnose CIPN. This figure shows two of the most common techniques (nerve conduction studies and thermotest) at evaluating the sensory function in suspected CIPN. a) the conventional sural nerve response, which is within normal limits (above) is compared with the more distal recording of the sural dorsal (below), which is clearly diminished; b) the thermode is applied at dorsum of the foot to test warm detection threshold (1–4 stimuli) and hot pain threshold (5–6 stimuli). Horizontal red line indicates normal values. The recording shows high thresholds to both, warm and pain. Note that detection of warm is near pain sensation because of the loss of function in C-fibers.

Other chemotherapy agents such us bortezomib or thalidomide produce a severe sensorimotor polyneuropathy with low amplitudes to all tested nerves. Despite axonopathy is the most frequent finding, in some cases a demyelinating pattern with reduced conduction velocities and prolonged proximal motor response (F-wave) may be possible (i.e., for example, 3 of 26 patients reported by Chaundhry [26]). The presence of signs of denervation in distal muscles at lower limbs is expected on EMG as well as atrophy of muscles together with weakness and instability to walk due to sensory deficits at feet.

6.2 Quantitative sensory testing (QST)

The measurement of sensory thresholds to thermal, vibration or mechanical stimulus indicates the loss or gain of function to each sensory modality. Commonly, temperature (cold and warm) detection and pain thresholds are evaluated distally in the dorsum of the hands and feet. At this sites, skin thickness-dependent delay and attenuation of temperature is reduced for contact heating (thermode) in comparison to glabrous skin [39]. Through QST examination we obtain functional information from small and large nerve fibers depending of the sensory modality examined.

One of the most common findings in QST is cold allodynia, that means early pain sensation at low temperatures (range from 10° to 25°C) frequently seen in oxaliplatin treated patients. Moreover, signs of sensory loss are present early in CIPN at hands and feet in comparison to other proximal sites (see an example in **Figure 3b**). Patients show high thresholds for warm and cold detection as well as for hot pain revealing deficient function of small nerve fibers [8, 10, 40].

In addition, the higher vibration and mechanical detection thresholds at upper and lower limbs reported by different authors indicates the coexistence with distal damage at large myelinated sensory fibers [38, 41, 42]. In fact, vibration detection threshold at tip of the big toe was found abnormal earlier than thermal QST [43]. However, QST has also important limitations that should be considered. First, it needs patient's cooperation. Second, a trained examiner should repeat stimuli to ensure consistency of responses. Finally, abnormal thresholds have been reported and considered a subclinical deficit for warm and cold sensations before receiving chemotherapy (at baseline) which makes difficult to detect a significant change related with starting of CIPN [10, 20, 21, 44].

6.3 Study of the autonomic nervous system

To evaluate the presence of dysautonomia, which is a failure of the sympathetic and/or parasympathetic nervous system, it may be possible to record the palmar and plantar sudomotor skin response. This is a change in the voltage measured from the surface of the skin which occurs after emotional or noxious stimuli, or following deep inspiration. The absence of response has been associated to axonal unmyelinated peripheral neuropathies [45]. More recently, the measurement of electrochemical skin conductance (Sudoscan) is an easy-use alternative that could have its role in future studies on CINP [46]. Parasympathetic function is assessed by measuring the variability of the R-R interval of heart's beat by different maneuvers (normal breathing, Valsalva, stand up). It requires more complex neurophysiological setting and the clinical relevance in CINP is still to be investigated.

7. Other non-neurophysiological techniques for early detection of CIPN

Skin biopsy allow us to examine directly under microscopy the free sensory nerve endings at skin. This is a well-recognize technique to quantify axonal damage occurring in sensory fibers with a minimal invasive punch biopsy. It provides support for diagnosing small fiber neuropathy [47] and is considered an early marker of more generalized (large and small) sensory polyneuropathy such us diabetic polyneuropathy. It makes skin biopsy presumably useful for early detection and monitoring patients receiving chemotherapy. Although a significant reduction in intraepidermal nerve fiber density has been reported by some authors after receiving oxaliplatin [42, 48], others have found cutaneous innervation more preserved [49]. In our experience, even when many patients show functional loss of small fibers (higher warm and cold detection thresholds at feet), the intraepidermal nerve fibers density seems to be partially preserved. Indeed, the rationale to less vulnerability of small neurons at DRG or higher capability to reinnervate the terminal small nerve fibers in contrast to myelinated receptors and fibers is still open.

Neuroimage is becoming available in different ways for providing signs of neurotoxicity in CIPN. Information by using these techniques is limited to few studies so far. Nerve high resolution ultrasound served to identify an increase in the cross-sectional area meaning a nerve enlargement at upper and lower limbs in patients receiving oxaliplatin [50] and taxanes [51]. By using magnetic resonance neurography has been also reported a significant hypertrophy of DRG [52] whereas other nerves, sciatic nerve, remain normal. In addition, changes at central nervous system, in dorsal columns at spinal cord, has been reported in patients affected by thalidomide-induced CIPN [53, 54].

Molecular biomarkers may also have a role in early detection of CIPN. They are in different categories, from pharmacogenomics to surrogate markers of neurotoxicity. Unfortunately, none has been established in clinical practice because of lack of large-scale and validation studies. The majority of genetic variants which has been candidates to indicate higher susceptibility of neurotoxicity showed controversial results (for example, see recent reviews [55, 56]. More is known about other molecules reflecting nerve damage which are available at blood analysis such us neurofilaments. Neurofilament light chain (NfL) is a cytoskeletal neuron-specific protein which has found increased after receiving vincristine and oxaliplatin [57]. Nerve Growth Factor (NGF) levels were also find higher in painful CIPN whereas they remained stable in patients with painless or absent CIPN [49]. Other metabolic parameters such us low hemoglobin or vitamin D levels or higher gamma-glutamyl transferase (GGT) have been identified as independent predictors associated to CIPN [58].

8. When CIPN is supposed to be resolved? Indicators of recovery

This is the main question in patient's mind which is difficult to answer. It depends on many factors, specially the severity of axonal loss at maximum of the neurotoxic effect of the drug. Complete recovery is calculated in about 40% of patients at 8–12 months after discontinuation of oxaliplatin whereas in almost 35% of patients is estimated to be persistent more than 5 years [59, 60]. Lower incidence has been reported for cisplatin which is estimated in 20% of patients at 12 months after therapy [27]. Patients treated with taxanes experience symptomatic sensory neuropathy distally at fingertips in hands and feet. It has been estimated in more than 70% of patients, being persistent in most of them longer than 5 years in some series [61]. Vincristine-induced neuropathy in pediatric population combines sensory and motor symptoms that are persistent in 27% of patients 2 years after treatment [62]. No correlation has been established between time until recovery and any clinical or neurophysiological parameter as far as I know. However, it is possible to said that low amplitudes at sensory nerve action potentials make prognosis for recovery very poor despite intraepidermal nerve fibers are partially preserved (personal observation).

9. Neuroprotection and other recommendations

Neuroprotectants have limited beneficial effects for preventing CIPN. The first step is to modify the chemotherapy regimen, such as dose reduction and longer interval between cycles, especially platinum agents like oxaliplatin or cisplatin and vincristine [63]. This is necessary in approximately 40% of patients based on average from different reports [64].

The intend to reduce oxidative-stress and the up-regulation of pro-inflammatory cytokines due to chemotherapy have led many authors to test antioxidant therapy. This is the case of vitamin B6, vitamin E and alpha-lipoic acid among others. Despite of contradictory results reported until now in different trials (see a recent review, [65]), the easiness to acquire these products for patients and their natural origin, most of them nutritional supplements, makes them a good choice in poor symptomatic CIPN or intermittent therapy between cycles of chemotherapy. Other pharmacological products such as the amifostine, glutathione, calcium/magnesium, minocycline or mangafodipir need further research.

Symptomatic treatment with antiepileptic drugs (pregabalin, gabapentin, oxcarbazepine) or antidepressants (duloxetine, amitriptyline) is recommended at low dose with a progressive increase until partial or total alleviation of sensory symptoms.

Regular exercise and lifestyle interventions help to prevent inactivity and improve body mass index [66]. Regular aerobic exercise training (30 minutes/day or 4 hours/week) and daily walking activity between 8000 to 10000 steps/day during 5 days/week are recommended (see https://www.foundationforpn.org). Indeed, they contribute to sensory and motor rehabilitation, improve self-confidence to walk previously diminished because of sensory loss in CIPN. Sensory feet stimulation with a rubber carpet of different textures as well as hand manipulation of soft tissue or lentils could be a form of manual therapy for neurorehabilitation after receiving chemotherapy treatment. An interdisciplinary team is also recommended to attend needs of persons with CIPN in every oncologic center [67].

10. Conclusion

This chapter reports on clinical assessment of CIPN in such a way to be easily understandable. The number of cancer survivors has been fortunately growing, so complications of neurotoxicity after chemotherapy has become a first order problem for clinicians that are searching a better quality of life for their patients. Mechanisms to produce CIPN are diverse depending of the drug and most of them converge on the same targets. The present manuscript emphasizes a comparison of different type of nerve fibers that lead to a wide spectrum of symptoms, mainly sensory, which are related to axonal damage at different type of nerve fibers. Selective techniques are necessary to detect sensory disfunction which seems to affect early distal vibration and warm perception. No indicators have found to predict patient's recovery so we have to assume that this process is possible, although perhaps partially, in all cases. The future will come to reduce toxic damage by personalized drug plans as well as multidisciplinary professional care to our patients.

Acknowledgements

This publication was supported by a grant from Instituto de Salud Carlos III through the project FI16/00894 (Co-funded by European Regional Development Fund (FEDER).

Conflict of interest

The author declares no conflict of interest.

Author details

Jordi Casanova-Mollà
Department of Neurology, Hospital Clínic of Barcelona, Institut d'Investigació Biomedica Agustí Pi Sunyer (IDIBAPS), University of Barcelona, Catalonia, Spain

*Address all correspondence to: jcasanov@clinic.cat; jcasanovamolla@gmail.com

References

[1] Seretny M, Currie GL, Sena ES, Ramnarine, Grant R, MacLeod MR, Colvin LE, Fallon M. *Incidence, prevalence, and pedictors of chemotherapy-induced peripheral neuropathy: A systematic review and meta-analysis;* Pain 2014; 155: 2461-2470.

[2] Lefaucher JP and Créange A. *Neurophysiological testing correlates with clinical examination according to fibre type involvement and severity in sensory neuropathy*; J Neurol Neurosurg Psychiatry 2004; 75: 417-422.

[3] Staff NP, Cavaletti G, Islam B, Lustberg M, Psimaras D, Tamburin S. *Platinum-induced peripheral neurotoxicity: from pathogenesis to treatment*; J Peripher Nerv Syst 2019; 245 (S2): S26-S39.

[4] Adelsberger H, Quasthoff S, Grosssakreutz J et al. *The chemotherapietuic oxaliplatin alters voltaje-gated (Na+) channel kinetics on rat sensory neurons.* Eur J Pharmacol 2000; 406:25-32.

[5] Heide R, Bostock H, Ventzel L, Grafe P, Bergmans J, Fuglsang-Frederiksen A, Finnerup NB, Tankisi H. *Axonal excitability changes and acute symptoms of oxaliplatin treatment: in vivo evidence for slowed sodium channel inactivation*. Clin Neurophysiol 2018; 129:694-706.

[6] Velasco R and Bruna J. *Oxaliplatin neurotoxicity*. Curr Colorectal Cancer Rep 2014 (online publication June 2014); DOI: 10.1007/s11888-014-0230-9.

[7] Tanishima H, Tominaga T, Kimura M, Maeda T, Shirai Y, Horiuchi T. *Hyperacute peripheral neuropathy is a predictor of oxaliplatin-induced persistent peripheral neuropathy*. Support Care Cancer 2017; 25:1383-1389.

[8] Attal N, Bouhassira D, Gautron M, Vaillant JN, Mitry E, Lepère, rougier P, Guirimand F. *Thermal hyperalgesia as a marker of oxaliplatin neurotoxicity: a prospective quantified sensory assessment study.* Pain 2009; 144:245-252.

[9] Pachman DR, Qin R, Seisler DK, Smith EML, Beutler AS, Ta LE, Lafky JM, Wagner-Johnston ND, Ruddy KJ, Dakhil S, Staff NP, Grothey A, Loprinzi CL. *Clinical course of oxaliplatin-induced neuropathy: results from the randomized phase III trial N08CB*. J Clin Oncol 2015; 33:3416-3422.

[10] Reddy SM, Vergo MT, Paice JA, Kwon N, Helenowski IB, Benson AB, Mulcahy MF, Nimeiri HS, Harden RN. *Quantitative sensory testing at baseline and during cycle 1 oxaliplatin infusion detects subclinical peripheral neuropathy and predicts clinically overt chronic neuropathy in gastrointestinal malignancies.* Clin Colorectal Cancer 2016; 15:37-46.

[11] Eeles R, Tait DM, Peckham MJ. *Lhermitte's sign as a complication of cisplatin-containing chemotherapy for testicular cancer*. Cancer Treat Rep 1986; 70:905-907.

[12] Loprizni CL, Reeves BN, Dakhil SR, Sloan JA, Wolf SL, Burger KN, Kamal A, Le-Lindqwister NA, Soori GS, Jaslowski AJ, Novotny PJ, Lachance. *Natural history of paclitaxel-associated acute pain syndrome: prospective cohort study NCCTG N08C1*. J Clin Oncol 2011; 29:1472-1478.

[13] Krarup-Hansen A, Helweg-Larsen S, Schmalbruch H, Rorth M, Krarup C. *Neuronal involvement in cisplatin neuropathy: prospective clincal and neurophysiological studies.* Brain 2007; 130:1076-1088.

[14] Screnci D, McKeage MJ, Galettis P, Hambley TW, Palmer BD, Baguley BC. *Relationship between hydrophobicity, reactivity, accumulation and peripheral*

nerve toxicity of a series of platinum drugs. Br J Cancer 2000; 82:966-972.

[15] Marini A, Bernardini A, Gigli GL, Valente M, Muñiz-Castrillo S, Honnorat J, Vogrig A. *Neurologic adverse events of immune checkpoint inhibitors: a systematic review*. Neurology 2021; 96:754-766.

[16] Montejo C, Navarro-Otano J, Mayà-Casalprim G, Campolo M, Casanova-Molla J. *Acute lumbar polyradiculoneuropathy as early sign of methtrexate intrathecal neurotoxicity: case report and literature review*. Clin Case Rep 2019; 7:638-643.

[17] Qweider M, Gilsbach JM, Rohde V. *Inadvertent intrathecal vincristine administration: a neurosurgical emergency. Case report*. J Neurosurg Spine 2007; 3:280-283.

[18] Glendenning JL, Barbachano Y, Norman AR, Dearnaley DP, Horwich A, Huddart RA. *Long-term neurologic and peripheral vascular toxicity after chemotherapy treatment of testicular cancer*. Cancer 2010; 116:2322-2331.

[19] Graf WD, Chance PF, Lensch MW, Eng LJ, Lipe HP, Bird TD. Severe vincristine neuropathy in Charcot-Marie-Tooth disease type 1A. Cancer 1996; 77:1356-1362.

[20] de Carvalho Barbosa M, Kosturakis AK, Eng C, Wendelschafer-Crabb G, Kennedy WR, Simone DA, Wang XS, Cleeland CS, Dougherty PM. *A quantitative sensory analysis of peripheral neuropathy in colorectal cancer and its exacerbation by oxaliplatin chemotherapy*. Cancer Res 2014; 74:5955-5962.

[21] Boyette-Davis JA, Eng C, Wang XS, Cleeland CS, Wendelschafer-Crabb G, Kennedy WR, Simone DA, Zhang H, Dougherty PM. *Subclinical peripheral neuropathy is a common finding in colorectal cancer patients prior to chemotherapy*. Clin Cancer Res 2012; 18:3180-3187.

[22] Lanzani F, Mattavelli L, Frigeni B, Rossini F, Cammarota S, Petrò D, Jann S, Cavaletti G. Role of a pre-existing neuropathy on the course of bortezomib-induced peripheral neuropathy. J Peripher Nerv Sys 2008; 13:267-274.

[23] Grunberg SM, Sonka S, Stevenson LL, Muggia FM. *Progressive paresthesias after cessation of therapy with very high-dose cisplatin*. Cancer Chemother Pharmacol 1989; 25:62-64.

[24] Besora S, Santos C, Izquierdo C, Martinez-Villacampa MM, Bruna J, Velasco R. Rechallenge with oxaliplatin and peripheral neuropathy in colorectal cancer patients. J Cancer Res Clin Oncol 2018; 144:1793-1801.

[25] Chaudhry V, Rowinsky EK, Sartorius SE, Donehower RC, Cornblath DR. Peripheral neuropathy from taxol and cisplatin combination chemotherapy clinical and electrophysiological studies. Ann Nerol 1994; 35:304-311.

[26] Chaudhry V, Cornblath DR, Polydefkis M, Ferguson A, Borrello I. *Characteristics of bortezomib- and thalidomide-induced peripheral neuropathy*. J Per Nerv Syst 2008; 13:275-282.

[27] Mollman JE, Hogan WM, Glover DJ, McCluskey. *Unusual presentation of cis-platinum neuropathy*. Neurology 1988; 38:488-490.

[28] Von Schlippe M, Fowler CJ, Harland SJ. *Cisplatin neurotoxicity in the treatment of metastasic germ cell tumour: time course and prognosis*. Br J Cancer 2001; 85:823-826.

[29] Lehcky TJ, Leonard GD, Wilson RH, Grem JL, Floeter MK. *Oxaliplatin-induced neurotoxicity: acute*

hyperexcitability and chronic neuropathy. Muscle Nerve 2004; 29:387-392.

[30] Choi J, Kong K, Mozaffar T, Holcombe RF. *Delayed oxaliplatin-associated neurotoxicity following adjuvant chemotherapy for stage III colon cancer*. Anticancer Drugs 2006; 17:103-105.

[31] National Cancer Institute-Common Terminology Criteria for Adverse Events [Internet]. Available from https://ctep.cancer.gov/protocolDevelopment/adverse_effects.htm

[32] Cavalleti G, Boglium G, Marzorati L, Zincone A, Piatti M, Colombo N, Parma G, Lissoni A, Fei F, Cundari S, Zanna C. *Grading of chemotherapy-induced peripheral neurotoxicity using the Total Neuropathy Scale*. Neurology 2003; 61:1297-1300.

[33] Cavalleti G, Frigeni B, Lanzani F et al; for the Italian NETox Group. *The Total Neuropathy Score as an assessment tool for grading the course of chemotherapy-induced peripheral neurotoxicity: comparison with the National Cancer Institute-Common Toxicity Scale*. J Peripher Nerv Syst 2007; 12:210-215.

[34] Postma TJ, Aaronson NK, Heimans JJ, Muller MJ, Hildebrand JG, Delattre JY, Hoang-Xuan K, Lantéri-Minet M, Grant R, Huddart R, Moynihan C, Maher J, Lucey R, EORTC Quality of Life Group. *The development of an EORTC quality of life questionnaire to assess chemotherapy-induced peripheral neuropathy: the QLQ-CIPN20*. Eur J Cancer 2005; 41:1135-1139.

[35] Preston DC and Shapiro BE. *Basic nerve conduction studies*. In: Electromyography and Neuromuscular Disorders. Clinical-Electrophysiologic correlations. 2nd ed. Elsevier Health Sciences; 2012. 664 p. DOI: 10.1016/B978-1-4557-2672-1.00003-9.

[36] Kokotis P, Schmelz M, Kostouros E, Karandreas N, Dimopoulos MA. *Oxaliplatin-induced neuropathy: a long-term clinical and neurophysiologic follow-up study*. Clin Colorectal Cancer 2016; 15:e133-e140. DOI: 10.1016/j.clcc.2016.02.009.

[37] Isak B, Tankisi H, Pugdahl K, Ventzel L, Finnerup NB, Fuglsang-Frederiksen A. *Neurophysiological assessment of small fiber damage in chemotherapy-induced peripheral neuropathy*. Clin Neurophysiol 2021; 1332:1947-1956.

[38] Bennedsgard K, Ventzel L, Andersen NT, Themistocleous AC, Bennet DL, Jensen TS, Tankisi H, Finnerup NB. *Oxaliplatin and docetaxel induced polyneuropathy: clinical and neurophysiological characteristics*. J Peripher Nerv Syst 2020; 25:377-387.

[39] Iannetti GD, Zambreanu L, Tracey I. *Similar nociceptive afferents mediate psychophysical and electrophysiological responses to heat stimulation of glabrous and hairy skin in humans.* J Physiol 2006; 577:235-248.

[40] Binder A, Stengel M, Maag R, Wasner G, Schoch R, Moosig F, Schommer B, Baron R. *Pain in oxaliplatin-induced neuropathy. Sensitization in the peripheral and central nociceptive system.* Eur J Cancer 2007; 43:2658-2663.

[41] Ventzel L, Madsen CS, Karlsson P, Tankisi H, Isak B, Fuglsang-Frederiksen A, Jensen AB, Jensen AR, Jensen TS, Finnerup NB. *Chronic pain and neuropathy following adjuvant chemotherapy*. Pain Medicine 2018; 19:1813-1824.

[42] Kroigart T, Schroder HD, Qvortrup C, Eckhoff L, Pfeiffer P, Gaist D, Sindrup SH. *Characterization and diagnostic evaluation of chronic polyneuropathies induced by oxaliplatin and docetaxel comparing skin biopsy to quatitative sensory testing and nerve conduction studies.* Eur J Neurol 2014; 21:623-629.

[43] Kroigard T, Svendsen TK, Wirenfeldt M, Schroder HD, Qvortrup C, Pfeiffer P, Gaist D, Sindrup SH. *Early changes in tests of peripheral nerve function during oxaliplatin treatment and their correlation with chemotherapy-induced polyneuropathy symptoms and signs.* Eur J Neurol 2020; 27:68-76.

[44] Delmotte JB, Beaussier H, Auzeil N, Massicot F, Laprévote O, Raymond E, Coudoré F. *Is quantitative sensory testing helpful in the management of oxaliplatin neuropathy? A two-year clinical study.* Cancer Treatment and Research Communications 2018, doi: 10.1016/j.ctarc.2018.10.002.

[45] Shahani BT, Halperin JJ, Boulu P, Cohen J. *Sympathetic skin response: a method of assessing unmyelinated axon dysfunction in peripheral neuropathies.* J Neurol Neurosurg Psy 1984; 47:536-542.

[46] Saad M, Psimaras D, Tafani C, Sallansonnet-Froment M, Calvet JH, Vilier A, Tigaud JM, Bompaire F, Lebouteux M, de Gresian T, Ceccaldi B, Poirier JM, Ferrand FR, Le Moulec S, Huillard O, Goldwasser F, Taillia H, Maisonobe T, Ricard D. *Quick, non-invasive and quantitative assessment of small fiber neuropathy in patients receiving chemotherapy.* J Neurooncol 2016; 127:373-380.

[47] Devigili G, Tugnoli V, Penza P, Camozzi F, Lombardi R, Melli G, Broglio L, Granieri E, Lauria G. *The diagnostic criteria for small fibre neuropathy: from symptoms to neuropathology.* Brain 2008; 131:1912-1925.

[48] Burakgazi AZ, Messersmith W, Vaidya D, Hauer P, Hoke A, Polydefkis M. *Longitudinal assessment of oxaliplatin-induced neuropathy.* Neurology 2011; 77:980-986.

[49] Velasco R, Navarro X, Gil-Gil M, Herrando-Grabulosa M, Calls A, Bruna J. *Neuropathic pain and Nerve Growth Factor in chemotherapy-induced peripheral neuropathy: prospective clinical-pathological study.* J Pain Symptom Manage 2017; 54: 815-825.

[50] Pitarokoili K, Höffken N, Lönneker N, Fisse AL, Trampe N, Gold R, Reinacher-Schick, Yoon MS. *Prospective study of the clinical, electrophysiologic and sonographic characteristics of oxaliplatin-induced neuropathy.* J Neuroimaging 2019; 29:133-139.

[51] Lycan TW, Hsu FG, Ahn CS, Thomas A, Walker FO, Sangueza OP, Shiozawa Y, Park SH, Peters CM, Romero-Sandoval EA, Melin SA, Sorscher S, Ansley K, Lesser GJ, Cartwright MS, Strowd RE. *Neuromuscular ultrasound for taxanes peripheral neuropathy in breast cancer.* Muscle Nerve 2020; 61:587-594.

[52] Apostolidis L, Schwarz D, Xia A, Weller M, Heckel A, Godel T, Heiland S, Schlemmer HP, Jäger D, Bendszus M, Bäumer P. *Dorsal root ganglia hypertrophy as in vivo correlate of oxaliplatin-induced polyneuropathy.* PLoS One 2017; 12(8):e0183845; DOI: 10.1371/journal.pone.0183845.

[53] Giannini F, Volpi N, Rossi S, Passero S, Fimiani M, Cerase A. *Thalidomide-induced neuropathy: a ganglionopathy?* Neurology 2003; 60:877-878.

[54] Isoardo G, Bergui M, Durelli L, Barbero P, Boccadoro M, Bertola A, Ciaramitaro P, Palumbo A, Bergamasco B, Cocito D. *Thalidomide neuropathy: clinical, electrophysiological and neuroradiological features.* Acta Neurol Scand 2004; 109:188-193.

[55] Alberti P. *A review of novel biomarkers and imaging techniques for assessing the severity of chemotherapy-induced peripheral neuropathy.* Expert

Opinion on Drug Metabolism & Toxicology 2020; 16:12, 1147-1158.

[56] Velasco R, Alemany M, Villagrán M, Argyriou AA. *Predictive biomarkers of oxaliplatin-induced peripheral neurotoxicity*. J Pers Med 2021; 11:669. DOI: 10.3390/jpm11070669.

[57] Kim SH, Choi MK, Park NY, Hyun JW, Lee MY, Kim HJ, Jung SK, Cha Y. Serum neurofilament light chain levels as a biomarker of neuroaxonal injury and severity of oxaliplatin-induced peripheral neuropathy. Sci Rep 2020; 10:7995.

[58] Yildirim N, Cengiz M. *Predictive clinical factors of chronic peripheral neuropathy induced by oxaliplatin.* Support Care Cancer 2020; 28:4781-4788.

[59] Pietrangeli A, Leandri M, Terzoli E, Jandolo B, Garufi C. *Persistence of high-dose oxaliplatin-induced neuropathy at long-term follow-up*. Eur Neurol 2006; 56:13-16.

[60] Brouwers EE, Huitema AD, Boogerd W, Beijnen JH, Schellens JH. *Persistent neuropathy after treatment with cisplatin and oxaliplatin*. Acta Oncol 2009; 48:832-841.

[61] Boyette-Davis J, Cata JP, Driver LC, Novy DM, Bruel BM, Mooring DL, Wendelschafer-Crabb G, Kennedy WR, Dougherty. *Persistent chemoneuropathy in patients receiving the plant alkaloids paclitaxel and vincristine.* Caner Chemother Pharmacol 2013; 71:619-626.

[62] Nama N, Barker MK, Kwan C, Sabarre C, Solimano V, Rankin A, Raabe J, Ross CJ, Carleton B, Zwicker JG, Rod Rassekh S. *Vincristine-induced peripheral neurotoxicity: a prospective cohort.* Ped Hem Oncol 2020; 37:15-28.

[63] Loprinzi CL, Lacchetti C, Bleeker J. *Prevention and management of chemotherapy-induced peripheral neuropathy in survivors of adult cancers: ASCO Guideline Update*. J Clin Oncol 2020; 14:01399.

[64] Hertz DL, Dockter TJ, Satele DV, Loprinzi CL, Le-Rademacher J. Neuropathy severity at the time of oxaliplatin treatment alteration in patients with colon cancer (Alliance A151912). Support Care Cancer 2021; Onlie ahead of print. DOI: 10.1007/s00520-021-06371-x.

[65] Starobova H, Vetter I. Pathophysiology of chemotherapy-induced peripheral neuropathy. Front Mol Neurosci 2017; 10:174.

[66] Tofthagen CS, Cheville AL, Loprinzi CL. *The physical consequences of chemotherapy-induced peripheral neuropathy.* Curr Oncol Rep 2020; 22:50.

[67] Tofthagen C, Visovsky C, Eckelman E, Clatterbuck B, Leggatt M, Buck H. *Starting a nurse-led clinic for patients with peripheral neuropathy.* Nursing 2018; 48:39-42.

Chapter 7

Neurotoxicity and Epileptogenesis

Carmen Rubio, Artemio Rosiles-Abonce, Elisa Taddei and Moisés Rubio-Osornio

Abstract

Many neurotoxic substances produce toxic effects on the nervous system. Given the neurotoxic substances found in the human body, certain people have been regarded as having a propensity to epileptic seizures. In many situations, the neurotransmission processes of these toxins are similar to the physiopathology of epilepsy. Epileptic models have been developed to induce seizures in animals, allowing researchers to study convulsive seizure mechanisms. Pentylenetetrazol, kainic acid, pilocarpine, penicillin, aluminum, bicuculline, picrotoxine, 4-aminopyridine, strictine, domoic acid, and other compounds fall under this category. However, there are some drugs used in clinical practice that can cause neurotoxicity as well. In this chapter, the predominant substances and drugs involved in epileptogenesis through neurotoxicity effects are reviewed. Throughout this chapter, we attempt to describe the mechanisms documented in the literature, in which epileptic seizures cause neurotoxicity in the brain by themselves, as shown with excitotoxicity mediated by glutamate and ions involved.

Keywords: Epilepsy, Epileptogenesis, Neurotoxic substances, Seizures

1. Introduction

The concept of toxicity refers to any substance capable of producing harm on livings organism. Hence, this chapter emphasizes on those compounds that harm the nervous system, particularly those capable of generating seizures. Within the pathophysiology of epilepsy, multiple mechanisms favor epileptogenesis, one of which is neurotoxicity. These excitotoxic mechanisms can exert their action through the glutamate receptors N-methyl-D-aspartate (NMDA); α-amino-2-3-dihydro-5-methyl-3-oxo-4-isoxazolepropionic acid (AMPA) and kainate, opening ionic channels permeable to calcium ($Ca2^+$), sodium ions (Na^+), that participate significantly in the neuronal damage derived from the excitotoxic effects. Though there are spontaneous inducers of epilepsy, different models that replicate seizures have been created to better understand the mechanisms underlying epileptic seizures. These models promote neurotoxicity in the brain and are triggered by certain substances, primarily agonists or antagonists of neurotransmitters involved in epileptic activity. In this review we aim to illustrate the neurotoxic potency of numerous agents administered in the brain with neurotoxic qualities, including medications used in clinical practice that can generate neurotoxicity.

Epileptic seizures, according to the World Health Organization, are defined as a neurological, chronic, recurrent, and repetitive condition of paroxysmal phenomena caused by an excessive abnormal discharge of groups of neurons, which can occur in different parts of the brain [1]. It is the result of synchronous electrical discharge from a group of hyper-excitable neurons, that when repeated consequently leads to neurotoxicity This hyperexcitability is due to an imbalance between the inhibitory processes given mainly by gamma-aminobutyric acid (GABA) and the excitatory ones of glutamate, which consequently modifies the function of ion channels regulated by Ca^{2+}, Na^{+}, and potassium (K^{+}) mainly, which finally play a crucial role between the timing and propagation of abnormal discharges, contributing to the epileptic process [2]. Glutamate release activates NMDA ionotropic receptors, causing a rapid entry of Na^{+} and a slow entry of Ca^{2+}. In epileptic seizures, with this massive entry of Ca^{2+}, there is an increase of mitochondrial Ca^{2+} producing, among other effects an excitotoxic effect, in addition to free radicals production, proteases activation, and synthesis of nitric oxide which, by acting as a retrograde messenger, enhances the excitotoxic effect on the cell by also increasing glutamate release from the presynaptic terminals [3]. This glutamate release also activates the AMPA receptors associated with non-voltage-dependent channels, responsible for depolarizing currents, due to the Na^{+} input. AMPA receptor antagonists are known to have been shown to markedly reduce or decrease epileptic activity [4].

Kainic acid (KA) glutamate agonist acts on glutamatergic receptors with a high affinity for KA which is associated with a Na^{+} ion channel, this depolarization in turn causes Na^{+} channels opening, which leads to Ca^{2+} channels aperture that further increases neuron excitability. Na^{+} channels' participation in epileptogenesis and their mutations in many epileptic disorders has been long studied. The Na^{+} channels classified as type Nav 1.1 and Nav 1.6 are over-expressed in mice administered NMDA, which leads to hyperexcitability. However, when these animals are given phenytoin Na^{+} channel blocker, electrographic excitability decreases. Ion involvement has been described as vital in seizures [5]. The neurotoxic effect of KA appears to exert its action on non-NMDA receptors, located in the postsynaptic region at the dendrites of neurons level or by acting on presynaptic ionotropic glutamate receptors (NMDA, AMPA, and kainate) [6, 7]. Other glutamate receptors are also activated, predominantly found in the membrane of neurons, performing an excitatory response to the cell that presents them. When acting on the cell, there are even injuries to the cytoplasmic membrane, cytoplasmic vacuolization, and edema in the mitochondria, which finally cause cell death [8]. Kainate Glutamate stimulates postsynaptic AMPA receptors. This depolarization is immediately reduced by the GABA receptor recurrent inhibition [9].

Activation of AMPA receptors, particularly NMDA receptors, triggers intracellular Ca^{2+} cascades. Ca^{2+} permeability studies indicate that there is also a low permeability of this ion through kainate receptors [10, 11]. Excessive Ca^{2+} intake, derived from a pathological condition such as epilepsy, contributes to an excitotoxic effect and subsequent neuronal death [12].

In epileptic seizures, glutamate elevation and GABA release are observed from the presynaptic terminals within the synaptic cleft. Astrocytes recapture these abnormally released neurotransmitters during the seizure, protecting neurons from excitotoxicity and eliminating excess glutamate. It is known that, derived from the epileptic processes, there is hypertrophy and significant changes in the ramifications and volume of the astrocyte soma. These changes undoubtedly impact the reuptake of neurotransmitters such as glutamate, allowing an excess of this in the synaptic space [13, 14].

It is worth noting that epilepsy research is so broad that despite not managing to control the neuropathology, some authors have claimed that studying the disease has allowed neuroscience to investigate more than just seizure disorders, but the brain regions not directly implicated in epilepsy, as well. This chapter, however, will concentrate only on epilepsy-related neurotoxicity.

2. Calcium channels and epilepsy

When Ca^{2+} enters, it produces hyperexcitability in the excitable neuron through voltage-dependent Ca^{2+} channels (VDCCs). Intracellular processes are initiated when Ca^{2+} enters the cell, such as membrane excitability regulation, which permits neurotransmitters to be released. The biophysical and pharmacological properties of six types of Ca^{2+} channels (T, L, N, P, Q, and R) have been characterized. Low-threshold channels have been classed as T-type channels, while the rest have been classified as high-threshold channels. The number of depolarizations required for their activation has led to this classification. All channels have four subunits referred to as I through IV, each of which is made up of six transmembrane segments referred to as S1, S2, S3, S4, S5, and S6. The N, P and Q type channels are particularly crucial in controlling the release of neurotransmitters like glutamate and GABA, which, as previously stated, play a key role in epilepsy. The fact that a decrease in extracellular Ca^{2+} concentration can cause hyperexcitability in neurons is evidence that VDCCs play a major role in the epileptic activity [15]. In epilepsy, this correlates with paroxysmal depolarizations. Which correlates with paroxysmal depolarizations in epilepsy. This phenomenon has been observed in the hippocampus's neurons and dendrites, particularly in the CA1 and CA3 neuroanatomical, critical regions in epileptic seizures. Ca^{2+} currents have been demonstrated to promote the development of epileptic seizures; this is thought to be due to an increase in postsynaptic responses triggered by excessive excitement, which then initiates an epileptic seizure. However, this type of activity also leads to neuronal death.

Epileptic activity can also be triggered by the input of extracellular Ca^{2+} into the neuron, which promotes neuronal membrane depolarization and action potential production, resulting in abnormal discharges and seizures. The rise in intracellular Ca^{2+} in the postsynaptic neuron has been linked to various factors that produce epileptogenesis, including persistent depolarization, inducing neurotoxicity. Animal models in mice (tottering, du-du, or stargazer) in which genes coding for Ca^{2+} channel subunits formation have been altered and made it possible to illustrate the role of Ca^{2+} in epileptogenesis, implying that channelopathies may be part of the substrate for abnormal activity. Because Ca^{2+} plays such a role in abnormal epileptic activity, drugs like ethosuximide have been developed to block T-type Ca^{2+} channels by reducing Ca^{2+} entry. Hence, neurotransmitter release is implicated in neuronal excitability [16–19].

3. Molecular signaling pathways for epileptogenesis

This chapter proposes several molecular signaling pathways that are involved in epileptogenesis. We described the most representative pathways in the epileptogenesis study. Until now, the complicated epileptogenesis pathophysiology and molecular processes that lead to seizures have remained a mystery. However, various anatomical pathways mechanisms, pathological pathways, and molecular interactions are known and have been explored based on the research available. Inhibitory and excitatory neurotransmission abnormalities have a big impact on neuron stability. Neuroinflammation and oxidative stress, for example, encourage the emergence of epileptic seizures and can potentially intensify them [20].

It has been claimed that the inflammatory state, and the elevation of its mediators, including IL-1ß, IL-6, high mobility group box TNF-α8, and cyclooxygenase-2. TNF-α produces endocytosis of GABA receptors through AMPA. Therefore, hyperexcitability in the hippocampus is boosted, resulting in seizures. Several studies have linked neuroinflammation to oxidative stress at the same time. The involvement of oxidative stress as a seizure generator is owing to an imbalance in the generation of reactive oxygen and nitrogen species, resulting in a deficiency in antioxidant mechanisms. The mitochondria are the body's principal generator of oxygen radicals [21]. Other free radicals, including nicotinamide adenine dinucleotide phosphate oxidase and xanthine oxidase, have been shown to act through glutamate receptors. The activation of the NMDA receptor is linked to epileptic activity [22].

Another pathway described in the study of epileptogenesis is the *Wnt* / β-Catenin pathway. *Wnt*/β-catenin is implicated in temporal lobe epilepsy. This pathway modulates, among other events, neuronal circuit formation and synaptic assemblages. Brain areas involved in epileptogenesis also play a key role in neuronal excitability modulation and neurotransmitter secretion. *Wnt* proteins dock with membrane receptors to initiate one of two major signal pathways: the canonical β-catenin pathway or the non-canonical pathway. β-catenin pathway manages transcriptional activity regulation and gene activation through the T-cell factor/ lymphoid enhancing factor pathway (TCF / LEF), that dictates cell determination, proliferation, and differentiation. *Wnt1*, *Wnt*3a, *Wnt*7a, and *Wn*t8 are most commonly found in β-catenin-dependent signaling. When one of these proteins binds to lipoprotein-related protein receptors, they lead to selective activation of the canonical pathway. Therefore, β-catenin dissociates from the degradation complex composed of axin, adenomatous polyposis coli protein (APC), casein kinase 1 (CK1), and glycogen synthase kinase 3 β (GSK3β). This promotes the accumulation of β-catenin in the cytosol, which is then translocated to the nucleus and associated with transcription factors of the TCF/LEF family to regulate *Wn*t-dependent gene expression. In the absence of the Fzd receptor by *Wnt*, the Axin and APC proteins boost phosphorylation of β-catenin through the kinases CK1 and GSK3-β. These proteins promote the ubiquitination and subsequent degradation of β-catenin by the proteasome [23].

Notoginsenoside R1 (NGR1, was recently discovered to upregulate mRNA levels of the proteins β-catenin, Dvl, and Fzd, as well as promote the proliferation of cultured cortical neurons. NGR1 has also been discovered to reduce persistent K^+ currents in hippocampus neurons, resulting in a reduced peak threshold. Treatment with a Wnt3a ligand, which activates the FZD receptor, caused K^+ channel internalization and enhanced β-catenin expression, according to a recent study. GSK-3β inhibition caused by *Wnt*/β-catenin activation resulted in a lack of phosphorylation of GSK on the surface of K^+ channels, resulting in internalization. This action lowers the current density of K^+ channels, preventing them from acting as hyperexcitability regulators. The non-canonical route refers to pathways that do not rely on β-catenin-TCF/LEF and instead rely on alternative downstream effectors to produce a transcription response. The *Wnt* /PCP (planar cell polarity) pathway, via *Wnt*-cGMP/Ca^{2+}, via *Wnt*/Via Ror, via *Wnt*-RYK, and via *Wn*t-mTOR are some of these pathways. Epileptogenesis has been linked to the mTOR signaling pathway. *Wnt*7a, a *Wnt* family ligand, is expressed in cerebellar granule cells and operates as a particular canonical signaling activator. *Wnt*7a is expressed in the developing hippocampus as well, particularly in the dentate gyrus and CA1 regions, as indicated by an increase in active β-catenin immunofluorescence after recombinant *Wnt*7a was applied. Other studies have shown that *Wnt*7a has a role in synapse formation, with an increase in the number of vesicular glutamate transporters puncta per dendritic area after hippocampal neurons were treated with recombinant *Wn*t7a, resulting in an increase in excitatory neurotransmitter. *Wnt*8a is also involved in synaptic terminal excitability modulation. Additionally, it is also involved in the regulation of synaptic terminal excitability. These findings show that *Wnt* impacts synaptic regions important in excitatory neurotransmitter release control and regulation and ligand-gated ion channels in the postsynaptic membrane via canonical activation. These physiological changes on the synaptic terminal of hippocampus neurons may play a role in the temporal lobe epilepsy pathophysiological pathway. The aforementioned is attributed to synaptic transmission imbalances between inhibitory and excitatory synapses [24].

In a previous study, a significant increase in β-catenin signaling in the cerebellar cortex of rats after kindling-induced generalized seizures was observed. β-catenin activation induces apoptosis through the expression of cMyc upregulation, a protein that negatively regulates anti-apoptotic proteins such as Bcl-2. This leads to a loss of mitochondria, membrane potential, releasing cytochrome-c and promoting activation of caspases 3 and 9, leading to neuronal death. The *Wnt*/β-catenin pathway participates not only in neuronal synchrony regulation. But also in NMDA receptor modulation, which, as previously described, plays an important role not only in epilepsy but also in epileptogenesis [25, 26].

4. Toxic substances that cause seizures

Exposure to toxins can trigger seizures due to their damaging effect on the nervous system through different mechanisms (**Table 1**). The ability of organophosphate insecticides to induce epileptic seizures is known through the inhibition of acetylcholinesterase due to its chemical structure that contain the groups carbamoyl and thiocarbamoyl, due to its capacity to phosphorylate and inactivate acetylcholinesterase and in addition to stimulating cholinergic receptors, these pesticides include parathion, chlorpyrifos, aldicarb, and carbaryl. Certain toxins present a dual mechanism for epileptic seizures production through the facilitation of the activation and the inhibition of voltage-gated Na^+ channels, how is the case for chemical and biological warfare agents like sarin and soman, as well as toxins such as scorpion venom and ciguatoxin that can lead to seizures by modulating ion flow through Na^+ channels. In other instance, anatoxin is a potent agent that causes seizures by the nicotinic receptor activation. The imbalance in inhibitory and excitatory neurotransmission is one of the mechanisms by which seizures occur. Par excellence GABA is the inhibitory neurotransmitter and glutamate is the excitatory neurotransmitter in the CNS, seizures are triggered by the activation of glutamate receptors by kainic acid and domoic acid, cyanide and azide both display the same process after cellular damage. Interference with the inhibition produced by GABA can trigger epileptic events, GABA receptor inhibition is caused by lindane, picrotoxin, strychnine, and tetramethylenedisulfotetramine [27–29].

Toxic substance	Mechanism
Parathion, chlorpyrifos, aldicarb, and carbaryl	Inhibiting acetylcholinesterase and hyperstimulation of cholinergic receptors
Sarin, soman, scorpion venom and ciguatoxin	Modulating ion flow through voltage-gated sodium channels
Anatoxin	Nicotinic receptor activation
Kainic acid and domoic acid	Activation of glutamate receptors
Lindane, picrotoxin and strychnine	GABA receptor inhibition

Table 1.
Toxic substances that can trigger seizures and their exerting mechanism.

5. Drugs associated with seizures

The administration of different drugs used therapeutically can predispose to epileptic seizures presence either by lowering the epileptogenic threshold, intoxication, or overdose of these. The main groups of antimicrobials that can cause seizures are beta-lactams, anti-tuberculous, and antimalarials. The pro epileptogenic effect of beta-lactams is related to high doses or their toxicity. Seizures related to drugs used to treat tuberculosis are mainly due to vitamin B6 deficiency. Mefloquine and chloroquine are reported antimalarial drugs that can lead to seizures. The proconvulsive effect of methylxanthines is thought to be due to A1 adenosine receptor inhibition. Paradoxically, it is known that carbamazepine can worsen generalized-onset seizures. As well as the withdrawal effect of benzodiazepines, which in some cases can lower the seizure threshold [30–34]. **Table 2** summarizes the main drugs associated with seizures. The following part reviews some of the toxic effects of the main antiepileptic drugs used in clinical practice.

5.1 Valproic acid

Since 1978, valproic acid or Na^+ valproate has been characterized as an antiepileptic drug that suppresses the neuronal excitation of different types of epilepsy, such as partial seizures and generalized seizures [35]. It appears that valproic acid exerts its inhibition by blocking the reuptake of the neurotransmitter GABA, the main inhibitory neurotransmitter. It also lowers glutamate levels and modifies K^+ conductance [36], exerting an inhibition through the voltage-dependent Na^+ channels. In this way, it reduces the excitement caused by epileptic seizures [37]. Once this drug reaches the central nervous system (CNS), it binds to plasma proteins and is distributed throughout the extracellular space [38]. It is metabolized in the liver and discharged through the urine. Although it is also eliminated with expirations in the form of CO2 [39]. However, this drug is known to have frequent toxic effects derived from the therapeutic dose in patients with toxic plasma levels greater than 120 μg/ml [40]. After an overdose, the patient may be lethargic and coma, most likely due

Category	Drugs associated with seizures
Sympathomimetics	Phenylephrine, pseudoephedrine, and anorexiants
Analgesics	Opioids
Anticancer drugs	Interferon alfa, methotrexate, mitoxantrone, nelarabine, platinum-based, cisplatin, vinblastine, vincristine, busulfan, chlorambucil, cytarabine, doxorubicin, etoposide, and fluorouracil
Antimicrobials	Carbapenems, cephalosporins, fluoroquinolones, isoniazid, and penicillin
Hypoglycemics	Any antidiabetic that causes hypoglycemia
Immunosuppressants	Cyclosporine, mycophenolate, tacrolimus, and azathioprine
Psychopharmaceuticals	Monoamine oxidase inhibitors, selective serotonin reuptake inhibitors, serotonin-norepinephrine reuptake inhibitors, serotonin modulators, tricyclic antidepressants, antipsychotics, atomoxetine, bupropion, buspirone, and lithium
Stimulants	Amphetamines and methylphenidate
Xanthine	Aminophylline and theophylline
Antiepileptics	Carbamazepine and benzodiazepines

Table 2.
Main drugs associated with drugs.

to inhibition produced in the CNS [41]. Another adverse situation that derives from the consumption of this antiepileptic drug is cerebral edema, probably caused by the overstimulation of the stimulation of NMDA receptors [42]. Cardiovascular alterations such as hypotension with tachycardia, gastric alterations such as pancreatitis, and hepatotoxicity have manifested with elevated transaminases, jaundice, and abdominal pain with inflammation, among others, may also occur [43].

5.2 Phenobarbital

Phenobarbital belongs to the family of barbiturates. These are characterized by providing the central nervous system with a depressant effect depending on the administered dose [44]. Its anticonvulsant mechanism is based on increasing the inhibitory activity of GABA, binding to the GABA receptor, and facilitating even more inhibitory neurotransmission. This inhibition reduces ATP levels, which causes the opening of Ca^{2+} channels associated with the NMDA receptor, coupled with the fact that a prolonged opening of these Ca^{2+} would lead to excitotoxic neuronal death [45]. The anticonvulsant dose ranges between 10 and 40 μg/ml. The administration of these doses and higher ones generates toxicity that is generally due to the increase in Ca^{2+} entry into the neuron [46]. Mitochondria are an intracellular target of barbiturates since they depolarize the mitochondrial membrane by inhibiting complex one of the electron transports chains and, furthermore, they could have an uncoupling effect on oxidative phosphorylation [47]. Its absorption of phenobarbital is gastric, which generates a decrease in peristaltic tone. Although it is metabolized in the liver and discharged through the kidneys and urine, it has a great fat solubility that crosses cell membranes, producing several alterations [48].

5.3 Carbamazepine

Carbamazepine is a mainly antiepileptic psychotropic drug whose mechanism of action is based on reducing glutamate release, reducing the permeability of neuronal membranes to Na^+ and K^+ ions, stabilizing neuronal membranes, and depressing dopamine and norepinephrine turnover, though an inhibitory effect on muscarinic and nicotinic receptors is also known [49]. When its therapeutic plasma concentrations are higher than 10 μg/ml, it produces toxic effects initially characterized by tachycardia, hypotension and hypertension, lethargy, ataxia, dysarthria, and nystagmus can occur, there are also gastric alterations such as vomiting and nausea. When intoxication is severe, it could even cause a coma [50]. Carbamazepine absorption is digestive, metabolized in the liver where it can cause liver dysfunction and, as its elimination is via the kidneys, adverse effects can also occur in this way [51].

5.4 Phenytoin

Phenytoin has been the most commonly used antiepileptic drug for patients with focal and generalized epilepsies since 1938 [52]. Its mechanism of action is exerted by inactivating voltage-gated Na^+ channels. It also acts by inhibiting the flow of Ca^{2+} through neuronal membranes, such as it is to be expected at the cardiac level, it also inhibits Na^+ channels, which is why it has toxic effects on the myocardium [53]. Phenytoin is bound to plasma proteins, such as albumin, which is metabolized in the liver, so it can cause liver diseases. Toxic effects are present even if the patient has adequate therapeutic levels, like at concentrations lower than 20 mg/Kg [54, 55]. Among the clinical toxic effects, patients may present nystagmus, ataxia, and numbness [56]. With more severe intoxications, in addition to the above: dysarthria, ataxia, the patient might not be able to walk, and may present hyperreflexia, besides consciousness usually being inhibited [57]. With higher doses, patients may even display a coma [58].

5.5 Lamotrigine

Lamotrigine is an antiepileptic drug principally used for generalized and partial seizures; it is also used in the adjunctive treatment of refractory crises [59]. Its action mechanism at the cellular level is based on blocking excitatory neurotransmitters, especially glutamate, through its NMDA receptors, as well as inhibiting voltage-dependent Na^+ currents [60]. The toxic effects on patients who take this drug above 600 mg are characterized primarily at the CNS level by difficulty in concentration, showing dysarthria, nystagmus, and blurred or double vision. Patients may even present a loss of balance or coordination [61]. Its absorption is intestinal, its elimination in the urine, metabolized in the liver. Thus, there is idiosyncratic hepatotoxicity that commonly requires liver transplantation [62].

5.6 Oxcarbazepine

Oxcarbazepine is a derivative of carbamazepine, approved as an antiepileptic drug in America in 2000 [63]. This drug is used in the treatment of any type of epileptic seizure. The cellular mechanism by which it exerts its antiepileptic effects is based on the fact that it blocks voltage-gated Na^+ channels, modulates the activity of Ca^{2+} channels, and increases K^+ conductance, which consequently produces a stabilization of hyperexcited neuronal membranes for epileptic seizures [64]. Oxcarbazepine is a drug that is metabolized like other antiepileptic drugs by the liver and excreted by the kidney [65]. Toxic effects when daily doses are above 30 mg/kg are basically characterized by gastric alterations: mainly nausea and vomiting. The alterations in the CNS are identified by headache, fatigue, drowsiness, and ataxia. It has also been reported that some patients may have vertigo and hyponatremia [66].

5.7 Ethosuximide

Ethosuximide is an anticonvulsant used to reduce the frequency of absence-type seizures. It exerts its mechanism by reducing Ca^{2+} currents antagonized by the T-type Ca^{2+} channels. Furthermore, linked to this drug, modulation of the function of voltage-activated Na^+ channels and Na^+/K^+ dendritic hyperpolarization-activated cyclic nucleotide-gated channel 1 channels has been suggested. It also reduces neuronal excitability by inhibiting the Na^+/K^+ pump [67]. However, ethosuximide is almost entirely absorbed in the digestive tract and metabolized in the liver, which can cause liver disease. The toxic effects of patients who consume above 25 mg/kg comprise gastric issues, nausea, vomiting, constipation, a state of sedation, headache, decreased alertness, drowsiness, and even comas have been reported at the CNS level [68]. Other adverse effects may include weight loss, as well as leukopenia [69].

5.8 Gabapentin

Gabapentin acts mainly by inhibiting partial and generalized seizures. Its mechanism of action is based on enhancing the inhibitory action of GABA [70]. A dose above 1,500 mg of gabapentin can cause hepatotoxicity, additionally, coupling various toxic effects like headaches, diplopia, nystagmus, diplopia, even involuntary movements have been described at the CNS level [71].

5.9 Topiramate

Topiramate is a drug used as an antiepileptic drug that acts by inhibiting partial and generalized seizures. Its action mechanism is exerted by blocking Na^+ channels. As an AMPA receptor antagonist, it reduces excitatory neurotransmission, in addition to enhancing the inhibitory action of GABA [72]. Topiramate taken at a dose above 50 mg produces toxic effects, including dizziness. At the CNS level, patients have headaches, drowsiness, decreased concentration, and even confusion. Nevertheless, other anomalies have also been reported [73].

6. Experimental models of epilepsy and neurotoxicity

As noted, before the development of epilepsy, experimental models have been crucial in the further research of a neurological disorder affecting approximately 1% of the worldwide population. Some drugs cause structural and metabolic alterations in the nervous system as demonstrated by experimental epileptic models, culminating in seizure generation [74]. Antiepileptic drugs that are conventionally used in clinical practice have been successfully tested in many of these models, even though certain models have neurotoxic consequences, as we will discuss below.

With the aluminum model, focal seizures are studied by directly applying the substance to the cerebral cortex of the animal under study, where it has been observed that this substance generates dendritic loss, gliosis, loss of GABAergic neurons, and a decrease in glutamate decarboxylase [75, 76]. This model has been used to study antiepileptic drugs including diphenylhydantoin and pentobarbital, both of which have shown positive outcomes in reducing epileptic seizures frequency [77].

Focal seizures have been researched using cobalt powder, which has been applied to the research animal's cortex or thalamus for epileptogenesis as part of the model development. This has reported GABA and glutamate decarboxylase enzyme production decreased, whereas neuronal death has been observed in the hippocampus. This cobalt model has also been suggested to interfere with Ca^{2+} signaling at NMDA glutamate receptors [78–80].

Similarly, using Zinc as an epilepsy model has been associated to neuronal death in the hippocampus, interference with $GABA_A$ receptors, and changes in the synapses of mossy fibers when there is a high concentration of this metal. It has also been observed to interfere with the responses of various receptors, including GABA, NMDA, and AMPA [81, 82]. While kainic acid, as an epileptic model, functions similarly to glutamate. The hippocampus is the most sensitive structure to this agent, with the highest number of receptors reported in the CA3 layer. This epilepsy model is used to examine focal seizures, with the hippocampus being the most sensitive structure to this substance. Changes in neuropeptide Y levels, hippocampus mossy fiber formation and a decrease in GABAB receptors are reported [83–85].

Pentylenetetrazol is used as an epileptic model to research generalized seizures. Shifts in the CA3 layer of the hippocampus, increased voltage in voltage-responsive K^+ receptors, and interactions with GABAA and NMDA receptors have all been documented [86, 87]. The model has been shown to be suppressed by phenytoin and pentobarbital [88, 89]. Flurothyl gas, on the other hand, can cause status epilepticus in laboratory animals. Although this gas has long been utilized to investigate generalized seizures, the exact mechanism through which it causes seizures is yet uncertain. However, alterations in the lipidic membranes of hippocampus, amygdala, and cerebral cortex cells have been reported. A decrease in GABA synthesis and activation of the c-Fos gene have also been reported [90–92].

On the other hand, penicillin, like cobalt, has been utilized as a model for focal seizures in epilepsy research, causing myoclonic seizures. The loss of GABAergic neurons, neuronal death, and an increase in mossy fibers in the hippocampus are the key abnormalities seen in this model [93–95]. While bicuculline is classified as a GABA antagonist, it causes generalized seizures when used. Edema has been found in the astrocytes of the cerebral cortex, where it interacts with Ca^{2+} and K^{+} channels [96, 97]. Tetanus toxin has also been employed as a model of epilepsy because of its effect on seizure induction. There are interactions with inhibitory neurotransmission, synapse formation, exocytosis blocking, and a decrease in GABAergic signaling threshold with this substance [98, 99].

Additionally, pilocarpine affects the muscarinic acetylcholine receptors. The increase in activation of these receptors in the hippocampus characterizes its epileptogenic effect. In experimental animals, it can even cause status epilepticus. Significant damage to nervous system structures has been observed, particularly the entorhinal and piriform cortex, olfactory bulb, amygdala, hippocampus, and thalamus, as well as abnormalities in the function of Na^{+}/K^{+} ATPase and NMDA receptors [100–103].

7. Conclusion

The described above has enabled us to identify the excitotoxic effect induced by epileptic seizures, whether clinical or experimental. Likewise, it illustrated some of the toxic effects of antiepileptic drugs. From what has been illustrated, it is necessary to conduct research that allows offering other therapeutic alternatives to reduce the toxic effects of seizures and pharmacological therapy. The proposal of alternative treatments to treat seizures is essential to boost anti-toxic defense mechanisms. It can be suggested to propose therapies that minimize neuronal death or treatments with substances that activate antiepileptic protein activity, such as the extrinsic and intrinsic *Wnt* pathway stimulation, or molecules that interact with the proteins involved in inflammatory and oxidative processes. The above mentioned could overall help reduce the interactions between the epileptic and pharmacological processes that ulteriorly lead to toxic effects on epileptic patients.

Appendices and nomenclature

NMDA	Glutamate receptors N-methyl-D-aspartate
AMPA	α-amino-2-3-dihydro-5-methyl-3-oxo-4-isoxazolepropionic acid
GABA	Gamma-aminobutyric acid
Ca^{2+}	Calcium
Na^{+}	Sodium ions
K^{+}	Potassium
CNS	Central nervous system
TCF/LEF	T-cell factor / lymphoid enhancing factor pathway
APC	Adenomatous polyposis coli protein
CK1	Casein kinase 1
GSK3β	Glycogen synthase kinase 3 β
NGR1	Notoginsenoside R1
NGR1	Notoginsenoside R1

Author details

Carmen Rubio[1], Artemio Rosiles-Abonce[1], Elisa Taddei[1]
and Moisés Rubio-Osornio[2]*

1 Department of Neurophysiology, National Institute of Neurology and Neurosurgery, Mexico

2 Department of Neurochemistry, National Institute of Neurology and Neurosurgery, Mexico

*Address all correspondence to: ruomon@gmail.com

References

[1] Epilepsy [Internet]. [cited 2021 Aug 21]. Available from: https://www.who.int/news-room/fact-sheets/detail/epilepsy

[2] An Introduction to Epilepsy [Internet] - PubMed [Internet]. [cited 2021 Aug 21]. Available from: https://pubmed.ncbi.nlm.nih.gov/20821849/

[3] Blanke ML, VanDongen AMJ. Activation Mechanisms of the NMDA Receptor. Biol NMDA Recept [Internet]. 2009 Jan 1 [cited 2021 Aug 21];283-312. Available from: https://www.ncbi.nlm.nih.gov/books/NBK5274/

[4] Boison D. New insights into the mechanisms of the ketogenic diet. Curr Opin Neurol [Internet]. 2017 Apr 1 [cited 2021 Aug 21];30(2):187. Available from: /pmc/articles/PMC5409832/

[5] J L, JM M. Kainate receptors in health and disease. Neuron [Internet]. 2013 Oct 16 [cited 2021 Aug 21];80(2):292-311. Available from: https://pubmed.ncbi.nlm.nih.gov/24139035/

[6] Garthwaite J, Garthwaite G. The mechanism of kainic acid neurotoxicity. Nat 1983 3055930 [Internet]. 1983 [cited 2021 Aug 21];305(5930):138-40. Available from: https://www.nature.com/articles/305138a0

[7] Y Y, J B, AJ B, ML M, AY L. Conformational analysis of NMDA receptor GluN1, GluN2, and GluN3 ligand-binding domains reveals subtype-specific characteristics. Structure [Internet]. 2013 Oct 8 [cited 2021 Aug 21];21(10):1788-99. Available from: https://pubmed.ncbi.nlm.nih.gov/23972471/

[8] SS W, S K. Glutamate, glutamate receptors, and downstream signaling pathways. Int J Biol Sci [Internet]. 2013 Sep 22 [cited 2021 Aug 21];9(9):948-59. Available from: https://pubmed.ncbi.nlm.nih.gov/24155668/

[9] MY M, DA R, DM K. Activation of AMPA, kainate, and metabotropic receptors at hippocampal mossy fiber synapses: role of glutamate diffusion. Neuron [Internet]. 1998 [cited 2021 Aug 21];21(3):561-70. Available from: https://pubmed.ncbi.nlm.nih.gov/9768842/

[10] Egebjerg J, Heinemann SF. Ca2+ permeability of unedited and edited versions of the kainate selective glutamate receptor GluR6. Proc Natl Acad Sci U S A [Internet]. 1993 Jan 15 [cited 2021 Aug 21];90(2):755. Available from: /pmc/articles/PMC45744/?report=abstract

[11] L VDB, W V, H K, E VH, W R. Ca(2+)-permeable AMPA receptors and selective vulnerability of motor neurons. J Neurol Sci [Internet]. 2000 Nov 1 [cited 2021 Aug 21];180(1-2):29-34. Available from: https://pubmed.ncbi.nlm.nih.gov/11090861/

[12] Rajakulendran S, Hanna MG. The Role of Calcium Channels in Epilepsy. Cold Spring Harb Perspect Med [Internet]. 2016 Jan 1 [cited 2021 Aug 21];6(1). Available from: /pmc/articles/PMC4691803/

[13] HF B. Glutamate, GABA and epilepsy. Prog Neurobiol [Internet]. 1995 [cited 2021 Aug 21];47(6):477-511. Available from: https://pubmed.ncbi.nlm.nih.gov/8787032/

[14] Traynelis SF, Wollmuth LP, McBain CJ, Menniti FS, Vance KM, Ogden KK, et al. Glutamate Receptor Ion Channels: Structure, Regulation, and Function. Pharmacol Rev [Internet]. 2010 Sep [cited 2021 Aug 21];62(3):405. Available from: /pmc/articles/PMC2964903/

[15] Catterall WA. Voltage-Gated Calcium Channels. Cold Spring Harb Perspect Biol [Internet]. 2011 [cited 2021 Sep 19];3(8):1-23. Available from: /pmc/articles/PMC3140680/

[16] Van Loo KMJ, Schaub C, Pitsch J, Kulbida R, Opitz T, Ekstein D, et al. Zinc regulates a key transcriptional pathway for epileptogenesis via metal-regulatory transcription factor 1. Nat Commun [Internet]. 2015 Oct 26 [cited 2021 Jun 12];6. Available from: https://pubmed.ncbi.nlm.nih.gov/26498180/

[17] Dezsi G, Ozturk E, Stanic D, Powell KL, Blumenfeld H, O'Brien TJ, et al. Ethosuximide reduces epileptogenesis and behavioral comorbidity in the GAERS model of genetic generalized epilepsy. Epilepsia [Internet]. 2013 Apr [cited 2021 Jun 12];54(4):635-43. Available from: https://pubmed.ncbi.nlm.nih.gov/23464801/

[18] Catterall WA, Kalume F, Oakley JC. NaV1.1 channels and epilepsy. Vol. 588, Journal of Physiology. 2010. p. 1849-59.

[19] Bondy SC. Intracellular calcium and neurotoxic events. Neurotoxicol Teratol. 1989 Nov 1;11(6):527-531.

[20] Rowley S, Patel M. Mitochondrial involvement and oxidative stress in temporal lobe epilepsy [Internet]. Vol. 62, Free Radical Biology and Medicine. Elsevier Inc.; 2013 [cited 2020 May 12]. p. 121-31. Available from: http://www.ncbi.nlm.nih.gov/pubmed/23411150

[21] Waldbaum S, Patel M. Mitochondria, oxidative stress, and temporal lobe epilepsy. Vol. 88, Epilepsy Research. 2010. p. 23-45.

[22] Zhu LJ, Chen Z, Zhang LS, Xu SJ, Xu AJ, Luo JH. Spatiotemporal changes of the N-methyl-D-aspartate receptor subunit levels in rats with pentylenetetrazole-induced seizures. Neurosci Lett [Internet]. 2004 Feb 6 [cited 2021 Jun 6];356(1):53-6. Available from: https://pubmed.ncbi.nlm.nih.gov/14746900/

[23] Rosiles A, Rubio C, Trejo C, Gutierrez J, Hernández L, Paz C. Commentary: Participation of Sox-1 Expression and Signaling of β-Catenin in the Pathophysiology of Generalized Seizures in Cerebellum of Rat. CNS Neurol Disord - Drug Targets. 2016;15(1):3-6.

[24] XT L, W M, XB W, Z L, JW Y, Y H, et al. Notoginsenoside R1 Promotes the Growth of Neonatal Rat Cortical Neurons via the Wnt/β-catenin Signaling Pathway. CNS Neurol Disord Drug Targets [Internet]. 2018 Jul 11 [cited 2021 Sep 19];17(7):547-56. Available from: https://pubmed.ncbi.nlm.nih.gov/29992896/

[25] Rubio C, Rosiles-Abonce A, Trejo-Solís C, Rubio-Osornio M, Mendoza C, Custodio V, et al. Increase signaling of Wnt/β-catenin pathway and presence of apoptosis in cerebellum of kindled rats. CNS Neurol Disord - Drug Targets. 2017;16(7).

[26] Rubio C, Luna R, Rosiles A, Rubio-Osornio M. Caloric Restriction and Ketogenic Diet Therapy for Epilepsy: A Molecular Approach Involving Wnt Pathway and KATP Channels. Front Neurol. 2020;11(November):1-17.

[27] Jett DA. Chemical toxins that cause seizures. Neurotoxicology [Internet]. 2012 Dec [cited 2021 Jun 12];33(6): 1473-5. Available from: https://pubmed.ncbi.nlm.nih.gov/23085523/

[28] Jett DA. Neurotoxic Pesticides and Neurologic Effects [Internet]. Vol. 29, Neurologic Clinics. Neurol Clin; 2011 [cited 2021 Jun 12]. p. 667-77. Available from: https://pubmed.ncbi.nlm.nih.gov/21803217/

[29] Assessment UENC for E. Handbook of neurotoxicology. 2009 Mar 15;

[30] Sutter R, Rüegg S, Tschudin-Sutter S. Seizures as adverse events of antibiotic drugs : A systematic review [Internet]. Vol. 85, Neurology. Lippincott Williams and Wilkins; 2015 [cited 2021 Jun 12]. p. 1332-41. Available from: https://pubmed.ncbi.nlm.nih.gov/26400582/

[31] Hitchings AW. Drugs that lower the seizure threshold. Adverse Drug React Bull. 2016 Jun 1;298(1):1151-1154.

[32] Kanner AM. Most antidepressant drugs are safe for patients with epilepsy at therapeutic doses: A review of the evidence [Internet]. Vol. 61, Epilepsy and Behavior. Academic Press Inc.; 2016 [cited 2021 Jun 12]. p. 282-6. Available from: https://pubmed.ncbi.nlm.nih.gov/27236241/

[33] Johannessen Landmark C, Henning O, Johannessen SI. Proconvulsant effects of antidepressants — What is the current evidence? [Internet]. Vol. 61, Epilepsy and Behavior. Academic Press Inc.; 2016 [cited 2021 Jun 12]. p. 287-91. Available from: https://pubmed.ncbi.nlm.nih.gov/26926001/

[34] Grill MF, Maganti RK. Neurotoxic effects associated with antibiotic use: Management considerations. Br J Clin Pharmacol [Internet]. 2011 Sep [cited 2021 Jun 12];72(3):381-93. Available from: https://pubmed.ncbi.nlm.nih.gov/21501212/

[35] N K, K G, A A, PS C, M T. Valproic acid as an antiepileptic drug: Is there a clinical relevance for the epilepsy surgeon? Epilepsy Res [Internet]. 2016 Nov 1 [cited 2021 Aug 21];127:191-4. Available from: https://pubmed.ncbi.nlm.nih.gov/27610748/

[36] Bourin M. Mechanism of Action of Valproic Acid and Its Derivatives. 2020 [cited 2021 Aug 21]; Available from: www.symbiosisonlinepublishing.com

[37] M R, P M, R D, S S, VE R, A V, et al. Valproic Acid and Epilepsy: From Molecular Mechanisms to Clinical Evidences. Curr Neuropharmacol [Internet]. 2019 Dec 28 [cited 2021 Aug 21];17(10):926-46. Available from: https://pubmed.ncbi.nlm.nih.gov/30592252/

[38] MM Z, HL L, LH S, XP C, J L, ZL Z. The pharmacogenomics of valproic acid. J Hum Genet [Internet]. 2017 Dec 1 [cited 2021 Aug 21];62(12):1009-14. Available from: https://pubmed.ncbi.nlm.nih.gov/28878340/

[39] Y G-P, CF T, JK L, JS L, W S, AK B, et al. Valproic acid pathway: pharmacokinetics and pharmacodynamics. Pharmacogenet Genomics [Internet]. 2013 [cited 2021 Aug 21];23(4):236-41. Available from: https://pubmed.ncbi.nlm.nih.gov/23407051/

[40] Diederich M, Chateauvieux S, Morceau F, Dicato M. Molecular and therapeutic potential and toxicity of valproic acid. J Biomed Biotechnol. 2010;2010.

[41] RM N, MG N. Adverse drug reactions induced by valproic acid. Clin Biochem [Internet]. 2013 Oct [cited 2021 Aug 21];46(15):1323-38. Available from: https://pubmed.ncbi.nlm.nih.gov/23792104/

[42] MD S. Valproic acid toxicity: overview and management. J Toxicol Clin Toxicol [Internet]. 2002 [cited 2021 Aug 21];40(6):789-801. Available from: https://pubmed.ncbi.nlm.nih.gov/12475192/

[43] V G, AK M, M K, B S, P G, M K. Valproic acid induced acute liver injury resulting in hepatic encephalopathy- a case report and literature review. J community Hosp Intern Med Perspect [Internet]. 2018 Sep 3 [cited 2021 Aug 21];8(5):311-4. Available from: https://pubmed.ncbi.nlm.nih.gov/30356994/

[44] GM P. Clinical Pharmacology of Phenobarbital in Neonates: Effects, Metabolism and Pharmacokinetics. Curr Pediatr Rev [Internet]. 2016 Feb 1 [cited 2021 Aug 21];12(1):48-54. Available from: https://pubmed.ncbi.nlm.nih.gov/26496779/

[45] N A-M, A S-R, S V, PA F. Neonatal phenobarbital exposure disrupts GABAergic synaptic maturation in rat CA1 neurons. Epilepsia [Internet]. 2018 Feb 1 [cited 2021 Aug 21];59(2):333-44. Available from: https://pubmed.ncbi.nlm.nih.gov/29315524/

[46] Cherian, Thomas S V. Status epilepticus. Ann Indian Acad Neurol [Internet]. 2009 Jul 1 [cited 2021 Aug 21];12(3):140. Available from: https://www.annalsofian.org/article.asp?issn=0972-2327;year=2009;volume=12;issue=3;spage=140;epage=153;aulast=Cherian

[47] Phenobarbital: biopharmacology - PubMed [Internet]. [cited 2021 Aug 21]. Available from: https://pubmed.ncbi.nlm.nih.gov/6990708/

[48] S K, RB S, JT D. Drug absorption. V. Influence of food on oral absorption of phenobarbital in rats. J Pharm Sci [Internet]. 1971 [cited 2021 Aug 21];60(11):1639-41. Available from: https://pubmed.ncbi.nlm.nih.gov/5133911/

[49] J G, M G, SR B. Carbamazepine-related antiepileptic drugs for the treatment of epilepsy - a comparative review. Expert Opin Pharmacother [Internet]. 2016 May 2 [cited 2021 Aug 21];17(7):885-8. Available from: https://pubmed.ncbi.nlm.nih.gov/26999402/

[50] Carbamazepine Toxicity - PubMed [Internet]. [cited 2021 Aug 21]. Available from: https://pubmed.ncbi.nlm.nih.gov/29939629/

[51] L B. Clinical pharmacokinetics of carbamazepine. Clin Pharmacokinet [Internet]. 1978 [cited 2021 Aug 21];3(2):128-43. Available from: https://pubmed.ncbi.nlm.nih.gov/346287/

[52] Gupta M, Tripp J. Phenytoin. Encycl Toxicol Third Ed [Internet]. 2021 Jul 25 [cited 2021 Aug 21];895-7. Available from: https://www.ncbi.nlm.nih.gov/books/NBK551520/

[53] Y Y, ME S, JH P. Phenytoin: mechanisms of its anticonvulsant action. Ann Neurol [Internet]. 1986 [cited 2021 Aug 21];20(2):171-84. Available from: https://pubmed.ncbi.nlm.nih.gov/2428283/

[54] Bochner F, Hooper WD, Tyrer JH, Eadie MJ. Effect of dosage increments on blood phenytoin concentrations. J Neurol Neurosurg Psychiatry [Internet]. 1972 [cited 2021 Aug 21];35(6):873. Available from: /pmc/articles/PMC494195/?report=abstract

[55] J P, Q W, E N, K K. Phenytoin - An anti-seizure drug: Overview of its chemistry, pharmacology and toxicology. Food Chem Toxicol [Internet]. 2020 Aug 1 [cited 2021 Aug 21];142. Available from: https://pubmed.ncbi.nlm.nih.gov/32376339/

[56] A I, BZ H. Phenytoin Toxicity. 2021 [cited 2021 Aug 21]; Available from: https://pubmed.ncbi.nlm.nih.gov/29494051/

[57] JM M, R M, O D. Phenytoin intoxication. South Med J [Internet]. 1991 [cited 2021 Aug 21];84(10):1199-204. Available from: https://pubmed.ncbi.nlm.nih.gov/1925719/

[58] Soderstrom J, Murray L, Little M, Daly FFS. Toxicology case of the month: carbamazepine overdose. Emerg Med J [Internet]. 2006 Nov [cited 2021 Aug 21];23(11):869. Available from: /pmc/articles/PMC2464388/

[59] Lamotrigine. An update of its pharmacology and therapeutic use in

epilepsy - PubMed [Internet]. [cited 2021 Aug 21]. Available from: https://pubmed.ncbi.nlm.nih.gov/8536554/

[60] Betchel NT, Fariba K, Saadabadi A. Lamotrigine. Essence Analg Analg [Internet]. 2021 Aug 6 [cited 2021 Aug 21];306-9. Available from: https://www.ncbi.nlm.nih.gov/books/NBK470442/

[61] G P. Risks associated with lamotrigine prescription: a review and personal observations. Australas Psychiatry [Internet]. 2018 Dec 1 [cited 2021 Aug 21];26(6):640-2. Available from: https://pubmed.ncbi.nlm.nih.gov/29480028/

[62] Lamotrigine | CAS#84057-84-1 | Anticonvulsant | MedKoo [Internet]. [cited 2021 Aug 21]. Available from: https://www.medkoo.com/products/8283

[63] MM K, NA H. Oxcarbazepine, an antiepileptic agent. Clin Ther [Internet]. 2001 [cited 2021 Aug 21];23(5):680-700. Available from: https://pubmed.ncbi.nlm.nih.gov/11394728/

[64] S S. Oxcarbazepine: a review. Seizure [Internet]. 2000 [cited 2021 Aug 21];9(2):75-9. Available from: https://pubmed.ncbi.nlm.nih.gov/10845729/

[65] EJ P, C S, M W-C, DJ M, HM D, W C, et al. Clinical Pharmacogenetics Implementation Consortium Guideline for HLA Genotype and Use of Carbamazepine and Oxcarbazepine: 2017 Update. Clin Pharmacol Ther [Internet]. 2018 Apr 1 [cited 2021 Aug 21];103(4):574-81. Available from: https://pubmed.ncbi.nlm.nih.gov/29392710/

[66] Hu X, Fu X, Jiang A, Yang X, Fang X, Gong G, et al. Multiomic analysis of mice epilepsy models suggest that MIR-21a expression modulates mRNA and protein levels related to seizure deterioration. Genet Res (Camb). 2015 Dec 22;97.

[67] JJ A. Use of antiepileptic drugs in hepatic and renal disease. Handb Clin Neurol [Internet]. 2014 [cited 2021 Aug 21];119:417-32. Available from: https://pubmed.ncbi.nlm.nih.gov/24365310/

[68] H S, M G, J O. Ethosuximide induced macroglossia and oropharyngeal edema. Int J Pediatr Otorhinolaryngol [Internet]. 2021 Jan 1 [cited 2021 Aug 21];140. Available from: https://pubmed.ncbi.nlm.nih.gov/33218689/

[69] T W, P C, J C. Ethosuximide-induced drug reaction with eosinophilia and systemic symptoms with mediastinal lymphadenopathy. Pediatr Dermatol [Internet]. 2019 Jul 1 [cited 2021 Aug 21];36(4):e99-101. Available from: https://pubmed.ncbi.nlm.nih.gov/31132165/

[70] S M, CC L, M U, S E. Pregabalin and gabapentin for pain. BMJ [Internet]. 2020 Apr 28 [cited 2021 Aug 21];369. Available from: https://pubmed.ncbi.nlm.nih.gov/32345589/

[71] KE E, JR C, AM P, L O, KE H. Reports of gabapentin and pregabalin abuse, misuse, dependence, or overdose: An analysis of the Food And Drug Administration Adverse Events Reporting System (FAERS). Res Social Adm Pharm [Internet]. 2019 Aug 1 [cited 2021 Aug 21];15(8):953-8. Available from: https://pubmed.ncbi.nlm.nih.gov/31303196/

[72] Bonifacio SL, VanMeurs K. Neuroprotective Therapies in Infants. Infect Dis Pharmacol. 2019 Jan 1;227-241.

[73] JP R, ALF C. Topiramate-Associated Movement Disorder: Case Series and Literature Review. Clin Neuropharmacol [Internet]. 2020 Jul 1 [cited 2021 Aug 21];43(4):116-20. Available from: https://pubmed.ncbi.nlm.nih.gov/32541330/

[74] Rubio C, Rubio-Osornio M, Retana-Marquez S, Lopez M, Custodio V, Paz C. In Vivo Experimental Models of Epilepsy. Cent Nerv Syst Agents Med Chem [Internet]. 2010 Dec 1 [cited 2020 May 12];10(4):298-309. Available from: http://www.eurekaselect.com/openurl/content.php?genre=article&issn=1871-5249&volume=10&issue=4&spage=298

[75] Jasper HH. E |An. O. Basic Mechanisms of the Epilepsies. Little, Brown and Company, 34 Beacon Street, Boston, Massachusetts 02106; 1969.

[76] Ribak CE, Harris AB, Vaughn JE, Roberts E. Inhibitory, GABAergic nerve terminals decrease at sites of focal epilepsy. Science (80-) [Internet]. 1979 [cited 2021 Jun 6];205(4402):211-4. Available from: https://pubmed.ncbi.nlm.nih.gov/109922/

[77] JS L, V U, LL D, JA F, BJ H. Efficacy of standard anticonvulsants in monkey model with spontaneous motor seizures. Epilepsia [Internet]. 1975 [cited 2021 Aug 21];16(2):301-17. Available from: https://pubmed.ncbi.nlm.nih.gov/1171007/

[78] Borbély S, Dobó E, Czégé D, Molnár E, Bakos M, Szucs B, et al. Modification of ionotropic glutamate receptor-mediated processes in the rat hippocampus following repeated, brief seizures. Neuroscience [Internet]. 2009 Mar 3 [cited 2021 Jun 6];159(1):358-68. Available from: https://pubmed.ncbi.nlm.nih.gov/19154779/

[79] Craig CR, Colasanti BK. GABA receptors, lipids, and gangliosides in cobalt epileptic focus. [Internet]. Vol. 44, Advances in neurology. 1986 [cited 2021 Jun 6]. p. 379-91. Available from: https://europepmc.org/article/med/3010678

[80] Tsuda T, Sugaya A, Ohguchi H, Kishida N, Sugaya E. Protective effects of peony root extract and its components on neuron damage in the hippocampus induced by the cobalt focus epilepsy model. Exp Neurol [Internet]. 1997 [cited 2021 Jun 6];146(2):518-25. Available from: https://pubmed.ncbi.nlm.nih.gov/9270063/

[81] Kapur J, Macdonald RL. Rapid Seizure-Induced Reduction of Benzodiazepine and Zn 2 Sensitivity of Hippocampal Dentate Granule Cell GABA A Receptors. 1997.

[82] Sørensen J, Slomianka L, Christensen J, Zimmer J. Zinc-containing telencephalic connections to the rat striatum: a combined Fluoro-Gold tracing and histochemical study. Exp Brain Res [Internet]. 1990 Feb 1 [cited 2021 Jun 6];105(3):370-82. Available from: http://link.springer.com/10.1007/BF00233037

[83] Furtinger S, Bettler B, Sperk G. Altered expression of GABAB receptors in the hippocampus after kainic-acid-induced seizures in rats. Mol Brain Res [Internet]. 2003 May 12 [cited 2021 Jun 6];113(1-2):107-15. Available from: https://pubmed.ncbi.nlm.nih.gov/12750012/

[84] Vezzani A, Sperk G, Colmers WF. Neuropeptide Y: Emerging evidence for a functional role in seizure modulation [Internet]. Vol. 22, Trends in Neurosciences. Elsevier Ltd; 1999 [cited 2021 Jun 6]. p. 25-30. Available from: https://pubmed.ncbi.nlm.nih.gov/10088996/

[85] Sperk G. Kainic acid seizures in the rat [Internet]. Vol. 42, Progress in Neurobiology. Prog Neurobiol; 1994 [cited 2021 Jun 6]. p. 1-32. Available from: https://pubmed.ncbi.nlm.nih.gov/7480784/

[86] Tian FF, Zeng C, Guo TH, Chen Y, Chen JM, Ma YF, et al. Mossy fiber sprouting, hippocampal damage and spontaneous recurrent seizures in

pentylenetetrazole kindling rat model. Acta Neurol Belg [Internet]. 2009 Dec 1 [cited 2021 Jun 6];109(4):298-304. Available from: https://europepmc.org/article/med/20120210

[87] Li X, Kuang H, Jiang N, Hu Y. Involvement of Scn1b and Kcna1 ion channels in audiogenic seizures and PTZ-induced epilepsy. Epilepsy Res [Internet]. 2005 [cited 2021 Jun 6];66(1-3):155-63. Available from: https://pubmed.ncbi.nlm.nih.gov/16157473/

[88] Clark CR. Comparative Anticonvulsant Activity and Neurotoxicity of 4-Amino-N-(2,6-dimethylphenyl) benzamide and Prototype Antiepileptic Drugs in Mice and Rats. Epilepsia [Internet]. 1988 Apr 1 [cited 2021 Aug 21];29(2):198-203. Available from: https://onlinelibrary.wiley.com/doi/full/10.1111/j.1528-1157.1988.tb04420.x

[89] RA U, AY C, EA S. Effects of gamma-aminobutyric acid (GABA) receptor agonists on the neurotoxicity and anticonvulsant activity of barbiturates in mice. J Pharmacol Exp Ther [Internet]. 1986 [cited 2021 Aug 21];237(2):468-72. Available from: https://pubmed.ncbi.nlm.nih.gov/3009786/

[90] Bertram EH, Lothman EW, Lenn NJ. The hippocampus in experimental chronic epilepsy: A morphometric analysis. Ann Neurol [Internet]. 1990 [cited 2021 Jun 6];27(1):43-8. Available from: https://pubmed.ncbi.nlm.nih.gov/2301927/

[91] Nevander G, Ingvar M, Auer R, Siesjö BK. Status epilepticus in well–oxygenated rats causes neuronal necrosis. Ann Neurol [Internet]. 1985 [cited 2021 Jun 6];18(3):281-90. Available from: https://pubmed.ncbi.nlm.nih.gov/4051457/

[92] Szot P, Weinshenker D, White SS, Robbins CA, Rust NC, Schwartzkroin PA, et al. Norepinephrine-deficient mice have increased susceptibility to seizure-inducing stimuli. J Neurosci [Internet]. 1999 Dec 15 [cited 2021 Jun 6];19(24):10985-92. Available from: https://pubmed.ncbi.nlm.nih.gov/10594079/

[93] Avoli M. Feline generalized penicillin epilepsy. Ital J Neurol Sci [Internet]. 1995 Mar [cited 2021 Jun 6];16(1-2):79-82. Available from: https://pubmed.ncbi.nlm.nih.gov/7642356/

[94] Akdogan I, Adiguzel E, Yilmaz I, Ozdemir MB, Sahiner M, Tufan AC. Penicillin-induced epilepsy model in rats: Dose-dependant effect on hippocampal volume and neuron number. Brain Res Bull [Internet]. 2008 Oct 22 [cited 2021 Jun 6];77(4):172-7. Available from: https://pubmed.ncbi.nlm.nih.gov/18762233/

[95] Ni H, Jiang Y wu, Tao L yuang, Cen J nong, Wu X ru. Effects of penicillin-induced developmental epilepticus on hippocampal regenerative sprouting, related gene expression and cognitive deficits in rats. Toxicol Lett [Internet]. 2009 Jul 24 [cited 2021 Jun 6];188(2):161-6. Available from: https://pubmed.ncbi.nlm.nih.gov/19446251/

[96] Söderfeldt B, Kalimo H, Olsson Y, Siesjö B. Pathogenesis of brain lesions caused by experimental epilepsy - Light- and electron-microscopic changes in the rat cerebral cortex following bicuculline-induced status epilepticus. Acta Neuropathol [Internet]. 1981 Sep 1 [cited 2021 Jun 6];54(3):219-31. Available from: https://europepmc.org/article/med/7257731

[97] Seutin V, Johnson SW. Recent advances in the pharmacology of quaternary salts of bicuculline [Internet]. Vol. 20, Trends in Pharmacological Sciences. Elsevier Ltd; 1999 [cited 2021 Jun 6]. p. 268-70.

Available from: https://pubmed.ncbi.nlm.nih.gov/10390643/

[98] Mitchell J, Gatherer M, Sundstrom LE. Aberrant Timm-stained fibres in the dentate gyrus following tetanus toxin-induced seizures in the rat. Neuropathol Appl Neurobiol [Internet]. 1996 Apr 1 [cited 2021 Jun 6];22(2):129-35. Available from: https://onlinelibrary.wiley.com/doi/full/10.1111/j.1365-2990.1996.tb00856.x

[99] Jordan SJ, Jefferys JGR. Sustained and selective block of IPSPs in brain slices from rats made epileptic by intrahippocampal tetanus toxin. Epilepsy Res. 1992 Apr 1;11(2):119-129.

[100] Cavalheiro EA, Leite JP, Bortolotto ZA, Turski WA, Ikonomidou C, Turski L. Long-Term Effects of Pilocarpine in Rats: Structural Damage of the Brain Triggers Kindling and Spontaneous I Recurrent Seizures. Epilepsia [Internet]. 1991 [cited 2021 Jun 6];32(6):778-82. Available from: https://pubmed.ncbi.nlm.nih.gov/1743148/

[101] Gibbs JW, Shumate MD, Coulter DA. Differential epilepsy-associated alterations in postsynaptic GABA(A) receptor function in dentate granule and CA1 neurons. J Neurophysiol [Internet]. 1997 [cited 2021 Jun 6];77(4):1924-38. Available from: https://pubmed.ncbi.nlm.nih.gov/9114245/

[102] Fernandes MJS, Naffah-Mazzacoratti MG, Cavalheiro EA. Na+K+ ATPase activity in the rat hippocampus: A study in the pilocarpine model of epilepsy. Neurochem Int [Internet]. 1996 [cited 2021 Jun 6];28(5-6):497-500. Available from: https://pubmed.ncbi.nlm.nih.gov/8792330/

[103] Scorza CA, Garrido YDC, Arida RM, Amado D, Cavalheiro EA, Naffah-Mazzacoratti MDG. Levels of the synaptic protein X11 alpha/mint1 are increased in hippocampus of rats with epilepsy. Epilepsy Res [Internet]. 2003 [cited 2021 Jun 6];57(1):49-57. Available from: https://pubmed.ncbi.nlm.nih.gov/14706732/

Section 3

Understanding of Neurotoxicity

Chapter 8

Multi-Omic Epigenetic-Based Model Reveals Key Molecular Mechanisms Associated with Palmitic Acid Lipotoxicity in Human Astrocyte

Felipe Rojas-Rodríguez, Andrés Pinzón, Daniel Fuenmayor, Tábata Barbosa, Diego Vesga Jimenez, Cynthia Martin, George E. Barreto, Andrés Aristizabal-Pachón and Janneth Gonzalez

Abstract

Astrocytes are critical for the metabolic, structural and functional modulatory support of the brain. Lipotoxicity or high levels of saturated fatty acid as Palmitate (PA) has been associated with neurotoxicity, the loss or change of astrocytic functionality, and the etiology and progression of neurodegenerative diseases such as Parkinson or Alzheimer. Several molecular mechanisms of PA's effect in astrocytes have been described, yet the role of epigenetic regulation and chromatin architecture have not been fully explored. In this study, we developed a multi-omic epigenetic-based model to identify the molecular mechanisms of lipotoxic PA activity in astrocytes. We used data from nine histone modifications, location of Topological Associated Domains (TADs) and transcriptional CTCF regions, where we identified the basal astrocyte epigenetic landscape. Moreover, we integrated transcriptomic data of astrocytic cellular response to PA with the epigenetic multi-omic model to identify lipotoxic-induced molecular mechanisms. The multi-omic model showed that chromatin conformation in astrocytes treated with PA have response genes located within shared topological domains, in which most of them also showed either repressive or enhancing marks in the Chip-Seq enrichment, reinforcing the idea that epigenetic regulation has a huge impact on the lipotoxic mechanisms of PA in the brain.

Keywords: epigenetic landscape, lipotoxicity, inflammation, astrocyte-neuron interaction, neurodegeneration

1. Introduction

Obesity is referred to as the excessive accumulation of body fat. It has become a worldwide public health issue which several studies have linked hormonal impairment to other diseases like coronary pathologies, diabetes, hypertension, atherosclerosis, and certain types of cancer among others [1, 2]. Studies using insulin growth factor-1 (IGF-1) receptor, insulin receptor substrate-1 (IRS-1), insulin receptor substrate-4 (IRS-4), glial fibrillary acidic protein, as well as an increase in β-actin protein have been associated with fatty acid excess in the brain [3]. Additionally, recent evidence has linked adiposity and high fatty acid concentrations to significant brain region-specific dysfunction, atrophy, inflammation, and cognitive decline [2, 4, 5], as well as an increased risk in developing the accumulation of amyloid β and Tau associated with Alzheimer's disease [3].

Astrocytes are the most versatile glial cells in the central nervous system (CNS) constituting from 20 to 40% of neuroglia, protecting the brain through so many signaling [6], demonstrating that these cells effectively engulf dead cells, synapses and protein aggregates of amyloid β (Aβ) and α-synuclein, typical of Alzheimer's disease (AD) and Parkinson's disease (PD), respectively. Additionally, astrocytes have been shown to regulate K+ levels [7] and prevent excitotoxicity in Huntington's disease (HD) [8–10]. Nonetheless, evidence suggests that elevated concentrations of fatty acids can trigger a pro-inflammatory response altering the correct functioning of astrocytes [11–13]. Recently, authors have proved that metabolic insults produced by fatty acids can trigger a pro-inflammatory response in astrocytes, due to their high recruitment and metabolic capacity. Among them is PA, a long-chain saturated fatty acid, that can trigger an increase in inflammatory cytokines [5] such as Interleukin (IL)-1B, IL-6 and tumor necrosis factor alpha (TNFα), leading to accelerated cognitive decline, decreased cell viability, increased endoplasmic reticulum stress, inhibition of autophagy, finally compromising the Blood–Brain Barrier (BBB) integrity and promoting dementia-like progression in humans and animal models [5, 7, 14, 15].

Recent evidence supports epigenetic responses in astrocytes followed by PA-lipotoxic exposure [10, 16]. Epigenetic transcriptional regulation such as chromatin accessibility by histone modifications and chromatin architecture modulate euchromatin/heterochromatin equilibrium has shown the great potential of providing groundbreaking insight into the effects of neurotoxic compounds such as PA [4, 17, 18]. Additionally, the epigenetic modulation in astrocytes produced by lipotoxic compounds like PA can trigger inflammation, neurotoxicity, astrocyte reactivity, and cell fate determination in the CNS [16, 19]. In this case, the epigenetic landscape regulatory role and its response in the PA-induced astrocyte lipotoxicity are both the key to comprehend the loss of cellular function. Furthermore, several authors have also demonstrated that multi-omic models have proved to be more efficient than conventional astrocytic models in the evaluation of non-linearity in chromatin regulation considering regulatory mechanisms such as enhancers, isolators, epigenetic marks, and non-coding RNA [20–22].

It has been demonstrated that epigenetic data such as Chip-Seq and Hi-C with transcriptomics allows the detailed identification of specific molecular mechanisms associated with impairment conditions. In the present study, we report a multi-omic model to describe the epigenetic baseline of astrocytes as well as the astrocytic response to PA-lipotoxicity over specific astrocytic processes such as inflammation, autophagy, endoplasmic reticulum stress, energetic metabolism, mitochondrial dysfunction, and astrocyte-neuron interaction pathways, herein described here as astrocytic PA response (APAR) mechanisms.

2. Materials and methods

2.1 Hi-C, ChiP-Seq and transcriptomics datasets acquisition

Hi-C has been adopted as a method to measure pairwise contacts between pairs of genomic loci and allows a mapping of the three-dimensional conformation of chromatin within a population of cells, as well as to detect the structural variation and corrects assembly of chromosomal missed junctions [23]. Chip-Seq data also allows the analysis of histone marks interaction with DNA in an activation/repression mechanism. In this study, we analyzed nine treatments which were controls, H3K36me3, H3K27me3, H3K9ac, H3K9me3, H3K79me2, H4K20me1, H3K4me1 and CTCF (entry: GSM733678, GSM733751, GSM733729, GSM1003534, GSM1003491, GSM1003490, GSM1003525, GSM733710 and GSM733765 respectively). Tissue-specific datasets for astrocyte Hi-C from cerebellum and spinal cord were downloaded from the Encyclopedia of DNA Elements (ENCODE), as part of the ENCODE project consortium with ID numbers 200105194 and 200105957, respectively [24–26]. From ChiP-Seq data we obtained nine astrocyte datasets from NHA cells culture from the ENCODE database. Moreover, the whole human genome GRC version hg19 was obtained from ENSEMBL (https://www.ensembl.org/index.html) to map and enrich all the datasets. Transcriptomic data was experimentally obtained in the laboratory of Experimental and Computational Biochemistry of the Pontificia Universidad Javeriana, Bogotá D.C, Colombia.

2.2 Transcriptomic data

We used Normal Human Astrocytes (NHA; Lonza, CC-2565) divided in three different batches (#0000612736, #00005656712, #0000514417), which were cultured according to the manufacturer's specifications. All batches were cultured in a supplemented medium with SingleQuots supplements. In order to induce PA toxicity, NHA cells were seeded in 48, 24, 12, and 6-well plates and incubated in a humidified incubator for 12 days at 37°C and 5% CO2. Then the NHA cells were washed with PBS 1x and starved in medium with serum-free DMEM without phenol red, L- and supplements (Lonza, Basel, Switzerland) for 6 h.

RNA extraction was performed using mini kit RNeasy (Qiagen, USA). The RNA quantification of the preparations was performed with NanoDrop (Thermo Fisher Scientific, Waltham, Ma, 174 USA). To remove possible DNA contamination, RNA was treated with DNase I. The RNA integrity (RIN) and 28S/18S ratio were determined with the RNA Nano 6000 Assay Kit of the Agilent Bioanalyzer 2100 system (Agilent Technologies, CA, USA). Transcriptomic datasets were obtained for NHA astrocytes treated in DMEM medium. RNA-seq libraries were prepared using the TruSeq Stranded mRNA library prep kit following the manufacturer's protocol (Illumina, Cat# RS-122-2101) [27, 28]. The RNA-seq libraries were sequenced in HiSeq platform (Illumina) using protocol 2x150bp paired-end configuration, single index per lane. Scores and nucleotide composition were assessed with FastQ to evaluate accuracy using the Nextflow (V18.10.1) pipeline QUARS (https://github.com/TainVelasco-Luquez/QUARS).

Salmon package was used for mapping and quantifying the expression level (https://combine-lab.github.io/salmon/, V0.13.1) on the genome assembly GRCh38 (patch 12) from the NCBI without ALT regions using Gencode [26, 29]. NOISeq was used to import data into R (V3.6.1) and assessed sequence plot quality diagnosis [5]. Gene level Ensembl IDs were used with tximport function to create the count matrix. We used DESeq2 for modeling the average expression in function of the treatments correcting for sex (design formula: ~ sex + condition) [30]. Moreover, DESeq2 was used for normalization by size, variance shrinkage, outliers filtering, and hypothesis testing. The Wald test was used for assessing genes differentially expressed above |LFC| > = 0.5 with an alpha cutoff at 0.05.

The overlap analysis was performed using Fisher's exact test using alpha at 0.05 implemented in the package GeneOverlap. To correct for multiple testing, p-values were adjusted using the Benjamini-Hochberg method [31]. Additionally, we leveraged the GeneOverlap's Odds Ratio and Jaccard Index as measures of the strength of association and the similarity, respectively. Odds ratio equal to or less than 1 means no associations and greater than 1 represents strong associations. Jaccard Index is a measure of similarity that varies between 0, no similarity, and 1, completely identical lists. The package WGCNA from the platform iDEP (V0.90) was used to perform the co-expression analysis, employing the 1000 more variable genes across all samples, with a soft threshold of 16 and minimum module size of 20 [32]. The Pearson's correlation was used on the count matrix, normalized and regularized using the log transformation of the DESeq2 library.

2.3 Epigenetics data analysis

To create the multi-layer model, first we obtained the ChIP-Seq data of an astrocyte in homeostatic conditions from the ENCODE database, then re-analyzed the BED/BAM files using ChIP-Seq model-based analysis implemented in MACS2. We integrated H3K4me3, H3K27ac, H3K27me3, H3K9ac, H3K4me1, H4K20me1, H3K36me3, and H3K79me2 to the human genome, in order to identify the core active regulatory and repressed genes in astrocyte, H3K27me3, H4K20me1 and H3K9me3. The active genes were also identified by the integration of H3K4me3, H3K4me1, H3K79me, 2H3K9ac, H3K27me3, and H3K27ac [33] to the same genome (hg19) and those who shared both repressing and enhancing modifications were identified as bivalent genes. All the individual samples, the core activation, repression and bivalent samples were enriched using the cutoff p-value set at 0.01 for both molecular function and biological process excluding redundant gene ontology (GO) terms.

Hi-C data was obtained from the ENCODE database. In this database, it can be found up to 80% of the annotated genome, in which for the interest of the investigation cerebellum and spinal cord data with ID numbers 200105194 and 200105957 respectively [24]. Hi-C data of spinal cord and cerebellum were compared to identify the potential tissue-specific differences in astrocyte functioning. All the individual samples, the core activation, repression, and bivalent samples were enriched using the cutoff p value set at 0.01. Molecular enrichment was performed using ShinyGO [34].

2.4 Data integration

In order to identify euchromatin and heterochromatin regions in astrocyte, we overlapped all activation/repression specific histone modifications covering regions. With this approach, it was possible to identify activation, repression and bivalent core genomic regions. Thus, both the omic and epigenetic integrations were performed through the adjudication of the data described above into a multi-omic model. The model consisted in three different layers of the Chip-seq and Hi-C of an astrocyte under homeostatic conditions and the transcriptomic data of an astrocyte under the lipotoxic effects of PA, where these three layers were used to make an inference about the possible epigenetic effects of PA in an astrocyte. Considering that there are no Hi-C or Chip-Seq data for astrocytes under the effects of PA, the integration of the transcriptomic data allows the identification and analysis of genes associated with PA response. Accordingly, the identification of changes in the epigenetic regulation of genes was performed as follows: first the differentially expressed genes in the transcriptome presented within the TADs of euchromatin and with the groups of genes were identified. Then, the proteomic data was sought to identify whether gene expression patterns are correlated with histone modification data sets [35–37]. Also, both the core regions and the specific histone marks with the Hi-C were overlapped with the TADs of an astrocyte in order to identify patterns between chromatin architecture and modulation of histone expression [37, 38]. Later, the Chip-Seq core regions integrated with TADs were compared with gene expression and proteomic data.

To identify the role of chromatin conformation in the expression and the effect of TADs in PA activity, gene expression and gene localization were associated with each other. This approach allowed us to identify additional epigenetic regulatory events related with TAD genes [39]. Subsequently non-coding regions such as enhancers and promoter regions were identified to be able to explain the patterns of expression of PA lipotoxicity. All data analysis was developed using R-Bioconductor suite (https://www.bioconductor.org/) as well as publicly available databases to ensure reproducibility and robustness. All the resulting sets of genes were enriched for molecular processes and biological functions.

3. Results

3.1 Chromatin/Histone expression regulation

Considering the functional importance of histone modifications in the cellular behavior [40], we identified a set of 34852 genes with known activation roles across the seven ChiP-Seq samples. Histone marks H3K4me3, H3K27ac, H3K9ac, H3K4me1, H4K20me1, H3K36me3, and H3K79me2 and the number of genes per activation mark were 2432, 3034, 3773, 5133, 8228, 6766 and 5486, respectively, with a non-homogenous pattern. We obtained a set of 11214 genes enhanced between the 7 studied active histone modifications with at least each gene included in two or more of the samples. Moreover, samples H3K27me3 and H3K9me3 showed 6276 and 6747 repressed genes, respectively. We identified a set of 9796 genes repressed in astrocytes based on H3K27me3 and H3K9me3 data with the condition that each gene should be present in at least one of the ChiP samples. Considering that a bivalent region is due to the presence of a repressor and an enhancer in the modifications of histones H3K4me3 and H3K27me3, we identified 7608 genes in bivalent sites. Moreover, shared genes for both activation and repression were identified as coding regions present in at least one of the mark datasets in each group for the specific markers [33].

In general, we performed a functional enrichment of the dataset where it was possible to identify the biological process and molecular functions associated with GO terms. As a result, 30 biological processes relevant to APAR biological mechanisms were presented (**Table 1**). Among these biological processes identified for the activation of ChIP-Seq datasets, glutamate-cysteine ligase activity, CD4 receptor binding, ion channel binding, and extracellular matrix binding were the top-enriched functions. Besides, functional groups associated with the homeostatic astrocytic activity were identified as highlighting transferase activity, carbohydrate derivative binding, hydrolase activity, DNA-binding transcription factor activity, molecular function regulator, transporter activity, oxidoreductase activity, enzyme regulator activity, transmembrane transporter activity, signaling receptor activity, extracellular matrix structural constituent, lipid binding, extracellular matrix binding, electron transfer activity, and lyase/ligase activity. The genes that encode the molecular functions mentioned above, are associated with metabolic support in astrocytic activity and neural functionality present in euchromatin regions.

It was also possible to identify active coding regions tightly regulated for cellular ion maintenance and response to stimuli that are essential for astrocytes well-functioning [7]. Additionally, we were able to associate the presence of constant euchromatin regions with genes that encode for metabolic and cellular exchange mechanisms necessary for astrocyte function [41]. Therefore, the model demonstrated that the presence of genes in regular euchromatin regions are often associated with many regulatory elements such as promoters, enhancers, insulators and silencers, all related with cell adhesion, support and exchange processes [42, 43].

Category	Process	Gene number
Function	Regulation of biological quality	4319
	Homeostatic processes	2004
	Ion homeostasis	836
	Response to nutrients	730
	Regulation of membrane potential	450
	Apoptotic mitochondrial changes	130
	Membrane depolarization	88
	Regulation of membrane depolarization	44
	Mitochondrial depolarization	24
	Regulation of mitochondrial depolarization	21
	Non-ribosomal peptide biosynthetic process	19
	Glutathione biosynthetic process	17
Group	Immune response	45
	Regulation of biological quality	32
	Response to stress	23
	Regulation of response to stimulus	20
	Regulation of molecular function	20
	Response to external stimulus	17
	Regulation of signaling	15
	Cell adhesion	11
	Catabolic processes	11

Table 1.
Top biological processes associated with the core activation dataset from the histone markers H3K4me3, H3K27ac, H3K9ac, H3K4me1, H4K20me1, H3K36me3, and H3K79me2. Accordingly, biological processes were separated into functions and groups, in terms associated with GO for a more detailed analysis.

In the case of bivalent expression regions, 30 biological processes were identified corresponding with APAR mechanisms, highlighting transcription regulation, sequence-specific DNA binding, RNA polymerase II/III distal enhancer, regulatory region, and proximal promoter sequence-specific DNA binding, gamma-aminobutyric acid transmembrane transporter activity, nerve growth factor binding, ubiquitin-protein transferase activator activity, mannosyl-transferase activity and cofactor, corepressor and coactivator transcription binding (**Table 2**). Additionally, these same genes that were also associated with specific functional groups such as macromolecule binding (*i.e.,* carbohydrates, sulfurates, lipids, amides), DNA-binding transcription factor activity, cofactor binding, extracellular matrix structural constituent, structural constituent of ribosome, structural constituent of cytoskeleton, extracellular matrix binding, neurotransmitter binding and structural constituent of myelin sheath and activity of hydrolase, transferase, peroxidase, oxidoreductase, isomerase, lyase/ligase signaling, transmembrane transporters, enzyme regulation, antioxidant, electron transfer, neurotransmitter transport, cytochrome-c oxidase, MAPKK, and glutathione dehydrogenase functionality.

Further, we identified all the specific genes associated with the APAR mechanisms in astrocytes under homeostatic conditions (**Figure 1**). It was possible to clarify the epigenetic basal response of astrocytes and identify the gene activation/expression profiling under homeostatic conditions of these cells to elucidate the potential response to PA detrimental conditions. Both activation and bivalent processes and functions made it possible to understand the expression and regulatory mechanisms associated with an epigenetic chromatin landscape in astrocytes [4]. For both activation and bivalent datasets, the biological processes and functions were consistent with the basal astrocytic activity (**Tables 1** and **2**).

Category	Process	Gene number
Function	Positive regulation of biosynthetic process	4091
	Positive regulation of nucleic acid-templated transcription	3293
	Positive regulation of cellular biosynthetic process	2082
	Positive regulation of RNA metabolic process	1789
	Positive regulation of RNA biosynthetic process	1695
	Extracellular matrix assembly	28
	Negative regulation of autophagy of mitochondrion	9
	Interleukin-23-mediated signaling pathway	9
	Positive regulation of axon extension involved in axon guidance	7
Group	Regulation of response to stimulus	1409
	Regulation of biological quality	1360
	Response to stress	1312
	Regulation of signaling	1242
	Immune system process	973
	Catabolic process	863
	Response to external stimulus	793
	Cell proliferation	708

Table 2.
Biological processes associated with histone markers H3K4me3 and H3K27me3 were separated between functions and groups. All the terms were associated with GO terms for further analysis [33].

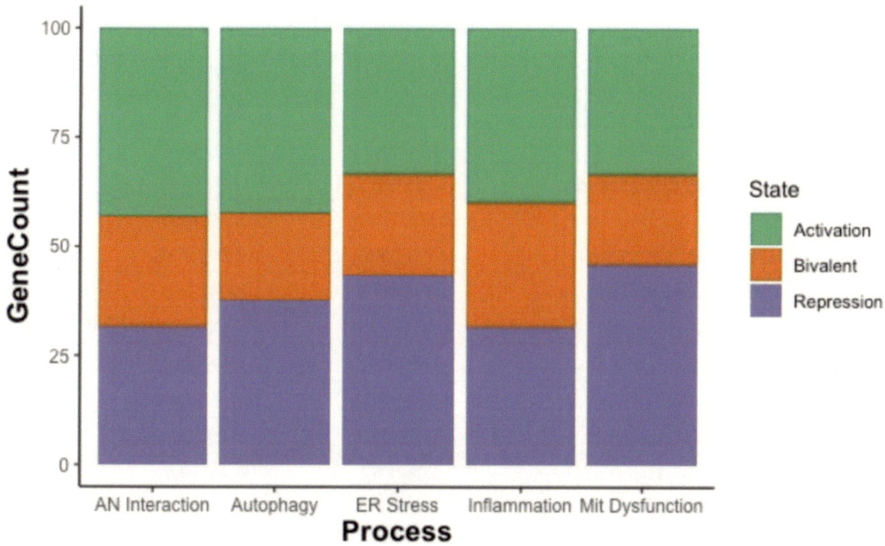

Figure 1.
Graphical representation of activation, repression, and bivalent genes present in every APAR categories. Specifically, AN interaction has 42%, 25% and 31%; autophagy has 42%, 20% and 37%; ER Stress has 33%, 23% and 43%; inflammation has 39%, 28% and 31% all for activation, bivalent and repression genes respectively. Note: the colors correspond to Green-Activation, Orange-Bivalent, and Purple-Repression.

3.2 Chromatin architecture involvement in APAR

Overexpressed genes in NHA astrocytes exposed to lipotoxic PA concentrations were fully integrated to ChIP-Seq data, APAR-related data and the chromatin conformation in order to identify co-regulated genomic regions in astrocytes [44]. We identified 328 molecular processes that were found overexpressed when astrocytes are exposed to PA, of which 27 molecular APAR associated processes were selected based on the role and significance (**Table 3**).

Although comparing specific TAD regions from Hi-C experiments and differentially expressed genes associated with APAR mechanisms in astrocytes, we identified clusters sharing the same TAD (**Table A1**). In this regard, we identified 3039 and 3048 TAD regions for spinal cord and cerebellum astrocytes, respectively. We focused on differentially expressed genes present among the APAR gene sets, located in the corresponding TAD regions to identify co-regulated genes or regulatory profiles. Moreover, due to the CTCF role in the conformation of chromatin folding architecture,

Molecular process	Adjusted p-value	Negative log10 adjusted p-value	Gene number
Inflammatory response	1.0487E-16	15.979344	53
Response to external stimulus	9.8873E-13	12.0049202	101
Response to lipid	1.8892E-11	10.7237215	51
Response to stress	8.5056E-11	10.070294	121
Response to stimulus	3.438E-09	8.46369645	205
Regulation of lipid metabolic process	4.1334E-08	7.38369637	29
Cellular response to stimulus	1.0314E-05	4.98659017	169
Regulation of biological quality	1.8704E-05	4.72806228	107
Regulation of immune response	0.0001047	3.98004731	43
Regulation of cell activation	0.00018219	3.73947057	30
Positive regulation of inflammatory response	0.00029935	3.52381953	14
Regulation of inflammatory response	0.00057697	3.23884686	22
Regulation of response to stress	0.00213314	2.67098006	50
Cellular lipid metabolic process	0.00528208	2.27719528	38
Positive regulation of biological process	0.00848563	2.07131588	136
Neuroinflammatory response	0.0114169	1.94245175	9
Regulation of ERK1 and ERK2 cascade	0.01342102	1.8722145	17
Glial cell activation	0.01563567	1.8058835	8
Interleukin-1 secretion	0.01762805	1.75379577	8
Positive regulation of metabolic process	0.01849939	1.7328425	89
Regulation of response to stimulus	0.02555143	1.59258475	101
ERK1 and ERK2 cascade	0.0278352	1.55540561	17
Positive regulation of immune response	0.03214889	1.49283399	32
Hippocampal neuron apoptotic process	0.0381717	1.41825855	3
Regulation of hippocampal neuron apoptotic process	0.0381717	1.41825855	3
Negative regulation of transport	0.04292557	1.36728396	23
Synapse pruning	0.04548992	1.34208479	4

Table 3.
Differentially expressed biological processes associated with the APAR mechanisms of PA-lipotoxicity in astrocytes. All considered processes have $p > 0.05$ as a threshold value of significance.

TAD regions were overlapped with CTCF in order to identify true TAD regions. In this sense, these results elucidated some of the potential role of epigenetic modulation in the APAR molecular mechanisms in astrocytes in response to PA-lipotoxicity [45–47].

4. Discussion

In the present study, our model showed that astrocytes regulate enzymatic and protein activity from the genomic to the protein level, considering the protein functional modulation at different molecular levels. Additionally, during normal conditions, the enzymatic activity of hydrolase, transferase, peroxidase, oxidoreductase, isomerase and lyase/ligase were identified as constantly regulated due to elevated metabolic rates and plasticity in astrocytes [48, 49]. In this case, metabolic maintenance and support are not permanently regulated by epigenetic processes due to a dynamic environmental-dependent mechanism in astrocytes. Nevertheless, the presence of metabolic processes in bivalent regions implies the presence of highly active metabolic processes that change across time due to the fact that a genomic region can present both marks and become active or repressed [43, 50]. In terms of astrocyte-neuron interaction, we identified the presence of antioxidant activity associated with glutathione biosynthetic processes, reductase activity, as well as the activity of structural constituents of myelin sheath [51, 52]. Relationship between astrocytes and neurons in the context of antioxidant defense to ensuring neuronal well-being during pathological conditions play a significant role in metabolic support by neuroprotective capacity from oxidative stress, supply of glutathione to neurons, modulation of the extracellular matrix assembly, among others [52, 53].

To examine the molecular response to PA or APAR mechanism in astrocytes, we integrated the epigenetic data with the transcriptomic data from NHA to elucidate the potential damaging conditions by the PA activity in the brain. The shared TAD regions from both cerebellum and spinal cord astrocyte Hi-C data were compared to each other in order to establish the differences and possible considerations associated with tissue-specific stimuli. Thus, our multi-omic model showed that during PA lipotoxicity in astrocytes, inflammatory and stress responses are overexpressed. Our results also indicated that lipid droplets are epigenetically regulated in order to respond to free fatty acid concentrations in homeostatic conditions by the presence of apolipoprotein-E (APOE) gene in euchromatin regions [4, 40]. For instance, recent evidence has shown that maintenance of the homeostasis between astrocytes and neurons mitigate the lipotoxic effects of fatty acids as well as modulating APOE-lipid particles becomes of vital importance [54].

The presence of PA is associated with the overexpression of biological processes such as response to cellular lipid metabolism, which can lead to disease [5, 55]. Moreover, high concentrations of PA induce the expression of markers involved in pro-inflammatory response where the secretion of IL-1 activates endothelial cells and astrocytes to propagate the inflammatory signals in CNS [56, 57]. Overall, IL-1 is a typical biomarker associated with lipotoxicity and inflammation in astrocytes, as LC3-II, p62, or TLR2 have been directly linked to the astrocytic response to PA [5, 11, 58]. Likewise, IL-1 supports mechanisms as extracellular matrix binding modulation and regulation obtained in experimental studies that are essential for the response to mechanical stimuli in astrocytes [41]. In this sense, our results support the involvement of epigenetic regulation over cellular functional determinants in astrocytes during neurodegeneration but are necessary to develop more precise algorithms associated with gene screening [4].

Moreover, our model shows and support evidence from experimental studies, highlighting the expression and regulation of transporters such as the glutamate and lactate shuttle, redox stress reduction, transfer mitochondrial, among others, which are associated with the APAR mechanisms. Many of these biological functions associated with the response of astrocytes seem to be regulated by some of the tested histone modifications. Also, the response to external stimulus can be associated with the presence of neurotransmitter receptors, evidencing the neuron-astrocyte interaction beyond the metabolic support. Interestingly, we also report the presence of genes involved in the biosynthetic process of glutathione in the euchromatin regions, meaning a recurrent antioxidant activity process in astrocytes. Glutathione biosynthesis and release have been associated as a strategy for the balance and detoxify of the neural activity mediated by mitochondrial reactive oxygen species (ROS) in neurons linked to neurotransmission, neuroinflammation, neural disease etiology and progression [59, 60]. Glutathione biosynthesis is related to astrocytes antioxidant defense activity during pathological and non-pathological conditions.

Transcriptomic data, epigenetic landscape of TDAs, and histone modification regions data allowed the identification of APAR genes in the transcriptomic dataset and their localization (bivalent activation) [61]. TNFRSF1B, IL1R2, IL18RAP, IL1A, IL5RA, CXCL10, IL5, PIK3CG, IL10RA, and CCL8 genes were identified and associated with APAR mechanisms in astrocytes. Recently it has been demonstrated that during non-stimulating conditions, astrocytes secrete cytokines such as GM-CSF, CXCL1, CCL2, CXCL8, IL-6, and IL-8, all of those displayed at different levels [22, 37]. Moreover, administration of IL-1B and TNF activates astrocytes response with the production of cytokines IL-1B, IL-1RA, TNFA, CXCL10, CCL3, CCL5 and IL6 [62–64], being IL-6 response more efficient at higher concentration [65, 66].

Chromatin conformation in astrocytes has shown that PA response genes were located within shared TADs. During inflammation interleukin-1 receptor type II (IL1R2) has been described as a key receptor of which the expression reduces IL1A and IL1B activity [9]. On the other hand, the interleukin 18 receptor accessory protein (IL18RAP) that is associated with the pro-inflammatory response of IL18 by intracellular signaling was located in the same TAD region, suggesting that they share the same regulatory response when inflammatory processes occur in astrocyte [67]. Additionally, this TAD region also contains IL1R1 which is a key molecular mechanism associated with astrocytic response to inflammation by interaction with IL1A, IL1B and IL1R-agonists. Likewise, the TAD contains IL1RL2, and IL18R1, both interleukin receptors related to inflammatory cellular processes [5, 68, 69].

The coregulation of certain gene groups can also be associated with either master regulatory regions in TADs or architecture proximity regulation in the nucleus [70]. It is plausible that PA-lipotoxic responses in regulation of astrocytes by activating TAD regions depends upon extracellular signaling. This is possible because of the proximity of TAD to nucleus for cooperative organized regulation of genomic regions [44, 71]. Our results finally suggest that epigenetic modulation has an important role in the regulation of APAR mechanisms, yet further experiments are necessary to explore the TAD proximity involved in APAR regulation.

5. Conclusions

We present the first comprehensive data integration of epigenetic involvement in the astrocytic response to PA through the analysis from Hi-C, ChIP-Seq, and transcriptomic data in a multi-omic level. We described the role of epigenetics as a key mechanism of astrocytic PA response within which we found histones markers with bivalent capacity associated with repression of genomic activity (H3K4me3 and H3K27me3). This finding determines the adaptability and response to environmental stress, provided through complex astrocyte metabolic plasticity networks. In addition, our results showed that markers as H3K4me3, H3K27ac, H3K9ac, H3K4me1, H4K20me1, H3K36me3 and H3K79me2 have regions associated with homeostatic processes linked to exchange processes, regulation of the extracellular matrix, protein maintenance and ion channels regulation. These processes were found in euchromatin regions, highlighting that it is associated with essential basal functions in astrocytes. Likewise, signaling pathways modulation (*i.e.,* PI3K/AKT), antioxidant activity (a recurrent mechanism in astrocytes), among others, were associated with glutathione biosynthesis processes, glutamate transport and glutamatergic neuronal support, identified as active basal coding regions.

APAR mechanisms proved to be highly regulated by histone modifications along the genome which is essential for the response to PA. Additionally, our results revealed the presence of highly regulatory regions in the TADs associated with IL1R2 and IL18RAP. Moreover, the location of genes encoding to interleukins in the genome and chromatin conformation revealed the putative epigenetic regulation of the inflammatory response. In this sense, our results support the involvement of APAR mechanisms on the lipotoxic effect of PA in astrocytes. While integrating transcriptomics with epigenetics data was possible to identify associated genes with APAR mechanisms and genes in response to PA located inside the topologically associated, genes found in the TAD region that shared the regulator responses linked to inflammatory processes were likely modulated by lipotoxicity actions. Additionally, it is possible to suggest that additional epigenetic mechanisms such as lncRNA, miRNA and extracellular signaling could be involved in the astrocytic response to PA. Considering that deterministic mechanisms of expression are still unknown for astrocytes in lipotoxic conditions, we suggest that epigenetic modulation is essential for an efficient and dynamic cellular response. This work is a novel approach that involves epigenetic regulation in the cellular response to PA-lipotoxicity in astrocytes. Therefore, it should be emphasized that it is recommended the development of new methodologies and algorithms for more accurate analysis associated especially to genetic encryption. Finally, an accurate investigation of this new multi-omic epigenetic-based model by integrating multiple underlying data sources about the cellular mechanisms of the response to PA-lipotoxicity in astrocytes, might help in the future to detect shared genetic patterns found in the TAD region among the neurodegenerative diseases, identifying biomarkers for differentiating disease states and thereby facilitating the decision-making process and treatment management.

Acknowledgements

We would like to acknowledge the members of the Computational and Experimental Biochemistry Group, whose help was indispensable for envisioning the research. RNA sequencing, and analysis were funded by Minciencias grants 8845, contract 886–2019, and 20304 awarded to the Pontificia Universidad Javeriana.

Conflict of interest

The authors declare no conflict of interest.

Abbreviations

PA	palmitic acid
TADs	topological associated domains

BBB	blood–brain barrier
ROS	reactive oxygen species
APAR	astrocytic PA response

Appendix

Gene (Regulation)	Location	TAD region	Genes in TAD
TNFRSF1B	chr1 12,166,949-12,209,228 [+Strand]	11,920,000-14,360,002	KIAA2013, PRAMEF13, KAZN, PLOD1, HNRNPCL2, AADACL3, PRAMEF5, MFN2, DHRS3, PRDM2, C1orf158, PRAMEF17, PRAMEF12, PRAMEF20, PRAMEF1, PRAMEF14, TNFRSF8, LRRC38, PRAMEF11, PDPN, HNRNPCL1, PRAMEF2, PRAMEF4, PRAMEF10, PRAMEF6, VPS13D, PRAMEF7, AADACL4, PRAMEF18, PRAMEF27, HNRNPCL3, PRAMEF25, PRAMEF26, HNRNPCL4, PRAMEF9, PRAMEF8, PRAMEF33, PRAMEF15
IL1R2	chr2 101,991,816-102,028,544 [+Strand]	101,880,002-102,560,000	SLC9A4, IL1R1, IL1RL1, IL1RL2, **IL18RAP**, IL18R1
IL18RAP	chr2 102,418,558-102,452,568 [+Strand]	101,880,002-102,560,000	SLC9A4, IL1R1, IL1RL1, IL1RL2, **IL1R2**, IL18R1
IL1A	chr2 112,773,915-112,785,394 [-Strand]	112,600,002-113,400,000	POLR1B, IL36G, PSD4, IL37, IL1F10, CHCHD5, IL36A, SLC20A1, IL36B, NT5DC4, IL36RN, CKAP2L, IL1B, IL1RN, PAX-AS1, PAX8
IL5RA	chr3 3,066,324-3,126,613 [-Strand]	2,360,002-3,160,000	CNTN4, TRNT1, CRBN
CXCL10	chr4 76,021,116-76,023,536 [-Strand]	75,760,002-76,440,000	USO1, NAAA, SCARB2, NUP54STBD1, PPEF2, CXCL11, SDAD1, FAM47E, CXCL9, FAM47E-STBD1, ART3, CCDC158
IL5	chr5 132,541,444-132,556,890 [-Strand]	132,440,002-133,360,000	IRF1-AS1, IL13, SOWAHA, CCNI2, KIF3AUQCRQ, FSTL4, SHROOM1, HSPA4, IRF1, GDF9, IL4, RAD50, SEPTIN8, LEAP2, AFF4, ZCCHC10
PIK3CG	chr7 106,865,278-106,908,980 [+Strand]	106,840,002-107,600,000	PRKAR2B, HBP1, COG5, GPR22, BCAP29, DUS4L
IL10RA	chr11 117,857,063-117,872,198 [+Strand]	117,240,002-118,320,000	DSCAML1, FXYD2, FYD6, CEP164, SMIM35, RNF214, PCSK7, PAFAH1B2, SIDT2, TAGLN, BACE1, TMPRSS13, TMPRSS4, SCN4B, SCN2B, JAML, MPZL3
CCL8	chr17 34,319,047-34,321,402 [+Strand]	33,520,002-35,720,000	ASIC2, CCL2, TMEM132E, FNDC8, CCL7, CCL11, CCT6B, PEX12, LIG3, CCL13, CCL1, ZNF830, NLE1, C17orf102, RFFL, AP2B1, RAD51D, UNC45B, SLC35G3, SLFN12L, SLFN5, SLFN13, SLFN11, SLFN14, SLFN12

Table A1.
Topological architecture of the differentially expressed genes associated with APAR mechanisms in astrocytes. All gene regions have been obtained from ENSEMBL (GRCh37/hg19). All the TAD described contained promoters, enhancers and promoter flanks.

Author details

Felipe Rojas-Rodríguez[1], Andrés Pinzón[2], Daniel Fuenmayor[3], Tábata Barbosa[3], Diego Vesga Jimenez[3], Cynthia Martin[4], George E. Barreto[5], Andrés Aristizabal-Pachón[3] and Janneth Gonzalez[3]*

1 Department of Molecular Pathology, Netherlands Cancer Institute (NKI), Amsterdam, Netherlands

2 Instituto de Genética, Universidad Nacional de Colombia, Colombia

3 Departamento de Nutrición y Bioquímica, Pontificia Universidad Javeriana, Bogota D.C, Colombia

4 Division of Neuropharmacology and Neurologic Diseases, Yerkes National Primate Research Center, Atlanta, GA, USA

5 Department of Biological Sciences, University of Limerick, Limerick, Ireland

*Address all correspondence to: janneth.gonzalez@gmail.com

References

[1] Naderali, Ebrahim K., Stuart H. Ratcliffe, and Mark C. Dale. 2009. "Review: Obesity and Alzheimer's Disease: A Link Between Body Weight and Cognitive Function in Old Age." *American Journal of Alzheimer's Disease & Other Dementiasr* 24 (6): 445-449. https://doi.org/10.1177/1533317509348208.

[2] Olsen, M. L., B. S. Khakh, S. N. Skatchkov, M. Zhou, C. J. Lee, and N. Rouach. 2015. "New Insights on Astrocyte Ion Channels: Critical for Homeostasis and Neuron–Glia Signaling." *Journal of Neuroscience* 35 (41): 13827-13835. https://doi.org/10.1523/JNEUROSCI.2603-15.2015.

[3] Shefer, Gabi, Yonit Marcus, and Naftali Stern. 2013. "Is Obesity a Brain Disease?" *Neuroscience & Biobehavioral Reviews* 37 (10): 2489-2503. https://doi.org/10.1016/j.neubiorev.2013.07.015.

[4] Neal, Matthew, and Jason R. Richardson. 2018. "Epigenetic Regulation of Astrocyte Function in Neuroinflammation and Neurodegeneration." *Biochimica et Biophysica Acta (BBA) - Molecular Basis of Disease* 1864 (2): 432-443. https://doi.org/10.1016/j.bbadis.2017.11.004.

[5] Ortiz-Rodriguez, Ana, Estefania Acaz-Fonseca, Patricia Boya, Maria Angeles Arevalo, and Luis M. Garcia-Segura. 2019. "Lipotoxic Effects of Palmitic Acid on Astrocytes Are Associated with Autophagy Impairment." *Molecular Neurobiology* 56 (3): 1665-1680. https://doi.org/10.1007/s12035-018-1183-9.

[6] Verkhratsky, Alexei, and Arthur Butt. 2018. "The History of the Decline and Fall of the Glial Numbers Legend." *Neuroglia* 1 (1): 188-192. https://doi.org/10.3390/neuroglia1010013.

[7] Verkhratsky, Alexei, Robert Zorec, and Vladimir Parpura. 2017. "Stratification of Astrocytes in Healthy and Diseased Brain: Astroglia in Health and Disease." *Brain Pathology* 27 (5): 629-644. https://doi.org/10.1111/bpa.12537.

[8] Cooper, Arthur J. L. 2013. "Quantitative Analysis of Neurotransmitter Pathways Under Steady State Conditions – A Perspective." *Frontiers in Endocrinology* 4. https://doi.org/10.3389/fendo.2013.00179.

[9] Lee, Eun Hye. 2018. "Epilepsy Syndromes during the First Year of Life and the Usefulness of an Epilepsy Gene Panel." *Clin Exp Pediatr* 61 (4): 101-107. https://doi.org/10.3345/kjp.2018.61.4.101.

[10] Schousboe, Arne. 2019. "Metabolic Signaling in the Brain and the Role of Astrocytes in Control of Glutamate and GABA Neurotransmission." *Neuroscience Letters* 689 (January): 11-13. https://doi.org/10.1016/j.neulet.2018.01.038.

[11] Hidalgo-Lanussa, Oscar, Eliana Baez-Jurado, Valentina Echeverria, Ghulam Md Ashraf, Amirhossein Sahebkar, Luis Miguel Garcia-Segura, Roberto C. Melcangi, and George E. Barreto. 2020. "Lipotoxicity, Neuroinflammation, Glial Cells and Oestrogenic Compounds." *Journal of Neuroendocrinology* 32 (1). https://doi.org/10.1111/jne.12776.

[12] Linnerbauer, Mathias, Michael A. Wheeler, and Francisco J. Quintana. 2020. "Astrocyte Crosstalk in CNS Inflammation." *Neuron* 108 (4): 608-622. https://doi.org/10.1016/j.neuron.2020.08.012.

[13] Ortiz-Rodriguez, Ana, and Maria-Angeles Arevalo. 2020. "The Contribution of Astrocyte Autophagy to Systemic Metabolism." *International*

Journal of Molecular Sciences 21 (7): 2479. https://doi.org/10.3390/ijms21072479.

[14] Bernaus, Ada, Sandra Blanco, and Ana Sevilla. 2020. "Glia Crosstalk in Neuroinflammatory Diseases." *Frontiers in Cellular Neuroscience* 14 (July): 209. https://doi.org/10.3389/fncel.2020.00209.

[15] Frago, Laura M., Sandra Canelles, Alejandra Freire-Regatillo, Pilar Argente-Arizón, Vicente Barrios, Jesús Argente, Luis M. Garcia-Segura, and Julie A. Chowen. 2017. "Estradiol Uses Different Mechanisms in Astrocytes from the Hippocampus of Male and Female Rats to Protect against Damage Induced by Palmitic Acid." *Frontiers in Molecular Neuroscience* 10 (October): 330. https://doi.org/10.3389/fnmol.2017.00330.

[16] Schönfeld, Peter, and Georg Reiser. 2016. "Brain Lipotoxicity of Phytanic Acid and Very Long-Chain Fatty Acids. Harmful Cellular/Mitochondrial Activities in Refsum Disease and X-Linked Adrenoleukodystrophy." *Aging and Disease* 7 (2): 136. https://doi.org/10.14336/AD.2015.0823.

[17] Nakagawa, Takumi, Yoshikuni Wada, Sayako Katada, and Yusuke Kishi. 2020. "Epigenetic Regulation for Acquiring Glial Identity by Neural Stem Cells during Cortical Development." *Glia* 68 (8): 1554-1567. https://doi.org/10.1002/glia.23818.

[18] Pavlou, Maria Angeliki S., Luc Grandbarbe, Noel J. Buckley, Simone P. Niclou, and Alessandro Michelucci. 2019. "Transcriptional and Epigenetic Mechanisms Underlying Astrocyte Identity." *Progress in Neurobiology* 174 (March): 36-52. https://doi.org/10.1016/j.pneurobio.2018.12.007.

[19] Tiwari, Neha, Abhijeet Pataskar, Sophie Péron, Sudhir Thakurela, Sanjeeb Kumar Sahu, María Figueres-Oñate, Nicolás Marichal, Laura López-Mascaraque, Vijay K. Tiwari, and Benedikt Berninger. 2018. "Stage-Specific Transcription Factors Drive Astrogliogenesis by Remodeling Gene Regulatory Landscapes." *Cell Stem Cell* 23 (4): 557-571.e8. https://doi.org/10.1016/j.stem.2018.09.008.

[20] Argelaguet, Ricard, Britta Velten, Damien Arnol, Sascha Dietrich, Thorsten Zenz, John C Marioni, Florian Buettner, Wolfgang Huber, and Oliver Stegle. 2018. "Multi-Omics Factor Analysis—a Framework for Unsupervised Integration of Multi-omics Data Sets." *Molecular Systems Biology* 14 (6). https://doi.org/10.15252/msb.20178124.

[21] Liu, Sixue, Zuyu Yang, Guanghao Li, Chunyan Li, Yanting Luo, Qiang Gong, Xin Wu, et al. 2019. "Multi-Omics Analysis of Primary Cell Culture Models Reveals Genetic and Epigenetic Basis of Intratumoral Phenotypic Diversity." *Genomics, Proteomics & Bioinformatics* 17 (6): 576-589. https://doi.org/10.1016/j.gpb.2018.07.008.

[22] Lundin, Elin, Chenglin Wu, Albin Widmark, Mikaela Behm, Jens Hjerling-Leffler, Chammiran Daniel, Marie Öhman, and Mats Nilsson. 2020. "Spatiotemporal Mapping of RNA Editing in the Developing Mouse Brain Using in Situ Sequencing Reveals Regional and Cell-Type-Specific Regulation." *BMC Biology* 18 (1): 6. https://doi.org/10.1186/s12915-019-0736-3.

[23] Pal, Koustav, Mattia Forcato, and Francesco Ferrari. 2019. "Hi-C Analysis: From Data Generation to Integration." *Biophysical Reviews* 11 (1): 67-78. https://doi.org/10.1007/s12551-018-0489-1.

[24] Lajoie, Bryan R, Job Dekker, and Noam Kaplan. 2016. "The Hitchhiker's Guide to Hi-C Analysis: Practical Guidelines," 28.

[25] The ENCODE Project Consortium. 2012. "An Integrated Encyclopedia of DNA Elements in the Human Genome." *Nature* 489 (7414): 57-74. https://doi.org/10.1038/nature11247.

[26] Harrow, J., A. Frankish, J. M. Gonzalez, E. Tapanari, M. Diekhans, F. Kokocinski, B. L. Aken, et al. 2012. "GENCODE: The Reference Human Genome Annotation for The ENCODE Project." *Genome Research* 22 (9): 1760-1774. https://doi.org/10.1101/gr.135350.111.

[27] Crowe, Elizabeth P., Ferit Tuzer, Brian D. Gregory, Greg Donahue, Sager J. Gosai, Justin Cohen, Yuk Y. Leung, et al. 2016. "Changes in the Transcriptome of Human Astrocytes Accompanying Oxidative Stress-Induced Senescence." *Frontiers in Aging Neuroscience* 8 (August). https://doi.org/10.3389/fnagi.2016.00208.

[28] Knight, V. Bleu, and Elba E. Serrano. 2017. "Hydrogel Scaffolds Promote Neural Gene Expression and Structural Reorganization in Human Astrocyte Cultures." *PeerJ* 5 (January): e2829. https://doi.org/10.7717/peerj.2829.

[29] Patro, Rob, Geet Duggal, Michael I Love, Rafael A Irizarry, and Carl Kingsford. 2017. "Salmon Provides Fast and Bias-Aware Quantification of Transcript Expression." *Nature Methods* 14 (4): 417-419. https://doi.org/10.1038/nmeth.4197.

[30] Love, Michael I, Wolfgang Huber, and Simon Anders. 2014. "Moderated Estimation of Fold Change and Dispersion for RNA-Seq Data with DESeq2." *Genome Biology* 15 (12): 550. https://doi.org/10.1186/s13059-014-0550-8.

[31] Birck, Cindy, Eric Koncina, Tony Heurtaux, Enrico Glaab, Alessandro Michelucci, Paul Heuschling, and Luc Grandbarbe. 2016. "Transcriptomic Analyses of Primary Astrocytes under TNFα Treatment." *Genomics Data* 7 (March): 7-11. https://doi.org/10.1016/j.gdata.2015.11.005.

[32] Langfelder, Peter, and Steve Horvath. 2008. "WGCNA: An R Package for Weighted Correlation Network Analysis." *BMC Bioinformatics* 9 (1): 559. https://doi.org/10.1186/1471-2105-9-559.

[33] Thalheim, Torsten, Maria Herberg, Markus Loeffler, and Joerg Galle. 2017. "The Regulatory Capacity of Bivalent Genes—A Theoretical Approach." *International Journal of Molecular Sciences* 18 (5): 1069. https://doi.org/10.3390/ijms18051069.

[34] Ge, Steven Xijin, and Dongmin Jung. 2018. "Shiny GO: A Graphical Enrichment Tool for Ani-Mals and Plants." Preprint. Bioinformatics. https://doi.org/10.1101/315150.

[35] Fraser, James, Iain Williamson, Wendy A. Bickmore, and Josée Dostie. 2015. "An Overview of Genome Organization and How We Got There: From FISH to Hi-C." *Microbiology and Molecular Biology Reviews* 79 (3): 347-372. https://doi.org/10.1128/MMBR.00006-15.

[36] Rocha, Pedro P, Ramya Raviram, Richard Bonneau, and Jane A Skok. 2015. "Breaking TADs: Insights into Hierarchical Genome Organization." *Epigenomics* 7 (4): 523-526. https://doi.org/10.2217/epi.15.25.

[37] Santiago, Ines de, and Thomas Carroll. 2018. "Analysis of ChIP-Seq Data in R/Bioconductor." In *Chromatin Immunoprecipitation*, edited by Neus Visa and Antonio Jordán-Pla, 1689:195-226. New York, NY: Springer New York. https://doi.org/10.1007/978-1-4939-7380-4_17.

[38] Cournac, Axel, Hervé Marie-Nelly, Martial Marbouty, Romain Koszul, and Julien Mozziconacci. 2012.

"Normalization of a Chromosomal Contact Map." *BMC Genomics* 13 (1): 436. https://doi.org/10.1186/1471-2164-13-436.

[39] Dixon, Jesse R., David U. Gorkin, and Bing Ren. 2016. "Chromatin Domains: The Unit of Chromosome Organization." *Molecular Cell* 62 (5): 668-680. https://doi.org/10.1016/j.molcel.2016.05.018.

[40] Moosavi, Azam, and Ali Motevalizadeh Ardekani. 2016. "Role of Epigenetics in Biology and Human Diseases." *Iranian Biomedical Journal*, no. 5 (November): 246-258. https://doi.org/10.22045/ibj.2016.01.

[41] Bylicky, Michelle A., Gregory P. Mueller, and Regina M. Day. 2018. "Mechanisms of Endogenous Neuroprotective Effects of Astrocytes in Brain Injury." *Oxidative Medicine and Cellular Longevity* 2018: 1-16. https://doi.org/10.1155/2018/6501031.

[42] Nagy, C, M Suderman, J Yang, M Szyf, N Mechawar, C Ernst, and G Turecki. 2015. "Astrocytic Abnormalities and Global DNA Methylation Patterns in Depression and Suicide." *Molecular Psychiatry* 20 (3): 320-328. https://doi.org/10.1038/mp.2014.21.

[43] Yadav, Tejas, Jean-Pierre Quivy, and Geneviève Almouzni. 2018. "Chromatin Plasticity: A Versatile Landscape That Underlies Cell Fate and Identity." *Science* 361 (6409): 1332-1336. https://doi.org/10.1126/science.aat8950.

[44] Phillips, Jennifer E., and Victor G. Corces. 2009. "CTCF: Master Weaver of the Genome." *Cell* 137 (7): 1194-1211. https://doi.org/10.1016/j.cell.2009.06.001.

[45] Galloway, Ashley, Adewale Adeluyi, Bernadette O'Donovan, Miranda L. Fisher, Chintada Nageswara Rao, Peyton Critchfield, Mathew Sajish, Jill R. Turner, and Pavel I. Ortinski. 2018. "Dopamine Triggers CTCF-Dependent Morphological and Genomic Remodeling of Astrocytes." *The Journal of Neuroscience* 38 (21): 4846-4858. https://doi.org/10.1523/JNEUROSCI.3349-17.2018.

[46] Merkenschlager, Matthias, and Duncan T. Odom. 2013. "CTCF and Cohesin: Linking Gene Regulatory Elements with Their Targets." *Cell* 152 (6): 1285-1297. https://doi.org/10.1016/j.cell.2013.02.029.

[47] Portovedo, Mariana, Letícia M. Ignacio-Souza, Bruna Bombassaro, Andressa Coope, Andressa Reginato, Daniela S. Razolli, Márcio A. Torsoni, et al. 2015. "Saturated Fatty Acids Modulate Autophagy's Proteins in the Hypothalamus." Edited by Marcia B. Aguila. *PLOS ONE* 10 (3): e0119850. https://doi.org/10.1371/journal.pone.0119850.

[48] Augusto-Oliveira, Marcus. 2020. "Astroglia-Specific Contributions to the Regulation of Synapses, Cognition and Behavior." *Neuroscience and Biobehavioral Reviews*, 27.

[49] Morita, Mitsuhiro, Hiroko Ikeshima-Kataoka, Marko Kreft, Nina Vardjan, Robert Zorec, and Mami Noda. 2019. "Metabolic Plasticity of Astrocytes and Aging of the Brain." *International Journal of Molecular Sciences* 20 (4): 941. https://doi.org/10.3390/ijms20040941.

[50] Mantsoki, Anna, Guillaume Devailly, and Anagha Joshi. 2015. "CpG Island Erosion, Polycomb Occupancy and Sequence Motif Enrichment at Bivalent Promoters in Mammalian Embryonic Stem Cells." *Scientific Reports* 5 (1): 16791. https://doi.org/10.1038/srep16791.

[51] Barreto, George E., Janneth Gonzalez, Yolima Torres, and L. Morales. 2011. "Astrocytic-Neuronal Crosstalk: Implications for Neuroprotection from Brain Injury."

Neuroscience Research 71 (2): 107-113. https://doi.org/10.1016/j.neures.2011.06.004.

[52] Gonzalez, Antonio. 2020. "Antioxidants and Neuron-Astrocyte Interplay in Brain Physiology: Melatonin, a Neighbor to Rely On." *Neurochemical Research*, January. https://doi.org/10.1007/s11064-020-02972-w.

[53] Feng, Jianxing, Tao Liu, Bo Qin, Yong Zhang, and Xiaole Shirley Liu. 2012. "Identifying ChIP-Seq Enrichment Using MACS." *Nature Protocols* 7 (9): 1728-1740. https://doi.org/10.1038/nprot.2012.101.

[54] Williams, Holden C., Brandon C. Farmer, Margaret A. Piron, Adeline E. Walsh, Ronald C. Bruntz, Matthew S. Gentry, Ramon C. Sun, and Lance A. Johnson. 2020. "APOE Alters Glucose Flux through Central Carbon Pathways in Astrocytes." *Neurobiology of Disease* 136 (March): 104742. https://doi.org/10.1016/j.nbd.2020.104742.

[55] Bennett, Michael V.L., Jorge E. Contreras, Feliksas F. Bukauskas, and Juan C. Sáez. 2003. "New Roles for Astrocytes: Gap Junction Hemichannels Have Something to Communicate." *Trends in Neurosciences* 26 (11): 610-617. https://doi.org/10.1016/j.tins.2003.09.008.

[56] Fatima, Sarwat, Xianjing Hu, Rui-Hong Gong, Chunhua Huang, Minting Chen, Hoi Leong Xavier Wong, Zhaoxiang Bian, and Hiu Yee Kwan. 2019. "Palmitic Acid Is an Intracellular Signaling Molecule Involved in Disease Development." *Cellular and Molecular Life Sciences* 76 (13): 2547-2557. https://doi.org/10.1007/s00018-019-03092-7.

[57] Zhu, Ling, Xiaoyu Liu, Daniel P. Nemeth, Damon J. DiSabato, Kristina G. Witcher, Daniel B. Mckim, Braedan Oliver, et al. 2019. "Interleukin-1 Causes CNS Inflammatory Cytokine Expression via Endothelia-Microglia Bi-Cellular Signaling." *Brain, Behavior, and Immunity* 81 (October): 292-304. https://doi.org/10.1016/j.bbi.2019.06.026.

[58] Cudaback, Eiron, Yue Yang, Thomas J. Montine, and C. Dirk Keene. 2015. "*APOE* Genotype-Dependent Modulation of Astrocyte Chemokine CCL3 Production: Astrocytic Chemokine Modulation by APOE." *Glia* 63 (1): 51-65. https://doi.org/10.1002/glia.22732.

[59] Bolaños, Juan P. 2016. "Bioenergetics and Redox Adaptations of Astrocytes to Neuronal Activity." *Journal of Neurochemistry* 139 (October): 115-125. https://doi.org/10.1111/jnc.13486.

[60] McBean, Gethin. 2017. "Cysteine, Glutathione, and Thiol Redox Balance in Astrocytes." *Antioxidants* 6 (3): 62. https://doi.org/10.3390/antiox6030062.

[61] Merienne, Nicolas, Cécile Meunier, Anne Schneider, Jonathan Seguin, Satish S. Nair, Anne B. Rocher, Stéphanie Le Gras, et al. 2019. "Cell-Type-Specific Gene Expression Profiling in Adult Mouse Brain Reveals Normal and Disease-State Signatures." *Cell Reports* 26 (9): 2477-2493.e9. https://doi.org/10.1016/j.celrep.2019.02.003.

[62] Cho, Seo-Hyun, Jason A. Chen, Faten Sayed, Michael E. Ward, Fuying Gao, Thi A. Nguyen, Grietje Krabbe, et al. 2015. "SIRT1 Deficiency in Microglia Contributes to Cognitive Decline in Aging and Neurodegeneration via Epigenetic Regulation of IL-1β." *The Journal of Neuroscience* 35 (2): 807-818. https://doi.org/10.1523/JNEUROSCI.2939-14.2015.

[63] Choi, Sung S., Hong J. Lee, Inja Lim, Jun-ichi Satoh, and Seung U. Kim. 2014. "Human Astrocytes: Secretome Profiles of Cytokines and Chemokines." Edited by Cesar V. Borlongan. *PLoS ONE* 9 (4): e92325. https://doi.org/10.1371/journal.pone.0092325.

[64] Thelin, Eric Peter, Claire E. Hall, Giulia E. Tyzack, Arvid Frostell, Susan Giorgi-Coll, Aftab Alam, Keri L.H. Carpenter, et al. 2020. "Delineating Astrocytic Cytokine Responses in a Human Stem Cell Model of Neural Trauma." *Journal of Neurotrauma* 37 (1): 93-105. https://doi.org/10.1089/neu.2019.6480.

[65] Lundin, Anders, Louise Delsing, Maryam Clausen, Piero Ricchiuto, José Sanchez, Alan Sabirsh, Mei Ding, et al. 2018. "Human IPS-Derived Astroglia from a Stable Neural Precursor State Show Improved Functionality Compared with Conventional Astrocytic Models." *Stem Cell Reports* 10 (3): 1030-1045. https://doi.org/10.1016/j.stemcr.2018.01.021.

[66] Sadick, Jessica S., and Shane A. Liddelow. 2019. "Do not Forget Astrocytes When Targeting Alzheimer's Disease." *British Journal of Pharmacology* 176 (18): 3585-3598. https://doi.org/10.1111/bph.14568.

[67] Zhang, Xiang Yang, Wei Tang, Mei Hong Xiu, Da Chun Chen, Fu De Yang, Yun Long Tan, Zhi Ren Wang, et al. 2013. "Interleukin 18 and Cognitive Impairment in First Episode and Drug Naïve Schizophrenia versus Healthy Controls." *Brain, Behavior, and Immunity* 32 (August): 105-111. https://doi.org/10.1016/j.bbi.2013.03.001.

[68] Alboni, Silvia, Davide Cervia, Shuei Sugama, and Bruno Conti. 2010. "Interleukin 18 in the CNS." *Journal of Neuroinflammation* 7 (1): 9. https://doi.org/10.1186/1742-2094-7-9.

[69] Berglöf, Elisabet, Ralph Andre, Blair R. Renshaw, Stuart M. Allan, Catherine B. Lawrence, Nancy J. Rothwell, and Emmanuel Pinteaux. 2003. "IL-1Rrp2 Expression and IL-1F9 (IL-1H1) Actions in Brain Cells." *Journal of Neuroimmunology* 139 (1-2): 36-43. https://doi.org/10.1016/S0165-5728(03)00130-9.

[70] Ibn-Salem, Jonas, Enrique M. Muro, and Miguel A. Andrade-Navarro. 2017. "Co-Regulation of Paralog Genes in the Three-Dimensional Chromatin Architecture." *Nucleic Acids Research* 45 (1): 81-91. https://doi.org/10.1093/nar/gkw813.

[71] Amberg, Nicole, Susanne Laukoter, and Simon Hippenmeyer. 2019. "Epigenetic Cues Modulating the Generation of Cell-type Diversity in the Cerebral Cortex." *Journal of Neurochemistry* 149 (1): 12-26. https://doi.org/10.1111/jnc.14601.

Chapter 9

Neurotoxicity, Types, Clinical Manifestations, Diagnosis and Treatment

Serap Bilge

Abstract

Neurotoxicity is a term that refers to the condition in which the nervous system is exposed to dangerous substances (neurotoxicants) either naturally occurring or created, impairing the nervous system's normal function. Few of these neurotoxins act directly on neural cells, whereas others impair metabolic processes heavily reliant on the neurological system. Neurotoxicity can occur as a side effect of chemotherapy, radiation therapy, drug therapies, organ transplantation, and vulnerability to heavy metals such as mercury and lead, certain foods, pesticides, industrial products, and solvents used in cleaning cosmetics, and pharmaceutical products. Additionally, there are a few naturally occurring compounds. Symptoms of intoxication may begin to develop immediately upon exposure or may take time to manifest. These symptoms may include encephalopathy, limb weakness or numbness, cognitive and behavioral impairments. Following the elimination or decrease of exposure to hazardous chemicals, symptomatic and supportive therapy is provided. The prognosis is highly variable and depends on the duration and depth of vulnerability and the degree of the neurological impairment. Neurotoxicant vulnerability can be lethal in rare instances. Patients may survive in some cases despite their failure to heal completely. In other cases, many individuals recover completely following treatment.

Keywords: neurotoxicity, neurotoxicants, nervous system

1. Introduction

Understanding brain and nerve poisons have been a long-standing tradition dating back to ancient times. By the turn of the twentieth century, contemporary physiological and biochemical investigations had elucidated a few of these poisons' mechanisms of action. *Neurotoxicity* is defined as any unfavorable effect on the central or peripheral nervous systems' chemistry, structure, or function induced by chemical or physical agents either at maturity or during development. Any impairment of normal function or adaptability to the surrounding environment is regarded as a side effect. Thus, even if functional and structural changes are minimal or reversible, the most prevalent morphological abnormalities, such as neurons, axonopathy, or myelinopathy, may be unfavorable [1].

Additionally, neurochemical alterations should be regarded as harmful even if they are reversible and transient and cause dysfunction. Neurotoxicity can also arise due to indirect effects, such as harm to the cardiovascular or hepatic systems or changes in the endocrine system. Numerous compounds function in various ways and can directly or indirectly affect the neurological system [2].

The nervous tissue present in the brain, spinal cord, and periphery includes an extraordinarily complex biological system that generally describes many of the original traits of individuals. However, as with any profoundly complex system, even minor disturbances to its environment can result in significant functional disturbances. Factors leading to the vulnerability of nervous tissue include a large surface area of neurons, a high lipid content that retains lipophilic toxins, high blood flow to the brain inducing increased effective toxin exposure, and persistence of neurons through an individual's lifetime, leading to the compounding of damages.

As the nervous system is more vulnerable to toxins, several mechanisms are designed to protect it from internal and external hazards, including the blood–brain barrier. The blood–brain barrier (BBB) and choroid plexus that provide a layer of protection against toxin absorption in the brain. The choroid plexuses are vascularized layers of tissue found in the brain's third, fourth, and lateral ventricles, which through the function of their ependymal cells, are responsible for the synthesis of cerebrospinal fluid (CSF). Importantly, through the selective passage of ions and nutrients and trapping heavy metals such as lead [1–3].

2. Mechanism of action in neurotoxicity

Many neurotoxicants function by inhibiting the $GABA_A$ receptor, resulting in prolonged closure of the chloride channel and excess nerve excitation (**Figure 1**). Cyclodiene, the organochlorine insecticide lindane, and some pyrethroid insecticides prove acute neurotoxicity, at least partly through this mechanism. Symptoms of GABA inhibition include dizziness, headache, nausea, vomiting, tremors, convulsions, and death. Other some acts via Na channel inhibitors (tetrodotoxin), K channel inhibitors (tetraethylammonium), Cl channel inhibitors (chlorotoxin), Ca channel inhibitors (conotoxin), inhibitors of synaptic vesicle release (botulinum toxin, tetanus toxin), receptor inhibitors (bungarotoxin), blood–brain barrier inhibitors (aluminum mercury), Ca-mediated cytotoxicity (lead), and toxins with multiple effects (ethanol). In some cases, the hemostasis of energy can be affected [2].

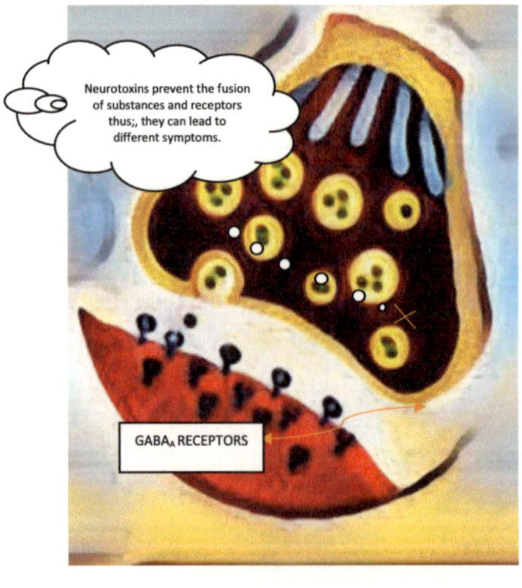

Figure 1.
The neurotoxins block the receptors, thus preventing the maintenance of proper physiological function.

3. Types of toxins and intoxications

Chemicals that disrupt the mammalian nervous system can occur naturally (neurotoxins) or be produced (neurotoxicants). While the term "neurotoxins" refers to substances with neurotoxic potential, this is not an inherent quality of the chemicals but rather a description of the effect that may occur when the tissue concentration surpasses a certain threshold. Neurotoxic biological substances usually demonstrate a high level of target selectivity and toxicity. Microorganisms, reptiles, and vertebrates exhibit direct or indirect neurotoxic effects that are well-understood mechanistically (**Table 1**) [3, 4].

Other naturally occurring compounds with less strong qualities have been shown to cause neurotoxicity when administered in high concentrations for a sustained length of time. Metals (arsenic, lead, and mercury) and other elements and compounds, such as selenium and vitamin B6, come into this category. While these chemicals are neurotoxic in high concentrations, they are required in trace levels to maintain proper physiological function, particularly in the nervous system. Natural enzymes (thiaminase) that metabolize necessary chemicals (thiamine) are also associated with neurological disorders in both animals and humans. Synthetic chemicals with neurotoxic potential are most frequently obtained through a

Life form	Substances with neurotoxic potential
Bacterium	Diphtheria, a toxin
Fungus	3-Nitropropionic acid
Plant	L-BOAA
Insect	Apamin
Reptile	Dendrotoxin
Bird	Batrachotoxin

Table 1.
Natural mammalian neurotoxic potential substances [3, 4].

Substance	Primary neurotoxic effects
Organophosphorus compounds (pesticides and warfare agents)	Cholinergic syndrome (certain compounds), peripheral neuropathy (certain compounds only), acetylcholinesterase İnhibition
Lead, inorganic	Peripheral neuropathy acute encephalopathy
Arsenic	Acute encephalopathy peripheral neuropathy
Mercury, inorganic	Cerebellar syndrome and psychological reactions (anxiety, personality changes, memory loss)
Methanol	Optic neuropathy extrapyramidal syndrome, retinopathy
Carbon monoxide	Encephalopathy/ parkinsonism(delayed), neuronal and tissue necrosis secondary to hypoxia
Phenytoin	Fetal phenytoin syndrome, cerebellar syndrome, chronic encephalopathy (cognitive dysfunction), extrapyramidal syndrome (chorea, dyskinesia), peripheral neuropathy
Arsenic	Acute severe encephalopathy, peripheral neuropathy
Tricyclic antidepressants	Seizure disorder (myoclonus), psychobiological reaction (serotonin syndrome, anticholinergic syndrome), tremor, extrapyramidal syndrome (dyskinesia)

Table 2.
Potentially neurotoxic heavy metals and synthetic substances [3, 4].

prescription (vincristine, ethambutol, isoniazid) and over-the-counter (bismuth preparations) pharmaceutical aisles; (pyridethione) products used in antidandruff shampoos; (2,6-dinitro-3-methoxy-4-tet-butyltoluene) fragrance raw materials; and (acrylamide) pyrolysis products used in broiled, baked. Others are associated with particular applications, such as chemical warfare in military and civilian settings (sarin). Directly neurotoxic substances are supplemented by medications that change neurological function due to their effects on another organ system on which the brain relies for proper operation. This class of medications includes those that target the lung, kidney, and liver particularly, as well as drugs that disrupt the nervous system's constant supply of oxygen (cyanide, azide) and glucose (glucose) (6-chloro-6-deoxyglucose). Chronic liver failure and manganese toxicity are associated with increased signal abnormalities in the basal ganglia on T1-weighted magnetic resonance images, implying that the metal accumulates due to the liver's general inability to eliminate it (**Table 2**) [3, 4].

4. Clinical manifestations of neurotoxicity

These manifestations include signs and symptoms in multiple parts of the central nervous system, including the central, peripheral, and autonomic nervous systems and skeletal muscle. They are typically accompanied by discomfort, altered sensations, such as taste and smell, decreased visual acuity, and hearing loss [5, 6].

4.1 Encephalopathy

Acute encephalopathies are a common occurrence. The majority are insignificant and dissipate within a few days. Headache, weariness, disorientation, loss of attention and short-term memory, lack of motor coordination, and the resulting gait irregularity, nausea, and dizziness are the most common indications and symptoms. Schaumburg identified several compounds (about 100) as possible causative factors, including aluminum, cannabis, cocaine, domoic acid, lead, organic solvents, and trimethyltin. While acute symptoms commonly resolve rapidly, chronic issues can significantly debilitating influence on job performance and productivity. There is a significant need for long-term follow-up and mental and psychological disorders assessment. Acute (moderate) encephalopathy rarely progresses to chronic (severe) encephalopathy with progressive cognitive and psychomotor impairment [5–7].

4.2 Movement disturbance

Cerebellar dysfunction, manifested by ataxia, intention tremor, and lack of coordination, is well documented due to chronic mercury exposure; however, overdose with various potentially lethal medications and substances, including 5-fluorouracil, lithium, and acrylamide, has also been reported. Cerebellar dysfunction is notoriously challenging to diagnose. Extrapyramidal syndromes such as parkinsonism, dystonias, dyskinesias, and tics are relatively well-defined toxic syndromes. While the destructive processes are unknown, they are frequently reversible, although symptoms can return years after the condition begins. Parkinsonism is arguably the most well-known form of Parkinson's disease, owing to an epidemic involving people exposed to MPTP (1-methyl-4-phenyl-1,2,3,6-tetrahydropyridine), a contaminant found in certain illicit substances. Most syndromes are induced by excessive medication use, particularly phenothiazines, rather than by exposure to non-therapeutic drugs [6–9].

4.3 Particular sensibilities

Loss of taste and smell and changes in smell and taste are common complaints that are difficult to quantify accurately, and quantitative procedures are not always practical. Despite the frequent involvement of organic solvents, this illness lacks a well-defined pathophysiological basis. Among the problems inherent in quantifying taste is that olfaction plays a significant role in detecting food's "flavor" and "perfume," even though many of us would categorize these as tastes. Changes in taste perception are frequently connected with administering a variety of therapeutic medicines. However, they are typically reversible. Although hearing loss has been associated with using organic solvents, particularly toluene, it is more usually associated with well-known ototoxic drugs such as aminoglycosides [6, 7].

4.4 Visual symptoms

Typically, vision loss occurs as a direct result of a toxic or corrosive material striking the cornea and conjunctiva or because the lens loses its transparency due to cataract formation. Direct attacks on the neuronal components of the visual system are less common than indirect attacks. Mydriasis and miosis are two distinct symptoms caused by exposure to or use of parasympathomimetic medications, anticholinesterase inhibitors, and parasympatholytics such as atropine. Nystagmus can develop as a side effect of certain medications, including phenytoin and antibiotics (aminoglycoside). Neurotoxic exposure is rarely associated with direct retinal injury despite a possible association with specific therapeutic medications. Both toluene (which induces demyelination) and hexachlorophene can cause optic nerve injury (leading to deformation of myelin). Alcohol addiction (methanol or ethanol) is also associated with widespread damage of the neuronal components of the visual system. Nonetheless, the etiology is suspected to be compounded by many chronic alcoholics' nutritional deficiencies [6, 7].

4.5 Peripheral nervous system neuropathies

These are frequently mistaken with axonopathies. However, the terms do not refer to the same thing. Peripheral neuropathy can develop within the neuron, resulting in the death or dysfunction of cells (in which case we call a neuronopathy). Axon degeneration (axonopathy) or loss of neuronal or axonal function may occur when the myelin sheath is disrupted. Channelopathy may develop from a change in the function of ion channels, or the toxin may target nerve terminals (leading to a neuromuscular transmission syndrome). Neuronopathies are easily recognized since they are much more likely to be sensory in origin and affect areas supplied by the injured neurons. The mechanisms by which they cause harm are not well understood. Methyl mercury is the neurotoxin most frequently connected with this illness. Proprioception may be compromised before or more severely than subsequent pain, whereas nerve conduction velocity and muscular strength are preserved. Healing is unpredictable, as neurons may survive or perish as a result of the toxic insult. Demyelinating neuropathies affect the peripheral nervous system when the Schwann cell or internode's myelin sheath is damaged. Diphtheria toxin can cause segmental demyelination by damaging the Schwann cell. Hexachlorophene and perhexiline have also been associated with myelin disturbance. Recovery is dependant upon the activation and replication of surviving Schwann cells. Regenerated internodes are slightly shorter than typical in length, myelin sheaths are thinner, and nodes can be somewhat longer than usual. Remyelinated axons conduct at a slower pace in general. Axonopathies are lesions of the peripheral nervous system produced by axon destruction. The presenting signs and symptoms typically manifest gradually and initially impact the long axons and distant locations. Sensory symptoms predominate over motor problems, and ankle reflexes degrade fast. The signs and symptoms then spread proximally for the duration of the axon's "regeneration." Healing occurs as a result of damaged axon regrowth. Recovery is often slow due to the 0.5–3.0 mm per day rate of axonal development. Numerous industrial chemicals, such as acrylamide, arsenic, carbon disulfide, n-hexane, lead, organic mercury, and thallium, have been shown to cause axon damage. While recovery is often uncomplicated, chronic ataxia, stiffness, and hyperreflexia can occur following severe poisoning. Axonal channelopathies are caused by aberrant ion channel activity and manifest as faulty axonal conduction. These are typically made up of natural toxins. The motor nerve terminal is a major target for a range of natural neurotoxins (clostridial toxins, cone snail toxins, snake, spider, and scorpion venoms), all of which induce harm to the nerve terminal. What is unknown is the involvement of the nerve terminal in the expression of toxic insult induced by a variety of harmful substances, including organophosphates and acrylamide, both of which have been shown to cause considerable nerve terminal damage. It is unsurprising that most axonopathies that die back originate at the nerve terminal [6, 7, 9].

4.6 Skeletal muscle

Skeletal muscle injury is rather infrequent. The bulk of toxicological problems in skeletal muscle is the result of genuine denervation. Several myotoxic substances, including clofibrate and related compounds such as insecticides and organophosphates, can cause substantial muscle loss by rhabdomyolysis. Diazacholesterols and herbicides containing chlorophenoxyisobutyric acid stimulate myotonic activity, whereas licorice, diuretics, and excessive alcohol use induce hypokalemic paralysis. Skeletal muscle regenerates rapidly following the removal of the causative factor. Rhabdomyolysis's most important acute clinical consequence is a significant risk of acute renal failure [6–9].

4.7 Psychiatric and Behavioral disorders

Depression is the most frequently reported symptom of neurotoxic diseases in patients. These individuals frequently express feelings of depression, anxiety, and forgetfulness. While the psychological signs of aluminum toxicity are normally mild, they can progress to severe dementia and parkinsonism/dementia syndrome. Lithium overdose with lysergic acid diethylamide may result in cerebellar ataxia, dementia, and severe psychotic illnesses (LSD). Due to widespread disdain for psychiatric/psychological disorders, there is a dearth of reliable knowledge regarding the diagnosis, management, and prognosis of mental health complaints associated with such intoxication. Additional study on the acute and chronic effects of neurotoxic drugs on cognitive function is necessary [6, 7].

5. Tests to detect neurotoxicity/Neurotoxicology screenings

While substances that lead to neurotoxic effects can be found by routine toxicity screening testings (e.g., chronic, acute, developmental/reproductive toxicity), specific standards exist to further evaluate compounds' potential neurotoxicity. The requirements established by the USEPA (the United States Environmental Protection Agency) are based on a functional observational battery, motor health assessments, and neuropathological examinations. Similarly, the OECD

(Organization for Economic Cooperation and Development) criteria emphasize clinical results, practical test findings (e.g., motor activity, sensory response to stimuli), and neuropathology. These batteries are intended to provide a Tier 1 screening for neurotoxicity, with positive findings necessitating additional testing (Tier 2), which may involve specialized behavioral tests in addition to electrophysiological and neurochemical data. Examples include memory and learning tests, nerve conduction velocity measurements, and biochemical tests linked to neurotransmission or indices of cell integrity or function. Specific recommendations for developmental neurotoxicity (DNT) testing have also been created in the United States of America and Europe. The mother is exposed to the test drugs from prenatal day 6 to postnatal day 10 or 21, ensuring exposure both in utero and via maternal milk. The examinations cover developmental milestones and reflexes, motor activity, hearing testing, learning and memory tests, and neuropathology. DNT has been demonstrated to be exceedingly practical and beneficial in detecting substances and agents that have the potential to cause developmental neurotoxicity during neurotoxicity testing. However, additional effort is needed to improve these tests, either because they are susceptible and generate a significant proportion of false positives or because they are insufficiently sensitive and thorough [8–11].

Additionally, concerns have been expressed about historical control data, toxicokinetic parameters, toxicity mediated by the mother versus direct effects, test selection, and their analysis and interpretation. Toxicologists have increasingly recognized the need for acceptable and accurate alternatives to conventional animal testing in recent years, highlighting the issues associated with rising costs and time requirements for toxicity assessment tests, the growing number of chemicals being developed, and commercializing the demand in response to recent legislation and efforts to reduce the number of animals used in toxicity testing. This, combined with efforts in the field of developmental neurotoxicity, has resulted in the development of alternative models, either using mammalian cells *in vitro* or nonmammalian model systems (using zebrafish), that may serve as valuable tools for neurotoxicity and developmental neurotoxicity testing, particularly for screening. These alternative tests should be utilized as Tier 1 testing for drugs and agents with an uncertain DNT potential. Given the complexity of the nervous system and the range of possible neurotoxic outcomes, developing a single test that covers the entire spectrum of neurotoxicity is challenging. Rather than that, a battery of tests should be explored that includes some *in vitro* experiments with mammalian cells and one or two tests using nonmammalian models. This can be augmented by applying computational approaches and procedures to develop a quantitative structure–activity relationship. Additionally, novel methodologies that are a component of "omics" technology can be applied in these endeavors. Alternative models for DNT must strive to reproduce a large number of events that occur *in vivo*, and given the complexity of the central nervous system (CNS), the approach for DNT is significantly more extensive than for other toxicity target organs [11–15].

6. Long-term effects of neurotoxicity/developmental neurotoxicity

Neurotoxic effects linked with developmental exposure during pregnancy, nursing, early childhood, and adolescence are frequently documented following a brief period of exposure. Nonetheless, evidence indicates that the insalubrious effects of toxicants may take months, if not years, to manifest clinically. The "silent" phase refers to the time period during which an individual may display no signs or symptoms of poisoning. Silent toxicity is a term that refers to continuing morphological or biochemical damage that is clinically undetected unless concealed by special techniques. Silent toxicity is comparable to carcinogenesis, in which cellular and molecular damage develop years, if not decades before clinical symptoms show. This area contains numerous instances of silent poisoning. Parkinsonism-dementia, frequently referred to as Guam's disease, is the most widespread kind, with a latency of several decades between supposed yet-undefined exposures and clinical manifestations. Another case of bovine spongiform encephalopathy (mad cow disease) is a form of Creutzfeld–Jacob disease with a documented latency of decades [8, 15–19]. The time interval between the onset of clinical symptoms and exposure to a neurotoxic event can be explained by a number of factors. For example, while a specific population of neurons may be injured, the brain's plasticity may compensate for this loss temporarily. Exogenous stressors (stress, illness, chemical exposure) or the normal aging process, on the other hand, may disclose the silent toxicity. Alternatively, an organism may be capable of compensating for a specific defect. Nevertheless, persistent loss of function may eventually exhaust the brain's functional reserve and plasticity. The likelihood of such a latent period occurring between exposure and clinical manifestation occurring throughout the development stage is significantly greater. David Barker was a pioneer in establishing the possibility that many adult disorders have fetal origins. The "Barker hypothesis" is the name given to this concept. Toxic substance exposure has the potential to directly destroy or modify developmental programming, resulting in later-life functional impairments [8, 9, 19–22]. Diethylstilbestrol is the most prominent example, which may contribute to an increase in vaginal adenocarcinoma around puberty as a result of in utero exposure. Perinatal exposure of rats to the Gram (–) bacteriotoxin lipopolysaccharide causes a 30% loss in dopaminergic neurons in the substantia nigra and persistent injury to the dopaminergic system, implying that, in humans, prenatal infections occurring at a specific gestational age may result in the birth of an individual with significantly fewer dopaminergic neurons. This could be an example of developmental neurotoxicity. This may seem minor, given that Parkinson's disease does not manifest clinically until around 80% of dopaminergic neurons are lost completely. When the aging process culminates in the typical progressive loss of dopaminergic neurons, this early-life lesion may play a substantial role in an individual's development of Parkinson's disease. Exposure to some pesticides during development, such as the herbicide paraquat and the fungicide maneb, both of which act on dopaminergic neurons, has also been related to the development of Parkinson's disease later in life. Similarly, developmental exposure to the now-banned organochlorine insecticide dieldrin has been found to cause significant and long-lasting alterations in the dopaminergic system, as well as a silent dopaminergic dysfunction. Rarely, modest and mild injuries may worsen as an individual develops and ages. In this manner, the neurotoxic effects of embryonic MeHg exposure do not manifest themselves for years. Microencephaly produced by uterine exposure to methyl azoxy methanol resulted in an early loss of cognitive abilities, and the neurotoxic consequences of neonatal exposure to triethyltin, a glial neurotoxicant, were increased with age. This cannot be the case in all other situations. Nonetheless, developmental exposure appears to have irreversible neurotoxic effects, and even if they do not deteriorate with age, they have long-term ramifications, as evidenced by perinatal lead exposure [23–28].

7. Treatment and Prognosis

The treatment of neurotoxicity involves terminating, eliminating, or reducing dangerous chemicals and commencing therapy to reduce symptoms and offer necessary support [2, 3].

The difficulty is that if biotoxicity or neurotoxicity is the underlying cause of the pain or sickness and the treatment plan does not include a detoxification regimen, the overall recovery will almost certainly be incomplete and take longer than necessary [2, 3].

Biotoxicity/neurotoxicity treatment protocol can also include acupuncture, herbal remedies & nutritional supplements, nutritional counseling, and prescription of medication. For example, the key factors in the initial management of acute arsenic intoxication are gut decontamination and hemodynamic stabilization in patients with suspected acute arsenic poisoning. Generally, in such neurotoxicity, rapid stabilization with fluid and electrolyte replacement in an intensive care setting is very important. Aggressive intravenous fluid replacement therapy maybe even life-saving in serious poisoning. Gastric lavage may also be useful soon after acute ingestion to prevent any further absorption. The efficacy of activated charcoal is controversial, but its administration together with a cathartic (such as sorbitol) is frequently recommended, but if profound diarrhea is present, cathartics must be withheld. Hemodialysis may be beneficial in a patient with concomitant renal failure. Chelating agents administered within hours of arsenic absorption can successfully prevent the full effects of arsenic toxicity. If patients are treated within several hours after arsenic ingestion, chelation is likely to be beneficial. Therefore, even if arsenic ingestion is only suspected but not confirmed, consultation with a clinical specialist with expertise in the treatment and management of arsenic poisoning is essential [29].

Generally, neurotoxicity has a prognosis and outcome that are determined by the extent and duration of toxic substance exposure and the extent of brain damage. In some cases, individuals die due to neurotoxins exposure, while others live but do not fully recover. The patient may recover entirely following the necessary treatment [2].

8. Innovations in the future

The potential threats to human health posed by hazardous chemicals in the surrounding environment have become a significant public health concern. It is critical to have the necessary abilities, tools, and facilities to study neurotoxicity in an individual. Treatment for patients exposed to environmental neurotoxins is not yet defined, and multidisciplinary teams will be necessary to manage the most severe cases. Diagnostic indicators for neurotoxic diseases based on rapid-response biomarkers should be identified and developed more efficiently to be used by all centers. Two essential variables should be considered—the severe effect on the developing fetus and newborn, the long-term health consequences of chronic exposure to low levels of environmental neurotoxins, and the long-term health consequences of severe acute poisoning in patients.

Additionally, a conclusive study is needed to address the frequent allegation that putative neurotoxins lack a "safe" limit, owing to our inadequate understanding of the lethal synergy that can occur when multiple toxins are exposed concurrently. Additionally, significant progress is anticipated in elucidating the relationship of harmful environmental chemicals and susceptibility risk factors in progressive neurodegenerative diseases such as motor neurons, Parkinson's disease, and Alzheimer's disease [2–4].

9. Conclusion

Neurotoxicity refers to the direct or indirect effect of chemicals that disrupt the nervous system. Neurotoxins can be found naturally in the environment, and they could be synthetic. Some neurotoxins act directly on neural cells; others interfere with metabolic processes on which the nervous system is primarily dependent— The effects of neurotoxicity can appear and disappear rapidly, evolve slowly over days or weeks, regress over months or years, or cause permanent deficits. Neurotoxicity is usually self-limiting after exposure ceases and rarely progressive in the absence of continued exposure. The treatment is terminating the toxins exposure and providing symptomatic treatment.

Author details

Serap Bilge
Pediatric Neurology Department, Çukurova University, Adana, Turkey

*Address all correspondence to: sarabsmustafa@hotmail.com

References

[1] Kostrzewa RM. Kostrzewa. Handbook of Neurotoxicity. New York, Heidelberg, Dordrecht, London: Springer; Library of Congress Control Number: 2014931656. ISBN: 978-1-4614-5835-7. ISBN: 978-1-4614-5836-4. (eBook) ISBN: 978-1-4614-7458-6 (print and electronic bundle) DOI: 10.1007/978-1-4614-5836-4

[2] Dai C, Xiao X, Li J, Ciccotosto GD, Cappai R, Tang S, et al. Molecular mechanisms of neurotoxicity induced by Polymyxins and chemoprevention. ACS Chemical Neuroscience. 2019; **10**(1):120-131

[3] Giordano G, Costa LG. Developmental neurotoxicity: Some old and new issues international scholarly research network. International Scholarly Research Network. ISRN Toxicology; 2012:**2012**:12. Article ID: 814795. DOI: 10.5402/2012/814795

[4] Spencer PS, Lein PJ. Neurotoxicity. Davis: University of California; 2014. DOI: 10.1016/B978-0-12-386454-3.00169-X

[5] Rice D, Barone S. Critical periods of vulnerability for the developing nervous system: Evidence from humans and animal models. Environmental Health Perspectives. 2000;**108**:511-533

[6] Costa LG. Neurotoxicity testing: A discussion of in vitro alternatives. Environmental Health Perspectives. 1998;**106**(supplement 2):505-510

[7] Feldman RG. Occupational and Environmental Neurotoxicology. Philadelphia, PA: Lippincott Raven; 1998

[8] Grandjean P, Landrigan PJ. Developmental neurotoxicity of industrial chemicals. Lancet. 2006;**368**:2167-2178

[9] Environmental Neurotoxicology Neurotoxicology Committee on Neurotoxicology and Models for Assessing Risk Board on Environmental Studies and Toxicology Commission on Life Sciences National Research Council

[10] ECETOC. Evaluation of the Neurotoxic Potential of Chemicals. Brussels, Belgium: European Center for Ecotoxicology and Toxicology of Chemicals; 1992

[11] Costa LG, Giordano G. Developmental neurotoxicity of polybrominated diphenyl ether (PBDE) flame retardants. Neurotoxicology. 2007;**28**(6):1047-1067

[12] OECD (Organization for Economic Co-operation and Development). Test guideline 424. OECD guideline for testing of chemicals. In: Neurotoxicity Study in Rodents. Paris, France: OECD; 1997

[13] Crofton KM. Thyroid disrupting chemicals: Mechanisms and mixtures. International Journal of Andrology. 2008;**31**(2):209-223

[14] USEPA (the United States Environmental Protection Agency). Health effects test guidelines. OPPTS 870.6200. In: Neurotoxicity Screening Battery. Washington, DC, USA: USEPA; 1998 8 ISRN Toxicology

[15] OECD (Organization for Economic Co-operation and Development). Test guideline 426. OECD guideline for testing of chemicals. In: Developmental Neurotoxicity Study. Paris, France: OECD; 2007

[16] USEPA (the United States Environmental Protection Agency). Health effects test guidelines. OPPTS 870.6300. In: Developmental Neurotoxicity Study. Washington, DC, USA: USEPA; 1998

[17] Claudio L, Kwa WC, Russell AL, Wallinga D. Testing methods for developmental neurotoxicity of

environmental chemicals. Toxicology and Applied Pharmacology. 2000;**164**(1):1-14

[18] Makris SL, Raffaele K, Allen S, et al. A retrospective performance assessment of the developmental neurotoxicity study in support of OECD test guideline 426. Environmental Health Perspectives. 2009;**117**(1):17-25

[19] Kaufmann W. Current status of developmental neurotoxicity: An industry perspective. Toxicology Letters. 2003;**140-141**:161-169

[20] Cory-Slechta DA, Crofton KM, Foran JA, et al. Methods to identify and characterize developmental neurotoxicity for human health risk assessment. I: Behavioral effects. Environmental Health Perspectives. 2001;**109**(supplement 1):79-91

[21] Li AA. Regulatory developmental neurotoxicology testing: Data evaluation for risk assessment purposes. Environmental Toxicology and Pharmacology. 2005;**19**(3):727-733

[22] Costa LG, Giordano G, Guizzetti M. Predictive models for neurotoxicity assessment. In: Xu JJ, Urban L, editors. Predictive Toxicology in Drug Safety. Cambridge: Cambridge University Press; 2011. pp. 135-152

[23] Bayer SA, Altman J, Russo RJ, Zhang X. Timetables of neurogenesis in the human brain based on experimentally determined patterns in the rat. Neurotoxicology. 1993;**14**(1): 83-144

[24] Rodier PM. Vulnerable periods and processes during central nervous system development. Environmental Health Perspectives. 1994;**102**(supplement 2): 121-124

[25] Myers GJ, Davidson PW, Cox C, et al. Prenatal methylmercury exposure from ocean fish consumption in the Seychelles child development study. The Lancet. 2003;**361**(9370):1686-1692

[26] Davidson PW, Myers GJ, Cox C, et al. Methylmercury and neurodevelopment: Longitudinal analysis of the Seychelles child development cohort. Neurotoxicology and Teratology. 2006;**28**(5):529-535

[27] Rice DC. Identification of functional domains affected by developmental exposure to methylmercury: Faroe islands and related studies. Neurotoxicology. 2000;**21**(6):1039-1044

[28] Clarkson TW, Strain JJ. Nutritional factors may modify the toxic action of methyl mercury in fish-eating populations. Journal of Nutrition. 2003;**133**(5, supplement 1):1539S-1543S

[29] Guha Mazumder DN, Santra A, Ghosh N, Das S, Lahiri S, Das T. Randomized placebo-controlled trial of 2,3-dimercapto-1-propane sulfonate (DMPS) in the therapy of chronic arsenicosis due to drinking arsenic-contaminated water. Journal of Toxicology. Clinical Toxicology. 2001;**39**(7):665-674